Atlas of Operative Proctology
Videos

Scan above QR and then
use this scratch code

to register for videos

VIDEO ▶

Includes Videos

Atlas of Operative Proctology

A Stepwise Approach

with

- 600+ illustrations
- 56 videos

VIDEO ▶
Includes Videos

Atlas of Operative Proctology

A Stepwise Approach

with
- 600+ illustrations
- 56 videos

Kamal Gupta MS FACS FAIS FACRSI
Consultant Colorectal Surgeon and Director
Karan Hospital, Jalandhar, India
Certified Trained Specialist in Laser Proctology, Berlin, Germany
Travelling Fellowship in Proctology, St. Mark's Hospital, London, UK
Fellow International Society of the University of Colon and Rectal Surgeons

Kushal Mital MS FACRSI
Consultant Surgeon and Director
Medicare Hospital, Thane and Govt CSMH, Kalwa, Thane, Mumbai

Niranjan Agarwal MS DNB FACRSI
Consultant, Laparoscopic and Colorectal Surgeon
Salasar Nursing Home, Bombay Hospital and Zen Multispecialty Hospital, Mumbai

CBSPD
CBS Publishers & Distributors Pvt Ltd
New Delhi • Bengaluru • Chennai • Kochi • Kolkata • Lucknow • Mumbai
Hyderabad • Jharkhand • Nagpur • Patna • Pune • Uttarakhand

Disclaimer

Science and technology are constantly changing fields. New research and experience broaden the scope of information and knowledge. The authors have tried their best in giving information available to them while preparing the material for this book. Although all efforts have been made to ensure optimum accuracy of the material, yet it is quite possible some errors might have been left uncorrected. The publisher, the printer and the authors will not be held responsible for any inadvertent errors, omissions or inaccuracies.

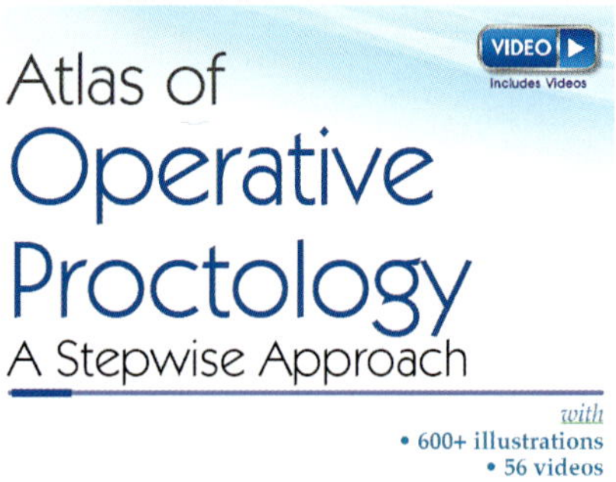

ISBN: 978-93-5466-749-7

First Edition 2024

Published by Satish Kumar Jain and produced by Varun Jain for
CBS Publishers & Distributors Pvt Ltd
4819/XI Prahlad Street, 24 Ansari Road, Daryaganj, New Delhi 110 002, India
Ph: 011-23289259, 23266861, 23266867 Website: www.cbspd.com
e-mail: delhi@cbspd.com

Corporate Office: 204 FIE, Industrial Area, Patparganj, Delhi 110 092, India
Ph: 011-49344934 Fax: 011-49344935
e-mail: publishing@cbspd.com; publicity@cbspd.com

Branches

- **Bengaluru:** Seema House 2975, 17th Cross, K.R. Road, Banasankari 2nd Stage, Bengaluru 560 070, Karnataka, India
  Ph: +91-80-26771678/79 Fax: +91-80-26771680 e-mail: bangalore@cbspd.com
- **Chennai:** 7, Subbaraya Street, Shenoy Nagar, Chennai 600 030, Tamil Nadu, India
  Ph: +91-44-26680620, 26681266 Fax: +91-44-42032115 e-mail: chennai@cbspd.com
- **Kochi:** 42/1325, 1326, Power House Road, Opposite KSEB, Power House, Ernakulum 682018, Kochi, Kerala, India
  Ph: +91-484-4059061–67 Fax: +91-484-4059065 e-mail: kochi@cbspd.com
- **Kolkata:** 147, Hind Ceramics Compound, 1st Floor, Nilgunj Road, Belghoria, Kolkata 700056, West Bengal, India
  Ph: +91-33-25330055/56 e-mail: kolkata@cbspd.com
- **Lucknow:** Basement, Khushuma Complex, 7 Meerabai Marg (behind Jawahar Bhawan), Lucknow 226001, UP, India
  Ph: +91-522-4000032 e-mail: tiwari.lucknow@cbspd.com
- **Mumbai:** PWD Shed, Gala No. 25/26, Ramchandra Bhatt Marg, Next JJ Hospital Gate No. 2, Opp. Union Bank of India, Noorbaug, Mumbai 400009, Maharashtra, India
  Ph: +91-22-66661880/89 e-mail: mumbai@cbspd.com

Representatives

- **Hyderabad** 0-9885175004
- **Jharkhand** 0-9811541605
- **Nagpur** 0-8692091830
- **Patna** 0-9334159340
- **Pune** 0-9664372571
- **Uttarakhand** 0-9716462459

Printed in India

Contributors List

Ganatra, Ashish MS
Sarvottam Surgical Hospital, Rajkot, Gujarat, India
Fistula Plug

Gore, Pravin MBBS, DNB (Gen.Surgery), FAIS, FACRSI
Laparoscopic Colon-Rectal Surgeon and Proctologist
GT Hospital Sir JJ Group of Govt Hospitals
CST-Mumbai, India
Botox in Anal Fissure

Jhawar, Nitish MS, FMAS, FIAGES, FALS, FACRSI
Laparoscopic and Colorectal Surgeon
Apollo Hospital, Navi Mumbai, India
Stapler Hemorrhoidopexy

Kaushal, Dhawal MBBS, MD
Fellowship in Diagnostic Neuroradiology
Fellowship in Obstetrics Ultrasound
Radiologist
MRI Fistulogram Images

Kukreja, Ajit Nanak Singh MBBS, MS, FICS, FACS, FIAGES, LLB
Gastrointestinal and Anorectal Surgeon
Ratandeep Surgical Hospital and Endoscopy Clinic
Ahmedabad, India
Doppler Guided Hemorrhoidal Artery Ligation

Nigam, SK MS, FICS, FAIS
Consultant Surgeon
Relief Day Care Centre
Fissurectomy with Mucosal Advancement Flap

Parthasarathi, R MS, FMAS, PhD
Consultant Laparoscopic and Colorectal Surgeon
GEM Hospital, Coimbatore, India
Ligation of Intersphincteric Fistula Tract (LIFT)

Pathak, DU MS, FACRSI
Consultant Anorectal Surgeon
Metro Hospital, Jabalpur, MP, India
Submucosal Ligation of the Fistula Tract (SLOFT)

Pratap, Brishank
Medical Illustrator
Goa, India
Medartica@gmail.com

Sharma, Pradeep
MS, MAMS, DNB, FICS, FAIS, FACRSI, FIAGES, FALS, FIMAS, FISCP
Advanced Laparoscopic, Gastrointestinal, Endocrine, Cancer Surgeon, Laser Surgeon
Ex-Professor in surgery, Bharti Vidya Peeth University, Pune
Jehangir Hospital and Medical Centre, Pune, India
President, Association of Colon and Rectal Surgeons of India
Surgical Management in the Pilonidal Sinus

Preface

When a subject is inadequately or poorly taught during the surgical residency days, it often has two consequences. Either the students lose interest, or after post-graduation, they start to hone their skills and seek guidance from an expert.

My journey shares a similar experience. *Atlas of Operative Proctology—A Stepwise Approach* is an outcome of this struggle. I have been fortunate to be trained in this specialized field by a few esteemed teachers based in India and overseas. In India, I learned the basic operative techniques used in anorectal disorders. While the use of Lasers in Proctology was introduced to me in Germany, I learned refined ways to perform a few procedures at St. Mark's, London.

After perusing through the publications of a few celebrated surgeons like Eisenhammer, Park and Hanley, I became an avid admirer of their work. Today, in my routine practice, where I use lasers to a great extent, I find myself following their techniques for all the hybrid procedures.

One day, I made the active choice to document all the procedures regularly conducted in our practice. I am blessed to have some great teachers and friends who are experts in proctology. I requested them to write a few procedures as they would have preferred to learn them. Beneath each procedure, readers will discover a section titled 'Tips and Tricks,' which delves into strategies for navigating challenging situations. Since this is an operative Atlas, the text has been kept to a minimum.

The Atlas comprises a variety of procedures practised worldwide. A corresponding image has been added for every procedural step to ensure better understanding. Since the anatomy is covered in the first part, *Atlas of Anatomy of Anal Canal—A Surgeon's Perspective*, the reader would gain a notable edge in understanding the surgical procedures if they were to review the initial Atlas before delving into the second one.

My earnest desire was to compile an Atlas that could serve as a practical reference for surgeons in the operating room. I sincerely wish an Atlas of this type existed during my initial learning years. Nevertheless, I am fortunate to have the opportunity to create an Atlas that can significantly help emerging colorectal surgeons. I also feel that learning is an ongoing process, and even after three decades of practice, every day offers new learning experiences for me. The Atlas of operative proctology is intended for colleagues who want to learn and enhance their skills continuously.

I want to take this opportunity to thank you all for appreciating my previous book, Lasers in Proctology, and making it a Bestselling Title.

Finally, I would like to thank Mr SK Verma (Vice President—Marketing and Operations, CBS Publishers and Distributors), for his innovative concept of creating video QR codes to enhance readers' comprehension.

As always, your suggestions are welcome, with the promise of integrating them into the forthcoming edition.

Kamal Gupta

Acknowledgements

The woods are lovely, dark and deep, but I have promises to keep, and miles to go before I sleep, and miles to go before I sleep.

—Robert Frost

This famous quote has forever been a source of inspiration for me. It is no surprise that soon after completing my first book, "Lasers in Proctology", my singular thought was, "What next?". My mind was crystal clear. It had to be a book on proctology, a subject close to my heart. The fruition of the currently published two Atlases, *The Atlas of Anatomy of Anal Canal—A Surgeon's Perspective* and *The Atlas of Operative Proctology – A Stepwise Approach*, can be attributed to the inspiration drawn from Robert Frost's inspirational words.

I have never quite been able to determine whether being the author of three books constitutes a significant honour or a profound responsibility. Once again, my teammate and life partner, Ruby, stepped up to assist me in pursuing my goal. Like before, she has done an outstanding job reviewing and proofreading the text. I am confident that without her steadfast support, I would not have been able to pursue my dream. The dictionary fails to describe the word I would have liked to use for her."Thank you" seems like such a small way to convey my gratitude. However, I would like to express my appreciation nonetheless for her patience and constructive feedback.

Blessings from my mentor, Dr Kushal Mital, and advice from my dear friend, Dr Niranjan Agarwal, are invaluable to me. I could not have wished for more when they willingly agreed to collaborate as coauthors for both Atlases upon my request.

I take this opportunity to thank all my friends and colleagues who have contributed to the various topics mentioned in the Atlas. I am confident that their decades of expertise in their respective fields will greatly assist readers in achieving a more precise understanding of the procedures.

I thank my assistant, Dr Neeru Sahni, for conducting extensive research and taking out pearls of wisdom from the publications crafted by a select group of brilliant minds, which were extremely helpful in understanding the anatomy and the surgical procedures. I want to thank my office manager, Riya Sharma, for maintaining a record of my procedures in the last decade, which allowed me to consolidate years of learning into the Atlas.

The credit for MRI images goes to the radiologist, Dr Dhawal Kaushal MD who is also a dear friend. He is an expert in MRI fistulograms.

While the Atlas includes some original hand-drawn illustrations, most have been sourced from the *Atlas of Anatomy*. Mr Brishank Pratap has done a remarkable job crafting this masterpiece. The images convey more than words can express.

Once again, the credit for allowing me to interact and engage with young minds throughout this enlightening journey goes to Dr Suchitra Bindoria, the director of IMMAST, Mumbai.

Lastly, I would like to thank CBS Publishers for publishing the Atlas and, through that, allowing the readers access to what I hope would offer a comprehensive understanding of the subject.

Kamal Gupta

List of Videos

Contents

Chapter

1

Pudendal Nerve Block

Pudendal nerve block temporarily numbs the perineal region by injecting an anaesthetic agent close to the pudendal nerve.

Indications

- To perform common benign anorectal surgeries under pudendal nerve block. The technique is an alternative to spinal or general anaesthesia.
- To reduce post-operative pain.

Absolute Indication

- To perform anorectal surgeries in cardiac patients where ejection fraction is low.

Principle

Pudendal nerve block temporarily interrupts nerve conduction in the pudendal nerve and relieves pain during various surgical procedures in the perineal area.

Routes of Administration

- Transperineal: It involves blockage of the pudendal nerve through the perineum.
- Transgluteal: It involves blockage of the pudendal nerve through the gluteal muscle.
- Transvaginal: The blockage is achieved by injecting the anaesthetic agent through the vaginal wall into the pudendal canal. This route is commonly used for gynaecological and obstetric procedures.

Palpation of the Ischial Tuberosity

- The surface marking of the ischial tuberosity is in the middle of the buttock at the level of the gluteal fold. The patient is asked to flex the hip as much as possible to displace the gluteus maximus superiorly away from the bony prominence (Fig. 1.1).
- In the lithotomy position, the ischial tuberosity can easily be palpated.

AGENTS USED FOR PUDENDAL NERVE BLOCK

Bupivacaine

Bupivacaine is a local anaesthetic agent. It blocks the generation of an action potential in the nerve cells by increasing the threshold for electrical excitation.

Mechanism of Action

Sodium channels are membrane proteins in the neurons and are essential for electrical signalling in the nervous system. Sodium channels initiate and propagate action potentials, which are electrical signals that travel along a neuron's length and allow it to communicate with other neurons. In other words, the sodium channels help transmit electric signals from one neuron to another.

Bupivacaine prevents sodium ions from entering the nerve fibres, which causes a temporary lack of sensation in the affected area.

Bupivacaine can be administered in three concentrations: 0.25%, 0.5%, and 0.75%.

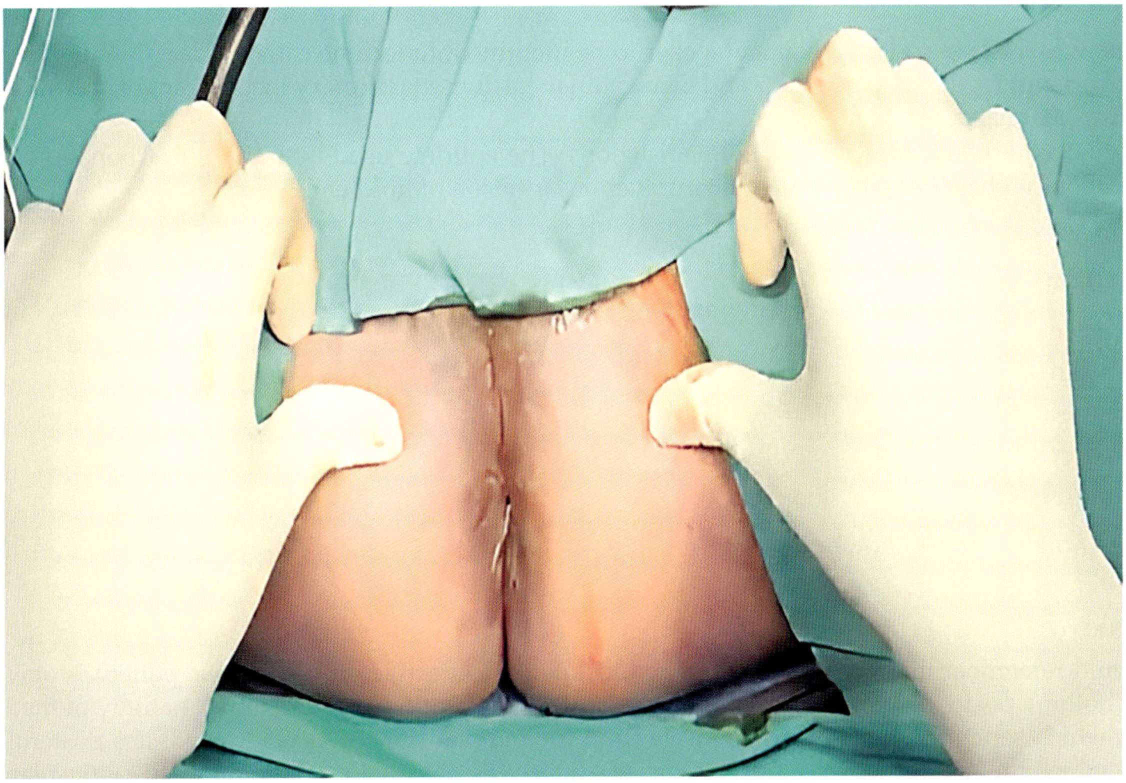

Fig. 1.1: Palpating ischial tuberosities

Lidocaine

Lidocaine was the first sodium channel blocker to be identified. Lidocaine can block sodium and potassium ion channels and regulate intracellular and extracellular calcium. Its primary mechanism of action is to block the sodium channels.

Rarely lidocaine can cause severe allergic reactions. The antidote used is sodium bicarbonate. The serum concentration can be lowered by giving an intravenous infusion of lipid emulsion.

INSTRUMENTATION (Fig. 1.2)

- Bupivacaine 0.5%
- 10 ml syringe
- Gauze piece
- Allis forceps
- Betadine

Position of the patient: Lithotomy

Technique

One should remember that the pudendal nerve block will be effective only when the patient is operated on in the lithotomy position. The technique used in our practice is entirely based on the anatomy of the Milligan septum, which separates the ischiorectal space from the perianal space. Alcock's canal lies posterolaterally, through which the pudendal nerve passes (Fig. 1.3). Once the anesthetic agent is released after piercing the Milligan septum, and with dispersion and gravity, it blocks the pudendal nerve.

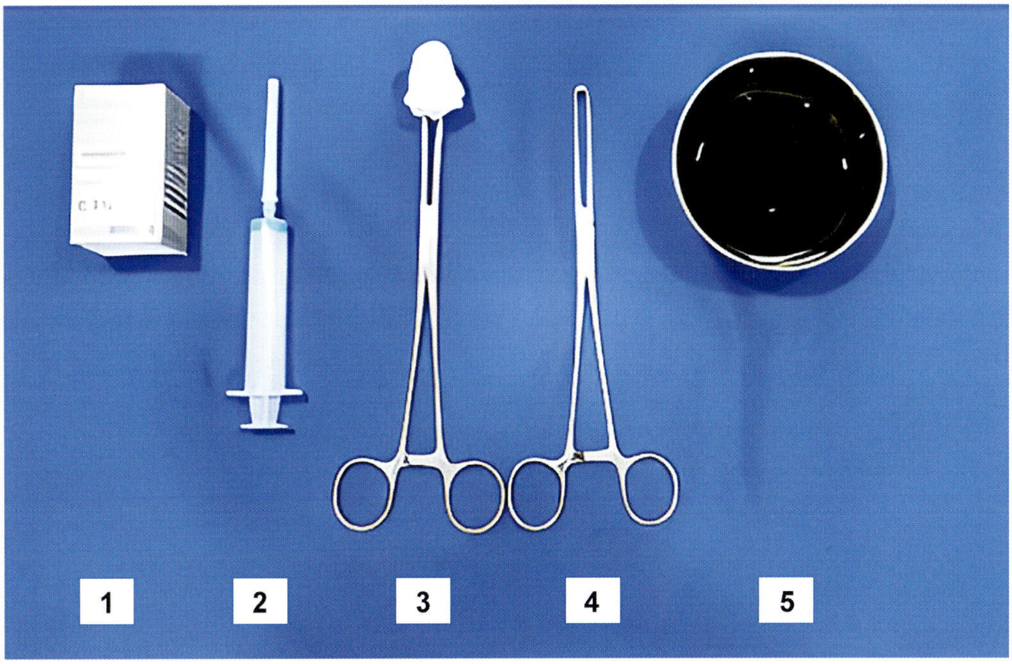

Fig. 1.2: 1) Bupivacaine 0.5%. 2) 10 ml syringe. 3) Gauze piece. 4) Allis forceps. 5) Betadine.

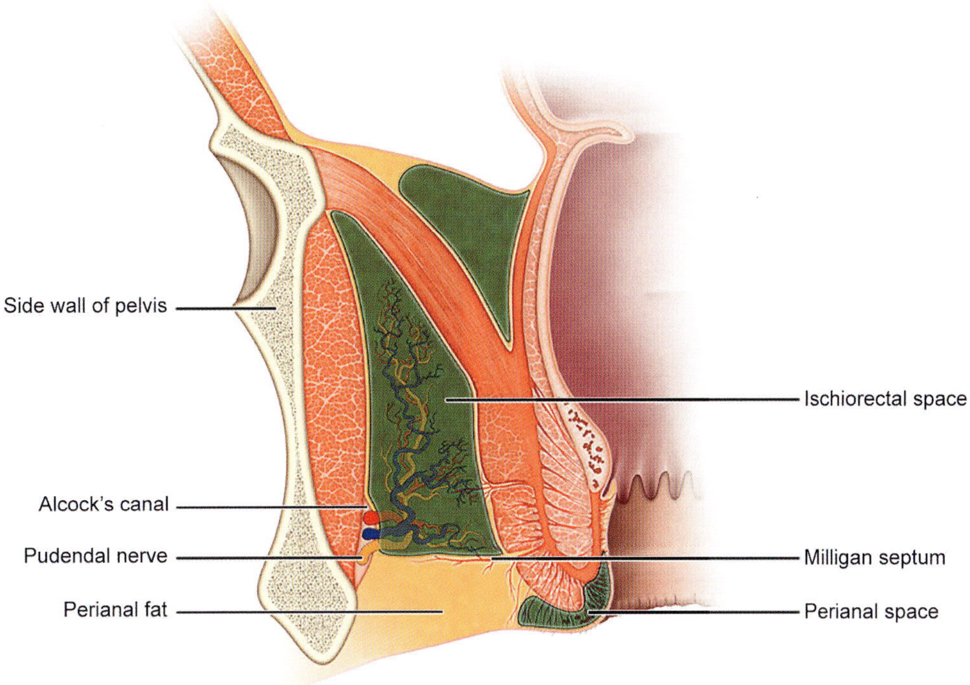

Fig. 1.3: Separation of ischiorectal fossa from perianal space by Milligan septum. Note the position of the Alcock's canal and the pudendal nerve.

Steps of the Procedure

Step 1: The ischiorectal area is cleaned using the povidone-iodine or chlorhexidine solution (Fig. 1.4A, B).

Step 2: To block the perineal branches of the pudendal nerve, 0.5% bupivacaine is injected all around the anal orifice (Fig. 1.4C).

Step 3: The ischial tuberosity is palpated, and the distance is marked from the outer boundary of the external anal sphincter (Fig. 1.4D). No attempt is made to palpate the ischial spine.

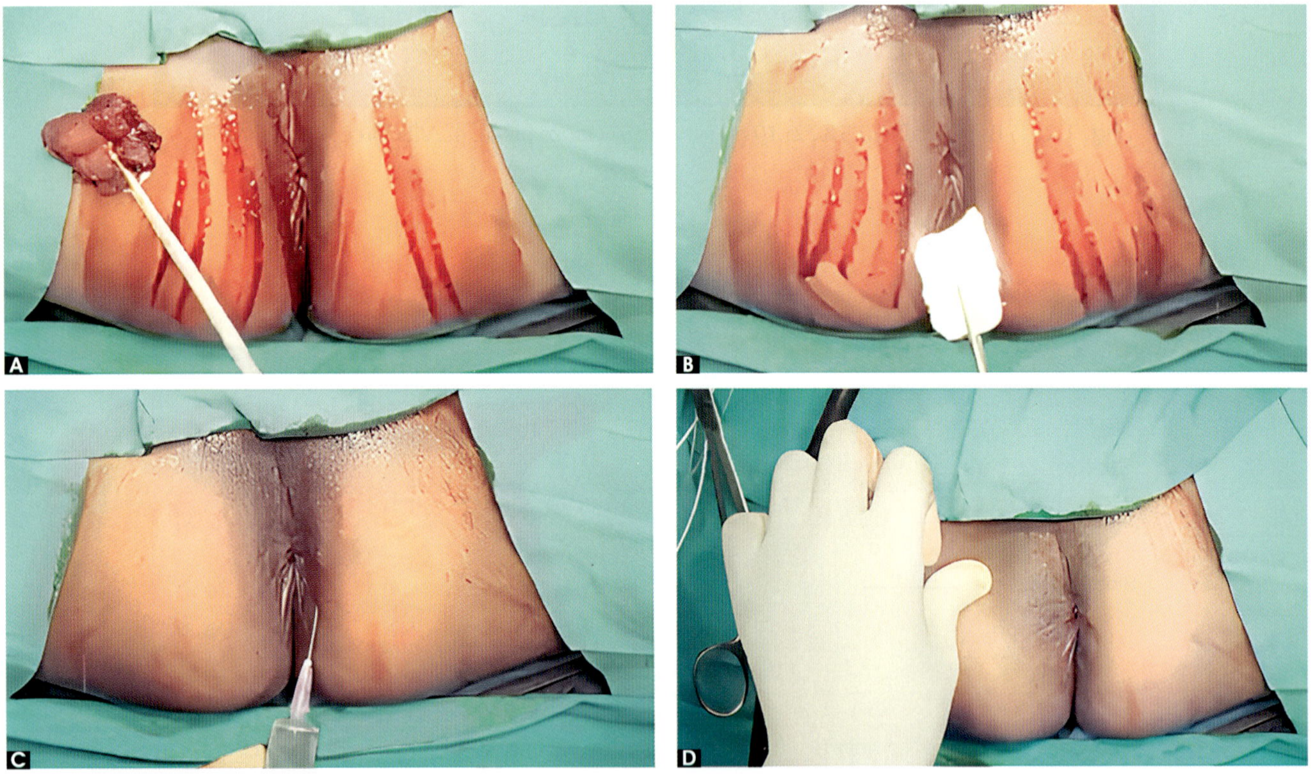

Fig. 1.4(A-D): Pudendal nerve block. A, B) Cleaning of the area with betadine. C) Injection of bupivacaine around the anal orifice. D) Palpation of the ischial tuberosity and injection of bupivacaine at 9 o'clock.

Step 4: 10 ml of 0.5% bupivacaine solution is injected between EAS's outer border and the ischial tuberosity at 9 o'clock using a 24G needle. The needle is pointed towards the right shoulder (Fig. 1.4E). The solution is released after piercing the Milligan septum, which lies just above the perianal space. With gravity and dispersion, the anaesthetic agent blocks the pudendal nerve in the Alcock's canal.

Step 5: The same procedure is repeated at 3 o'clock with the needle pointing towards the left shoulder (Fig. 1.4F, G). Figure 1.4H shows a diagrammatic representation of the pudendal nerve block.

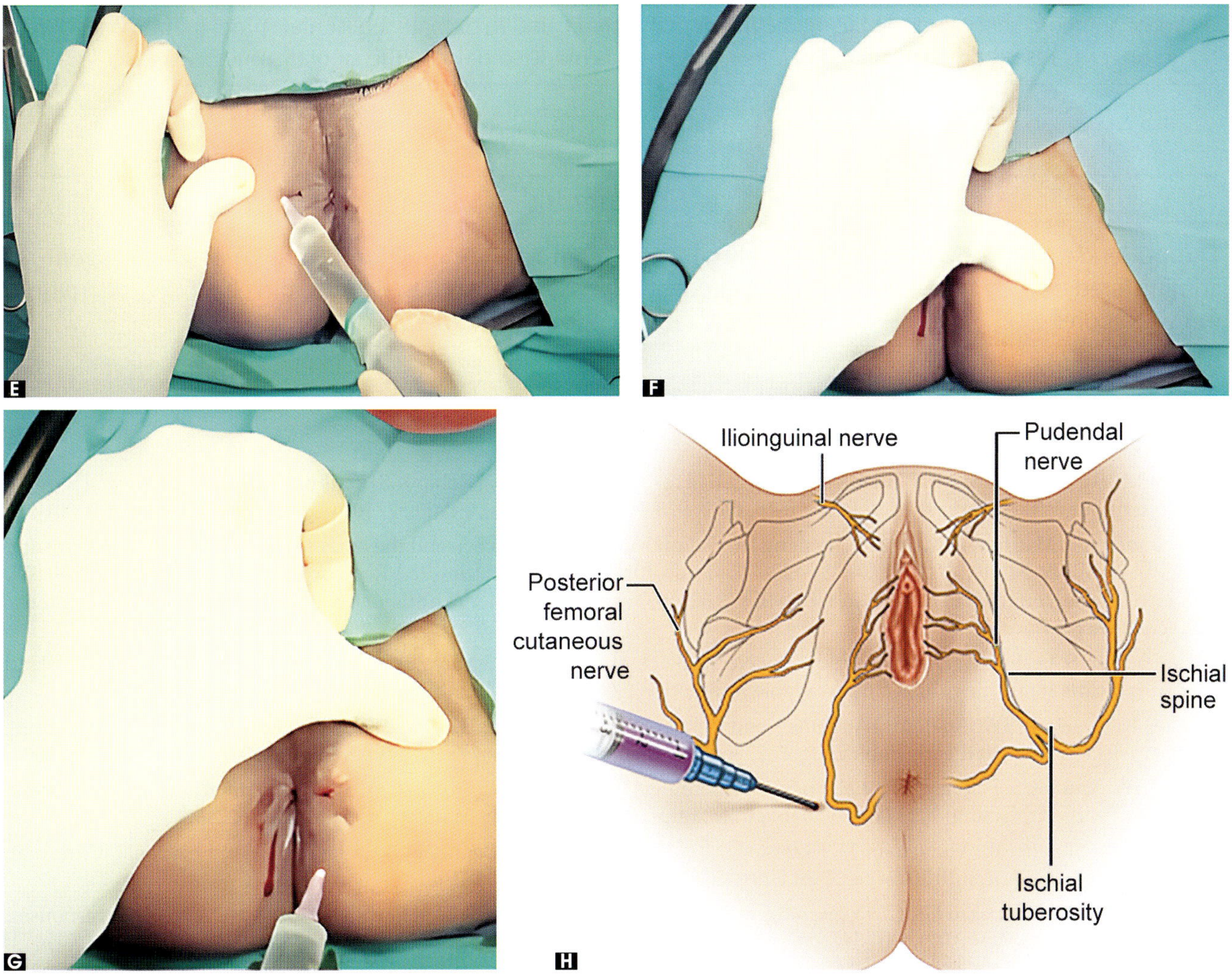

Fig. 1.4(E-H): Pudendal nerve block. E) Palpation of the ischial tuberosity and infiltration of bupivacaine at 9 o'clock. F, G) Palpation of the ischial tuberosity and infiltration of bupivacaine at 3 o'clock. H) Diagrammatic representation of pudendal nerve block.

Scan QR Code for Video on
Pudendal Nerve Block
VIDEO 1

Tips and Tricks

- Many surgeons use a lumber puncture needle for injecting a local anaesthetic agent to give the pudendal nerve block. Based on anatomy, one only requires a long needle to pierce the Miligam septum. A simple 24G needle is sufficient.
- Some surgeons recommend placing the finger in the anal canal to palpate the ischial spine. In this procedure, no finger is inserted in the anal canal, as no attempt is made to palpate the ischial spine.

Conclusion

The pudendal nerve block can effectively alleviate pain in the pelvic area. The anaesthetic agent is administered directly to the nerve site. The effect of bupivacaine lasts 6 to 8 hours and effectively decreases the VAS score.

FURTHER READING

- Alexis MP Schizas, Andrew B. Williams,1 - Anorectal investigation, Editor(s): Robin K.S. Phillips, Sue Clark, Colorectal Surgery (Fifth Edition), WB. Saunders, 2014, Pages 1–16, ISBN 9780702049651,https://doi.org/10.1016/B978-0-7020-4965-1.00001-9.
- Colebunders B, Matthew MK, Broer N, Persing JA, Dellon AL. Benjamin Alcock and the pudendal canal. J Reconstr Microsurg. 2011 Jul;27(6):349–54. doi: 10.1055/s-0031-1278705. Epub 2011 May 27. Erratum in: J Reconstr Microsurg. 2012 Oct;28(8):571. Broerm, Niclas [corrected to Broer, Niclas]. PMID: 21623563The Pudendal Nerve https://teachmeanatomy.info/pelvis/other/pudendal-nerve/
- Ghanavatian S, Leslie SW, Derian A. Pudendal Nerve Block. [Updated 2023 May 30]. In: StatPearls [Internet]. Treasure Island (FL): StatPearls Publishing; 2023 Jan-. Available from: https://www.ncbi.nlm.nih.gov/books/NBK551518/
- Kinter KJ, Newton BW. Anatomy, Abdomen and Pelvis, Pudendal Nerve. [Updated 2023 Feb 10]. In: StatPearls [Internet]. Treasure Island (FL): StatPearls Publishing; 2023 Jan-. Available from: https://www.ncbi.nlm.nih.gov/books/NBK554736/
- Leslie SW, Antolak S, Feloney MP, et al. Pudendal Neuralgia. [Updated 2022 Nov 28]. In: StatPearls [Internet]. Treasure Island (FL): StatPearls Publishing; 2023 Jan. Available from: https://www.ncbi.nlm.nih.gov/books/NBK562246/
- Oelhafen K, Shayota BJ, Muhleman M, Klaassen Z, Tubbs RS, Loukas M. Benjamin Alcock (1801-?) and his canal. Clin Anat. 2013 Sep;26(6):662–6. doi: 10.1002/ca.22080. Epub 2012 Apr 9. PMID: 22488487.
- Paganelli MA and Popescu GK (2015). Actions of bupivacaine, a widely used local anesthetic, on NMDA receptor responses. Journal of Neuroscience, 35(2), 831–842.
- Shafiei FT, McAllister RK, Lopez J. Bupivacaine. [Updated 2023 Jun 5]. In: StatPearls [Internet]. Treasure Island (FL): StatPearls Publishing; 2023 Jan-. Available from: https://www.ncbi.nlm.nih.gov/books/NBK532883/
- Weech D, Ameer MA, Ashurst JV. Anatomy, Abdomen and Pelvis, Penis Dorsal Nerve. [Updated 2022 Aug 8]. In: StatPearls [Internet]. Treasure Island (FL): StatPearls Publishing; 2023 Jan-. Available from: https://www.ncbi.nlm.nih.gov/books/NBK525966/
- Yang X, Wei X, Mu Y, Li Q, Liu J. A review of the mechanism of the central analgesic effect of lidocaine. Medicine (Baltimore). 2020 Apr;99(17):e19898. doi: 10.1097/MD.0000000000019898. PMID: 32332666; PMCID: PMC7440315.

Chapter

2

Office Procedures for Hemorrhoids

The management of hemorrhoids depends on the grading of hemorrhoids. Grade 1 to 2 hemorrhoids are best treated with office or ambulatory procedures. The most commonly performed procedures are:

- Infrared coagulation
- Sclerotherapy
- Rubber band ligation

INFRA-RED COAGULATION (IRC)

Infrared energy causes protein denaturation in the vessels leading to dearterialization followed by shrinkage of hemorrhoids.

Instrumentation (Fig. 2.1A-C)

- IRC equipment
- Transparent proctoscope with an obturator
- Lidocaine jelly 2%
- Allis forceps

Position of the patient: Lithotomy

Anaesthesia: No anaesthesia is required

Depth of the beam: 2.5 mm

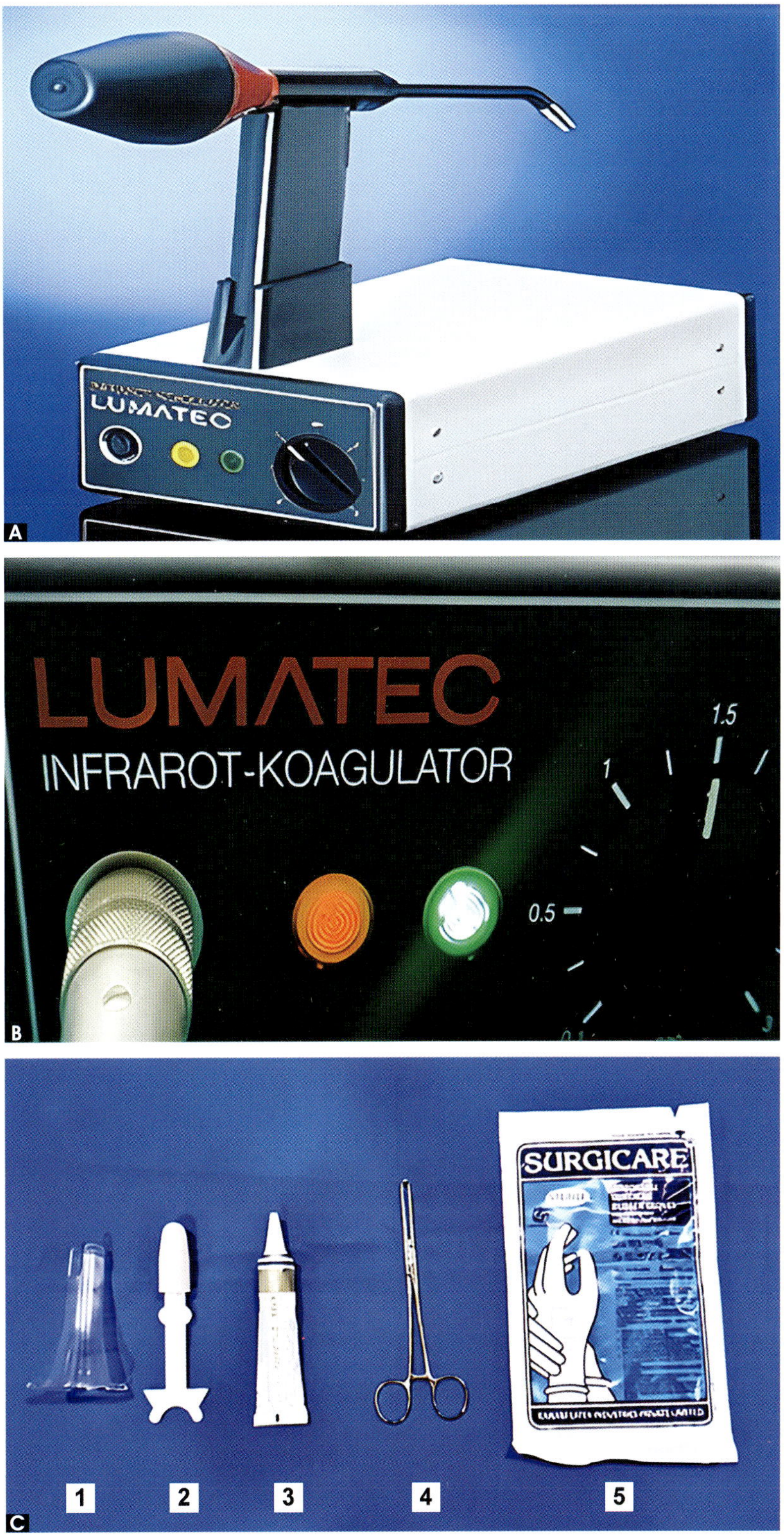

Fig. 2.1(A-C): A, B. IRC equipment, C. 1. Proctoscope 2. Obturator 3. Lubricant jelly 4. Allis forceps. 5. Gloves.

To check the beam of light: One should know how to check the beam of light of the IRC equipment. Take a mug filled with water, activate the equipment, and observe the reflection of the light within the water. A visible light circle indicates that the infrared beam is functioning correctly (Fig. 2.2).

Steps of the Procedure

Step 1: Proctoscopy Evaluation of Hemorrhoids

The routine proctoscope is replaced with a transparent proctoscope with an obturator. A well-lubricated proctoscope is inserted into the anal canal to assess the grade of haemorrhoids (Fig. 2.3). Bleeding may or may not be present in the case of a grade 1 haemorrhoid.

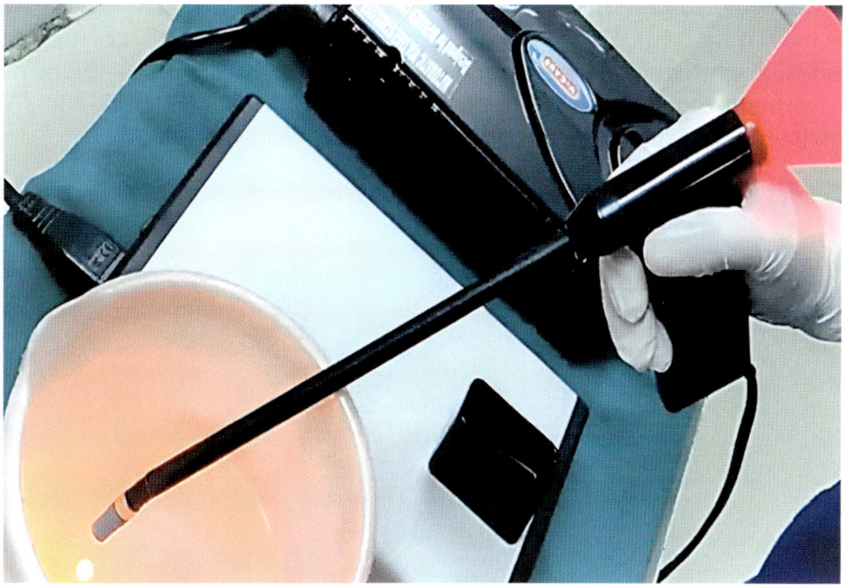

Fig. 2.2: The appearance of a small circle during the activation of IRC.

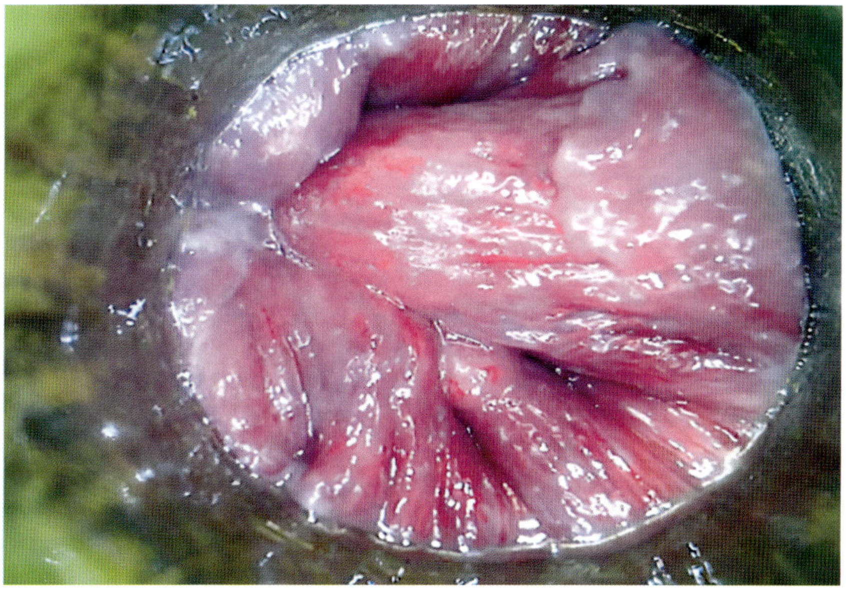

Fig. 2.3: Grade 1 hemorrhoids as seen through the proctoscope.

Step 2: Once inside the anal canal, the obturator is removed, and the proctoscope window is rotated towards 3 o'clock (Fig. 2.4A). The pile mass can be seen protruding out in the window.

Step 3: The rotatable infrared coagulation probe is inserted through the window and pressed along the mucosa at the apex of the pile mass (Fig. 2.4B). The probe is activated with a pulse of 1.5 seconds, and energy is released at the apex at three sites. A white eschar formation is seen at the apex caused by the infrared thermal energy, which occurs due to protein denaturation (Fig. 2.4C). The circle of white eschar is approximately 3 mm, corresponding to the diameter of the tip of the IRC probe.

Step 4: The same procedure is repeated at 7 and 11 o'clock (Fig. 2.4D).

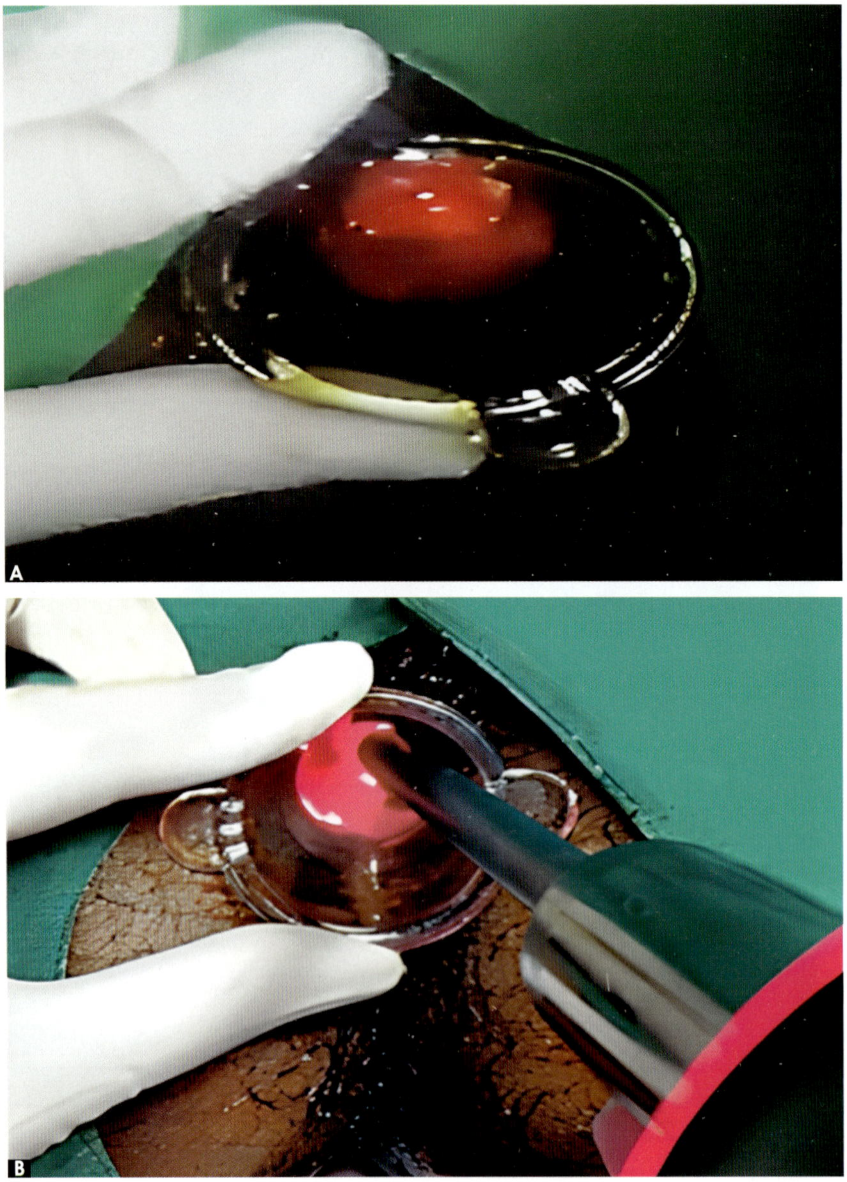

Fig. 2.4A and B: Technique of infra red coagulation. A) Transparent proctoscope inside the anal canal. B) Insertion and activation of IRC probe at 3 o'clock.

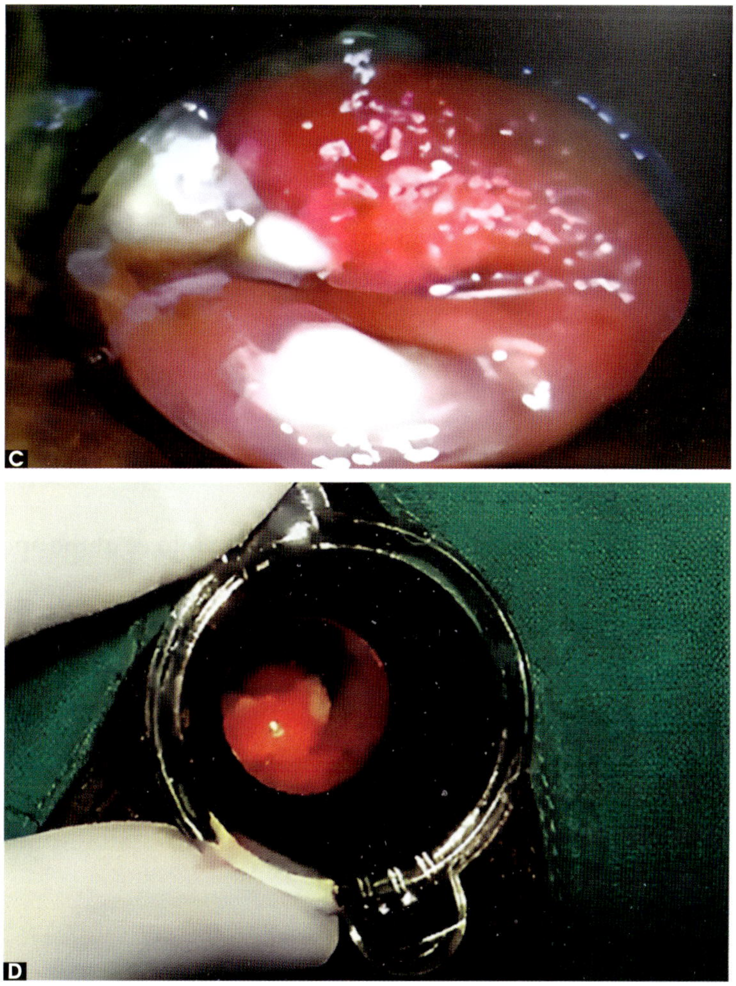

Fig. 2.4C and D: Technique of infra red coagulation. C) Appearance of white eschar at the end of the procedure seen at each pile mass. D) Repetition of procedure at 7 o'clock.

Scan QR Code for Video on
IRC
VIDEO 2

Tips and Tricks

- The energy should never be released at the dentate line as it can lead to pain.
- Sometimes bleeding can occur due to sloughing of the mucosa at the site of IRC. The bleeding can be controlled by giving antibiotics and tranexamic acid. MPFF can also be added as they reduce inflammation.
- A balloon tamponade can also be used to control bleeding. Those using lasers can spray energy using a bare laser fibre at a distance of 1 mm from the mucosa.

SCLEROTHERAPY

Sclerotherapy is the procedure in which a sclerosant is injected directly into or at the apex of the pile mass.

Instrumentation (Fig. 2.5)

- Three-way cannula
- Sclerosant
- LP needle
- Two syringes, each 5 ml
- Proctoscope with obturator
- Gloves

Position of the patient: Left lateral

Anaesthesia: No anaesthesia is required

Steps of the Procedure

Step 1: A well-lubricated proctoscope is inserted into the anal canal to assess the grade of the haemorrhoids. The obturator is then gradually pulled out. One can see the pile masses protruding into the proctoscope (Fig. 2.6).

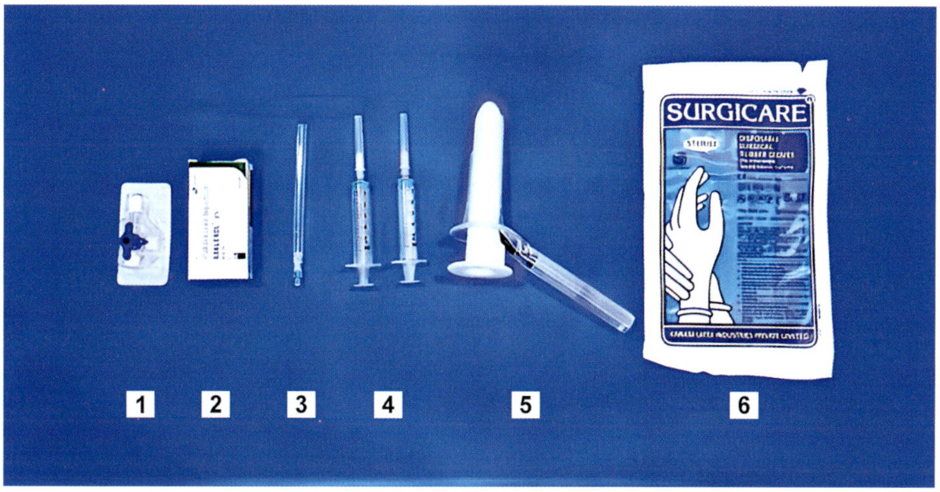

Fig. 2.5: 1) Three-way cannula. 2) Inj Polidocanol 3%. 3) LP needle. 4) 5 ml syringes. 5) Proctoscope. 6) Gloves.

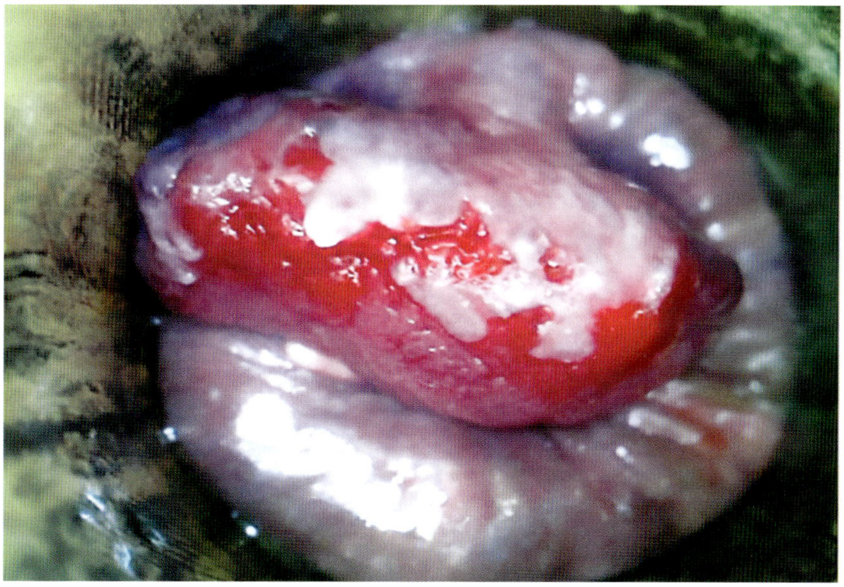

Fig. 2.6: Grade 2 hemorrhoids, as seen through the proctoscope.

Step 2: A lumber puncture needle is taken, and 0.5ml of polidocanol 3% is injected into each pile mass. One should withdraw the piston of the syringe to ensure that the needle is not in a blood vessel. After the injection, the needle is kept inside for a few seconds to prevent blood from oozing from the injection site. All three pile masses can be dealt with in a single sitting (Figs 2.7A–D). Instead of a concentrated polidocanol solution, foam can also be used.

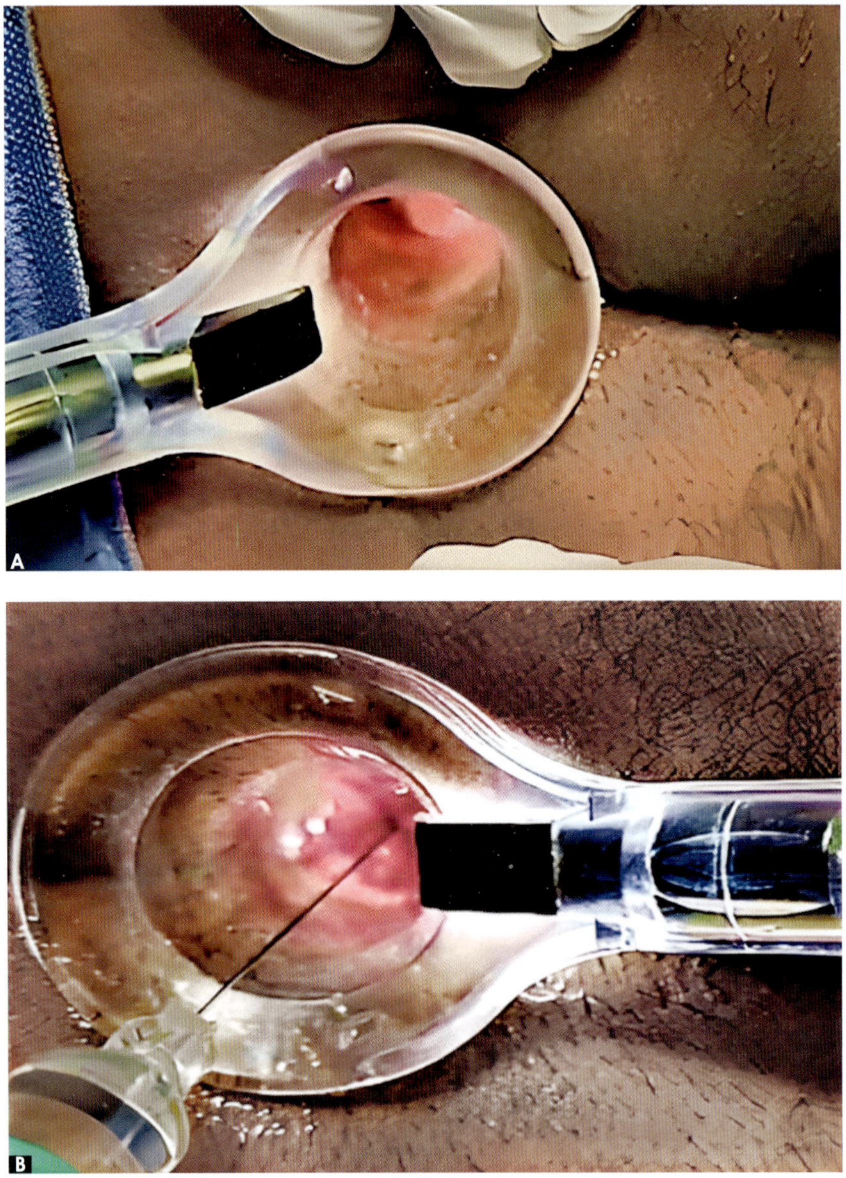

Fig. 2.7A and B: The technique of sclerotherapy. A) Insertion of a proctoscope. B) Injecting sclerosant at 3 o'clock.

Scan QR Code for Video on
Sclerotherapy

VIDEO 3

Step 3: After the injection of a sclerosant, the proctoscope is removed. A gloved finger is inserted, and the pile masses are massaged for uniform diffusion of the solution.

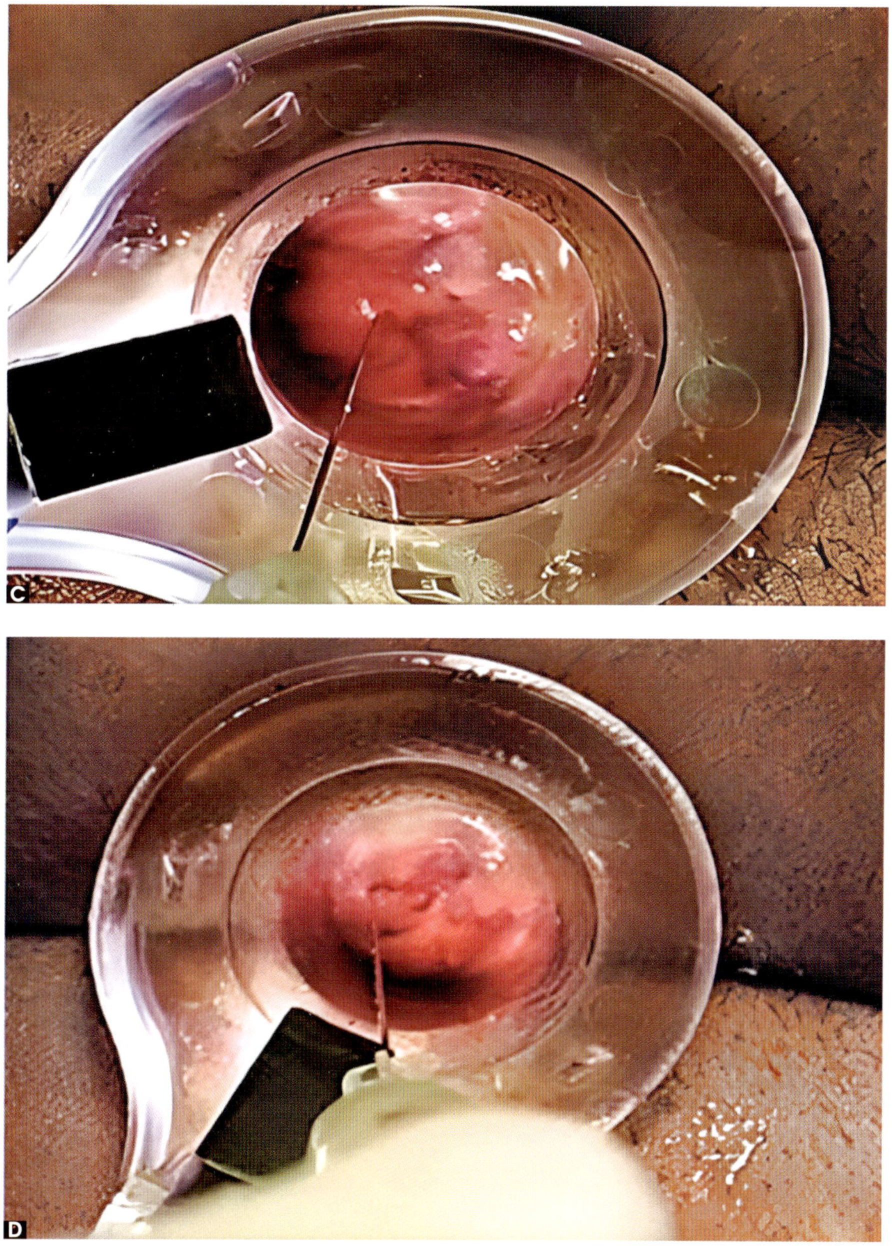

Fig. 2.7C and D: The technique of sclerotherapy. C) Injecting sclerosant at 11 o'clock. D) Wheal formation after sclerotherapy.

Tessari's Method

- Take a three-way cannula and two syringes (5 ml each).
- Mix 1 ml of polidocanol 3% solution with 4 ml of air by continuous withdrawing movements for 20 times (Fig. 2.8A, B).
- The foam produced is then injected into the hemorrhoids.

> **Tips and Tricks**
>
> - Never inject the solution close to the dentate line. It can cause severe pain.
> - Once the solution has been injected into the pile mass, look for wheal formation (Fig. 2.7C.) A bleb formation indicates that the solution is injected superficially into the mucosa.
> - If no bleb or a wheal is formed, it indicates the solution is injected deep into the sphincters.

Injections into the deeper plane may lead to infection and abscess formation. Sloughing can occur due to the following reasons:

- If the injection is too superficial.
- Too much solution is injected into a single hemorrhoid.
- A second injection is given into the hemorrhoids too soon after the first.

Ideally, the injection can be repeated if the bleeding recurs.

Scan QR Code for Video on
Tessari's Method

VIDEO 4

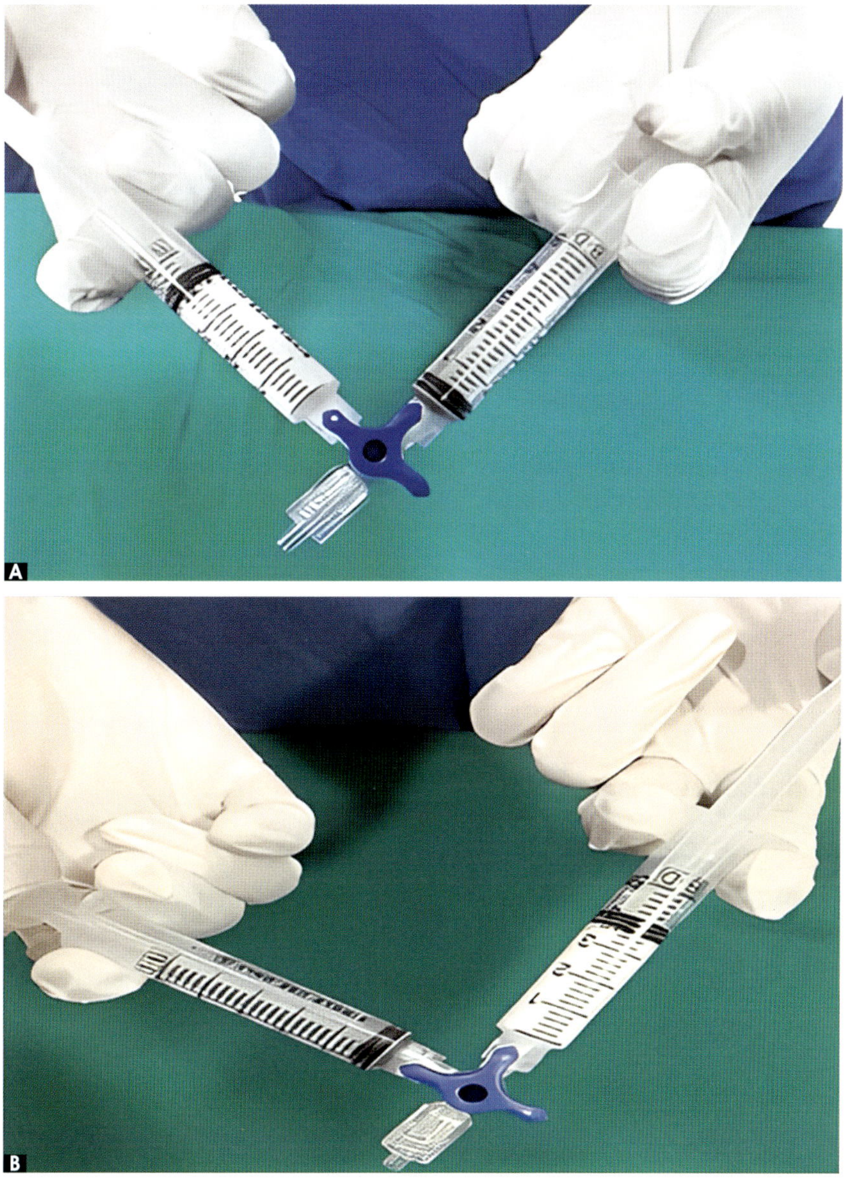

Fig. 2.8(A-B): Tessari's method. A, B. Mixing of the solution to make foam using a three-way cannula.

RUBBER BAND LIGATION

Rubber band ligation is a procedure commonly used to treat hemorrhoids by applying a rubber band around the base of the haemorrhoid to cut off its blood supply. Hemorrhoids shrink and fall off within a few days, usually without causing pain or discomfort.

Instrumentation

- Barron band ligator
- Grasping forceps
- Proctoscope (Fig. 2.9)

Position of the patient: Left lateral

Type of anaesthesia: No anaesthesia is required

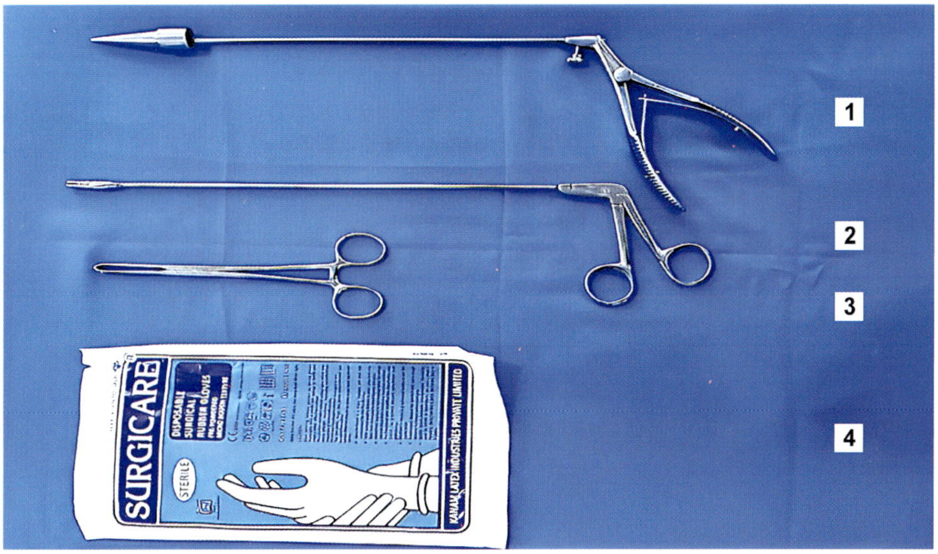

Fig. 2.9: 1) Barron band ligator. 2) Grasping forceps. 3) Allis forceps. 4) Gloves.

Steps of the Procedure

Step 1: A well-lubricated proctoscope is inserted into the anal canal to assess the grade of the hemorrhoids, and the obturator is pulled out. The pile masses gradually protrude into the proctoscope upon withdrawing the obturator (Fig. 2.10A).

Step 2: A rubber band is loaded on the Barrons band ligator and inserted through the proctoscope. The pile mass is gently held with a grasper and pulled out (Fig. 2.10B).

Step 3: The rubber band is released at the apex of the pile mass. All the pile masses can be ligated in a single sitting.

A pre-loaded band ligator with a suction port can also be used (Fig. 2.10C).

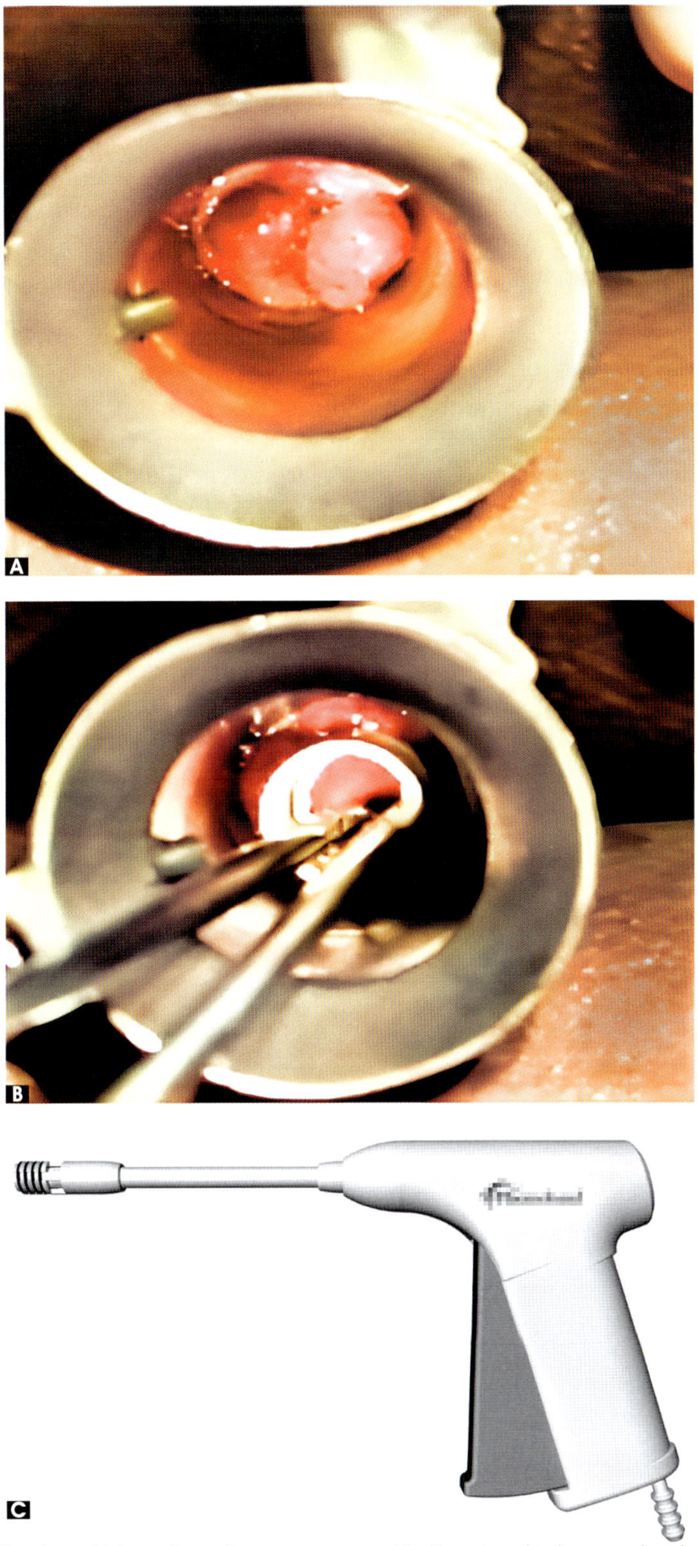

Fig. 2.10(A-C): Rubber band ligation. A) Insertion of a proctoscope. B) Grasping the haemorrhoid with forceps and release of the rubber band at the internal haemorrhoid base. C) Pre-loaded band ligator with suction tip. (Images A, B. *Courtesy:* Dr Parvez Sheikh).

Tips and Tricks

- One should refrain from releasing the band at the dentate line. If the patient complains of severe pain, the band should be immediately removed with suture-cutting scissors.
- If the pile mass is small, 1 ml of normal saline can be injected into the pile mass after the application of the band. It tightens the noose around the neck and prevents the band from slipping (Fig. 2.11).
- Bulk agents or stool softeners should be prescribed after ligation.
- A few drops of blood may be seen for 5–7 days after the banding.
- Patients can resume their regular diet after the procedure.

Note: The severe pain indicates that the band has been placed over the dentate line. Go for immediate band removal (Fig. 2.12A, B).

Conclusion

All office procedures are performed above the dentate line; the underlying principle is scar fibrosis. In infrared coagulation, dearterialization results in the reduction of hemorrhoids. Sclerotherapy leads to chemical ablation followed by scar fixation of the mucosa by fibrosis. In the rubber band, ligation of the hemorrhoidal tissue results in necrosis or ischemia of the prolapsing mucosa, followed by scar fixation in the rectal wall.

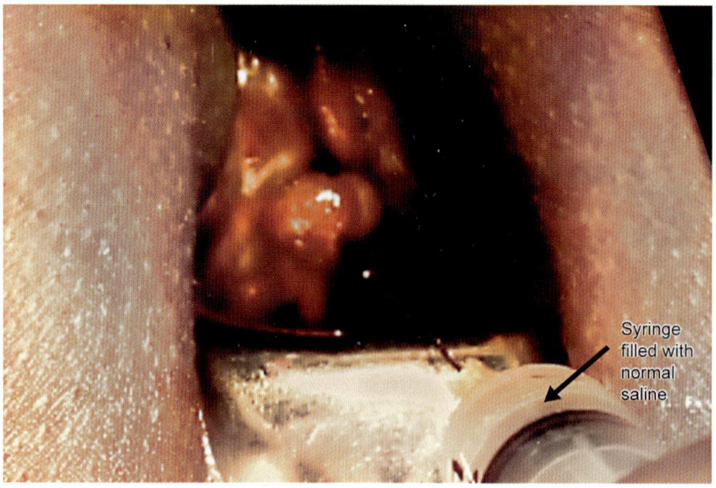

Fig. 2.11: Injecting the normal saline solution into the pile mass to increase its volume. (Images and video *Courtesy:* Dr. Parvez Sheikh).

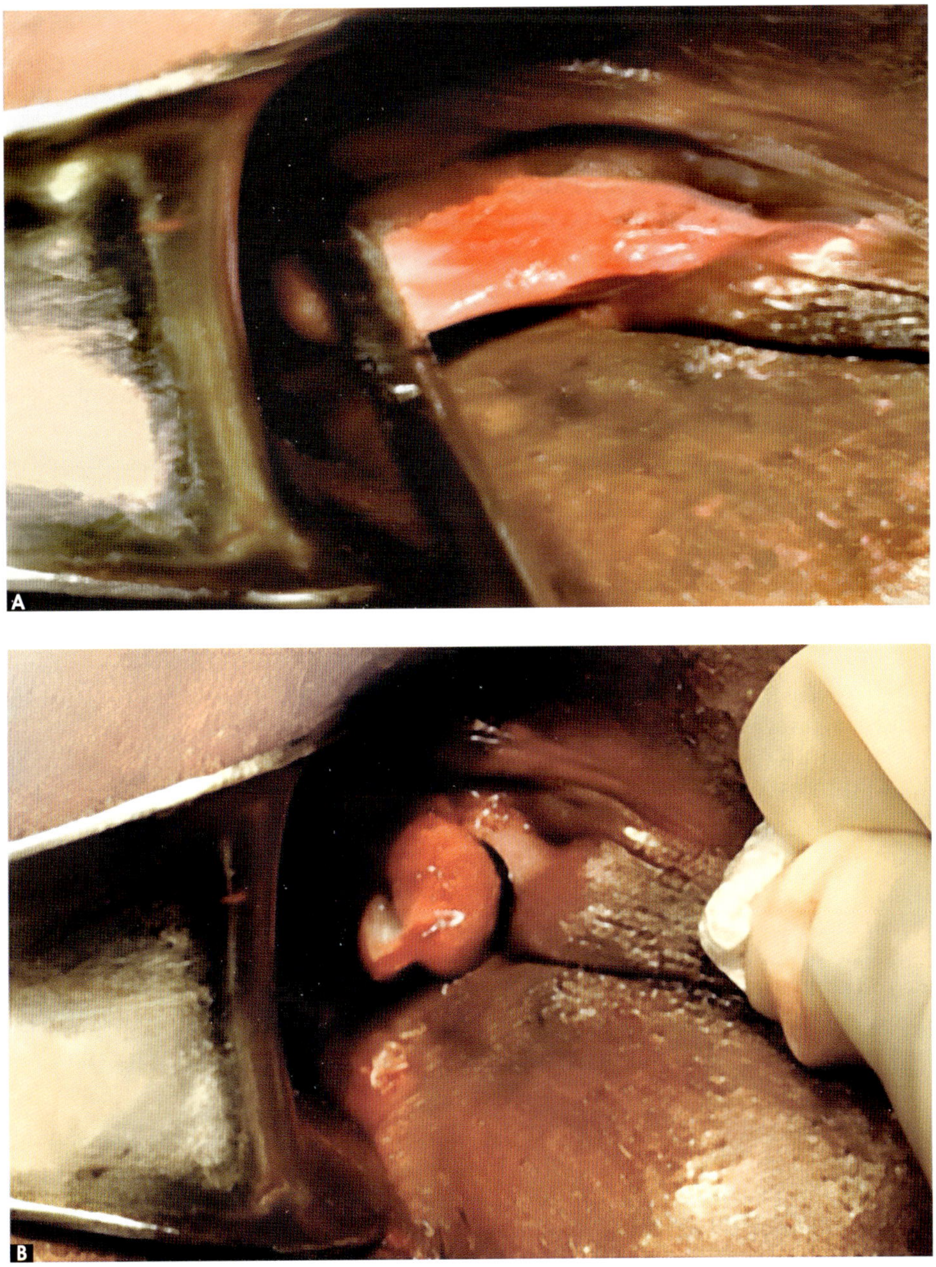

Fig. 2.12A, B: Wrongly placed rubber bands at the dentate line (Image *Courtesy:* Dr Parvez Sheikh).

Scan QR Code for Video on
RBL

VIDEO 5

FURTHER READING

- Agarwal N, Singh K, Sheikh P, Mittal K, Mathai V, Kumar A. Executive summary - The Association of Colon & Rectal Surgeons of India (ACRSI) practice guidelines for managing Hemorrhoids-2016. Indian J Surg. 2017;79(1):58–61. https://doi.org/10.1007/s12262-016-1578-7.
- Albuquerque A. Rubber band ligation of hemorrhoids: A guide for complications. World J Gastrointest Surg. 2016 Sep 27;8(9):614-620. doi: 10.4240/wjgs.v8.i9.614. PMID: 27721924; PMCID: PMC5037334.
- Bacon HE. The anus, rectum and sigmoid colon. 3rd ed. Philadelphia: Lippincott; 1949.
- Blanchard CE. Textbook of ambulant proctology. Youngstown: Ohio Medical Success Press; 1928. p. 134.
- Chew SS, Marshall L, Kalish L, Tham J, Grieve DA, Douglas PR, Newstead GL. Short-term and long-term results of combined sclerotherapy and rubber band ligation of hemorrhoids and mucosal prolapse. Dis Colon Rectum. 2003 Sep;46(9):1232–7. doi: 10.1007/s10350-004-6720-0. PMID: 12972968.
- Davis BR, Lee-Kong SA, Migaly J, Feingold DL, Steele SR. The American Society of Colon and Rectal Surgeons clinical practice guidelines for the management of hemorrhoids. Dis Colon Rectum. 2018;61(3):284–92.
- Gupta PJ. Infrared coagulation: a preferred option in treating early hemorrhoids. Acta Cir Bras. 2004;19(1):74–8.
- Iyer VS, Shrier I, Gordon PH. Long-term outcome of rubber band ligation for symptomatic primary and recurrent internal hemorrhoids. Dis Colon Rectum. 2004 Aug;47(8):1364–70. doi: 10.1007/s10350-004-0591-2. PMID: 15484351.
- Johanson JF, Rimm A. Optimal nonsurgical treatment of hemorrhoids: a comparative analysis of infrared coagulation, rubber band ligation, and injection sclerotherapy. Am J Gastroenterol. 1992 Nov;87(11):1600–6. PMID: 1442682.
- Kodilinye SM, & Kalloo AN. (2023). Endoscopic approaches to the management of hemorrhoids. Current Opinion in Gastroenterology, 10-1097.
- Lobascio P, Laforgia R, Novelli E, Perrone F, Di Salvo M, Pezzolla A, Trompetto M, Gallo G. Short-term results of sclerotherapy with 3% polidocanol foam for symptomatic second- and third-degree haemorrhoids.
- Longman RJ, Thomson WH. A prospective study of outcome from rubber band ligation of piles. Colorectal Dis. 2006 Feb;8(2):145–8. doi: 10.1111/j.1463-1318.2005.00873.x. PMID: 16412076.
- Mott T, Latimer K, Edwards C. Hemorrhoids: diagnosis and treatment options. Am Fam Physician. 2018;97(3):172–9. PMID: 29431977
- Nikshoar MR, Maleki Z, Nemati Honar B. The clinical efficacy of infrared photocoagulation versus closed hemorrhoidectomy in treatment of hemorrhoids. J Lasers Med Sci. 2018;9(1):23–6. https://doi. org/10.15171/jlms.2018.06.
- Rabe E, Breu FX, Flessenkämper I, et al. Sclerotherapy in the treatment of varicose veins. Hautarzt. 2021;72:23–36. https://doi.org/10.1007/ s00105-020-04705-0.
- Tomiki Y, Ono S, Aoki J, Takahashi R, Ishiyama S, Sugimoto K, et al. Treatment of internal hemorrhoids by endoscopic sclerotherapy with aluminium potassium sulfate and tannic acid. Diagn Ther Endosc. 2015;2015:517690.
- Weledji EP. Minor anorectal conditions in proctology. Austin J Surg. 2018;5(5):1142.
- Xu J, Wang YF, Chen AW, Wang T, Liu SH. A modified Tessari method for producing more foam. Springerplus. 2016;5:129. https://doi.org/10.1186/ s40064-016-1769-5.
- Yano T, Yano K. Comparison of injection sclerotherapy between 5% phenol in almond oil and aluminium potassium sulfate and tannic acid for grade 3 hemor- rhoids. Ann Coloproctol. 2015;31(3):103–5. https:// doi.org/10.3393/ac.2015.31.3.103.
- uk V, Š epanovi M, Krd i I, Keni M, Kova evi B, uk V. Where are we now in the treatment of hemorrhoids? Acta Medica Medianae. 2015;54(1):97–106.

Chapter

3

Surgical Management of Hemorrhoids Excisional Hemorrhoidectomy

Hemorrhoidectomy means "the excision of hemorrhoids." Though many techniques have been developed, the conventional Milligan-Morgan hemorrhoidectomy is considered a "Gold standard" for large, strangulated, or circumferential hemorrhoids.

This chapter focuses on the commonest operative techniques of excisional hemorrhoidectomy by Milligan Morgan and Ferguson.

Indications

- Grade 2 hemorrhoids (failure of medical management/office procedures)
- Grade 3 and 4 hemorrhoids
- Thrombosed internal hemorrhoids
- Strangulated hemorrhoids
- Interno-external hemorrhoids

Preoperative Preparation

Prepare the patient one night before the intervention by giving two bisacodyl tablets. Enema on the day of surgery is avoided to prevent a messy field during the procedure.

Instrumentation (Fig. 3.1)

- Self-retaining proctoscope
- Sim's speculum
- Half cut proctoscope
- Scissors
- Jelly
- Thread for ligation (Vicryl 2-0 and 3-0)
- Three Allis forceps
- Surgical cautery/Harmonic scalpel/Ligasure (depending on the surgeon's choice)

Position of the patient: Lithotomy/Jack-knife (Fig. 3.2).

Type of anaesthesia: Spinal/General/Pudendal nerve block

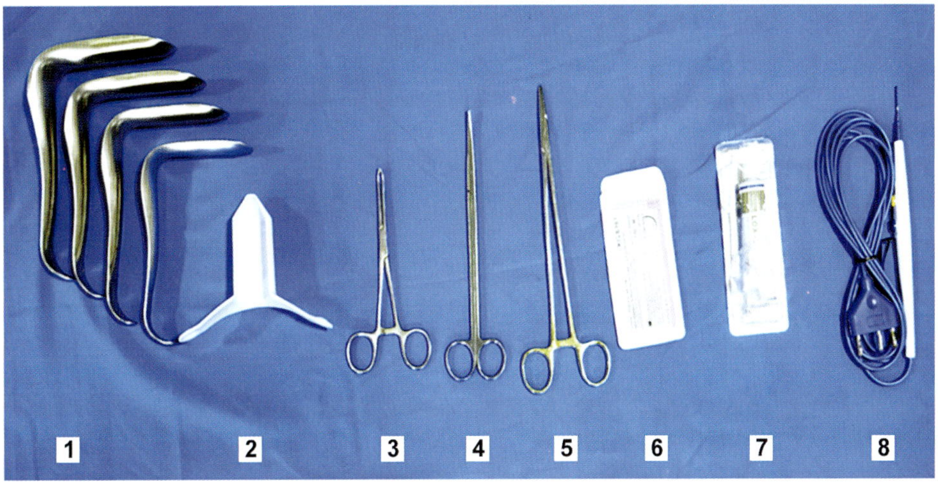

Fig. 3.1: 1) Sim's speculum. 2) Half-cut proctoscope. 3) Allis forceps. 4) Scissors. 5) Needle holder. 6) Vicryl 2-0 suture. 7) Lubricant jelly. 8) Surgical cautery.

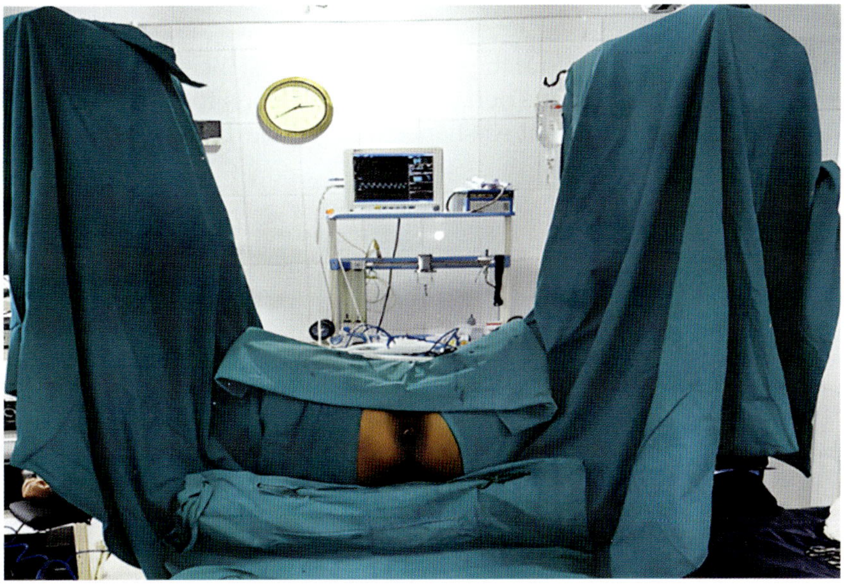

Fig. 3.2: Lithotomy position.

OPEN HEMORRHOIDECTOMY (MILLIGAN MORGAN)

Steps of Procedure

Step 1: After cleaning and draping, artery forceps are applied on the perianal skin at 3, 7 and 11 o'clock. Gentle traction is given outwards to visualize the internal hemorrhoids (Fig. 3.3A).

Step 2: A pedicle stitch using the Figure of 8 technique is taken at the apex of the pile mass, approximately at the anorectal junction. The suture used is polyglactin 2-0 (Fig. 3.3B). This helps in reducing the bleeding during surgical excision.

Step 3: A marking is done using the cautery tip at the site of the proposed incision to ensure that the least anoderm is excised. The V-shaped marking starts at the perianal skin. It extends towards the apex of the hemorrhoids (Fig. 3.3C). Alternatively, an hourglass or dumbbell-shaped marking can be done around the hemorrhoidal mass.

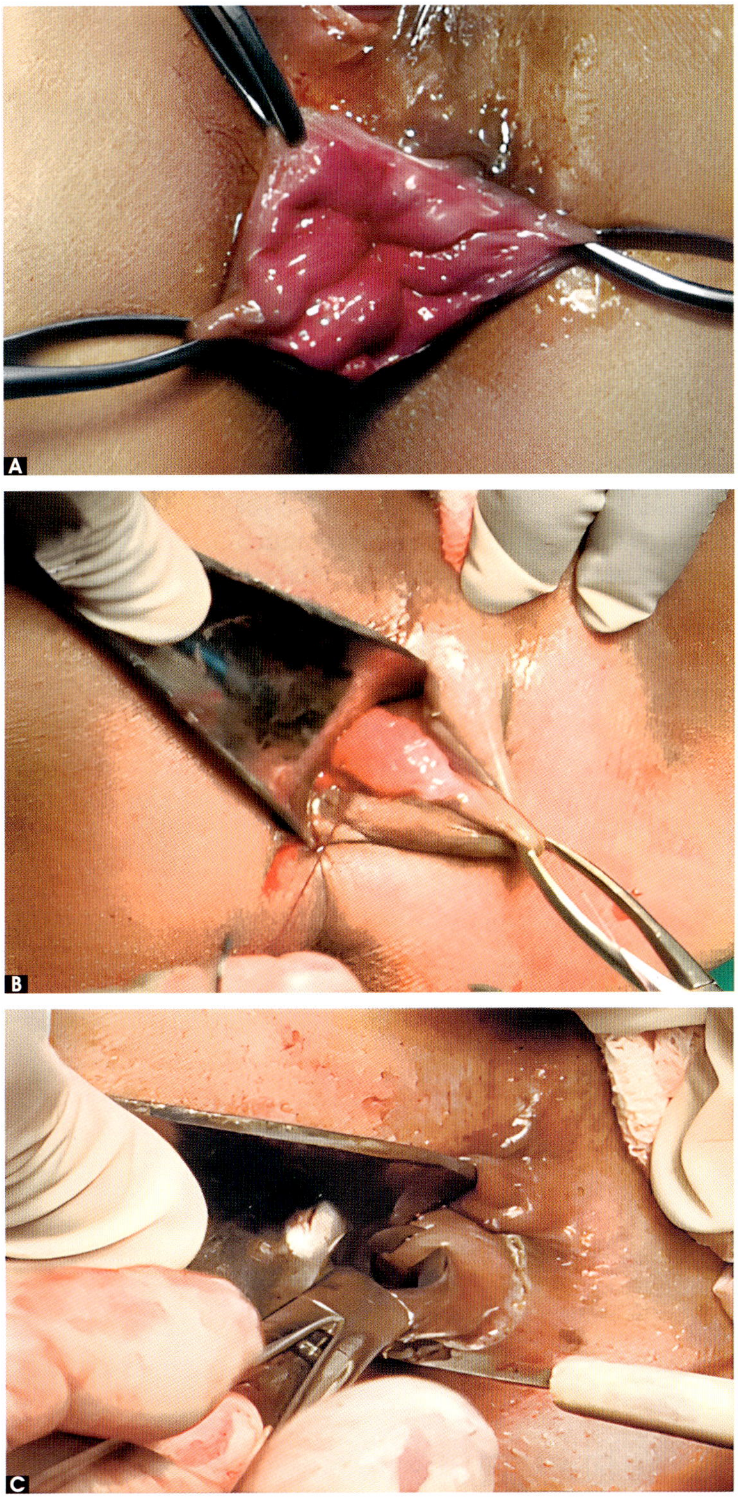

Fig. 3.3A–C: Milligan Morgan technique. A) Application of artery forceps at 3,7 and 11 o'clock positions. B, C) Milligan Morgan technique. B) Pedicle stitch using the Figure of 8 technique is taken at the apex of the pile mass. C) After marking V-shaped incision is given starting at the perianal skin.

Step 4: The dissection is started from the largest haemorrhoid, or if of similar size, with the one at 3 o'clock (Fig. 3.3D). During the dissection, one should stay in the submucosal plane. The plane can be easily identified during the dissection as one can see the fibres of the internal anal sphincter.

Step 5: Once the dissection is over, the pedicle is secured at the apex of the hemorrhoidal mass by an absorbable 2-0 polyglactin suture to prevent post-operative bleeding (Fig. 3.3E). The excised tissue is separated and sent for histopathology examination (Fig. 3.3F).

In this technique of excisional hemorrhoidectomy, after excision and ligation of the pedicle, the incision is kept open to heal by secondary intention. Usually, the raw area heals in 3 to 4 weeks.

All three hemorrhoids are excised similarly, ensuring adequate anoderm and mucosal tissue is retained between the excised hemorrhoids.

Tips and Tricks

- Since the position of the branches of SHA is not constant, it is advisable to palpate the vessel with the index finger before taking a suture to ensure proper ligation.
- It is crucial to preserve sufficient anoderm between the two excised hemorrhoids to prevent anal stenosis, especially while operating for circumferential hemorrhoids.

Scan QR Code for Video on

Milligan Morgan

VIDEO 6

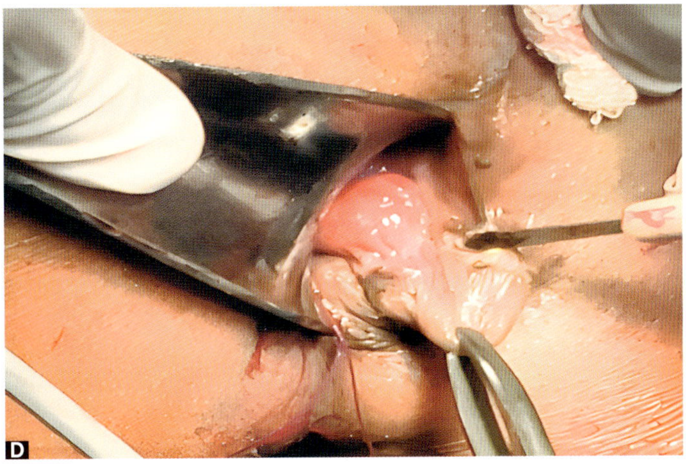

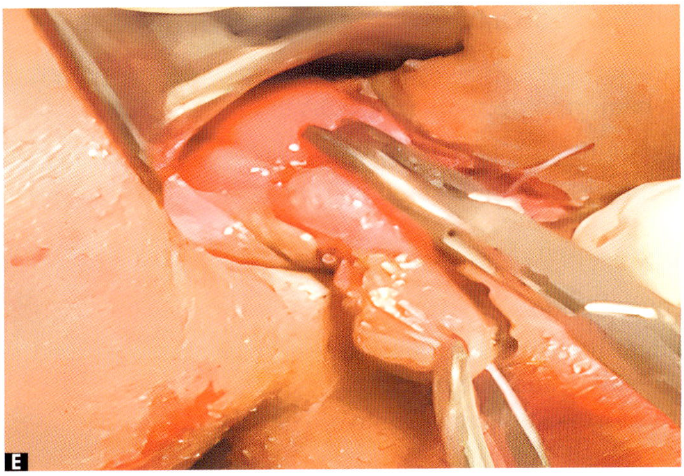

Fig. 3.3D and E: Milligan Morgan technique. D) Dissection starting at 3 o'clock, E) Securing of pedicle at the apex of the hemorrhoidal mass by an absorbable 2-0 polyglactin suture.

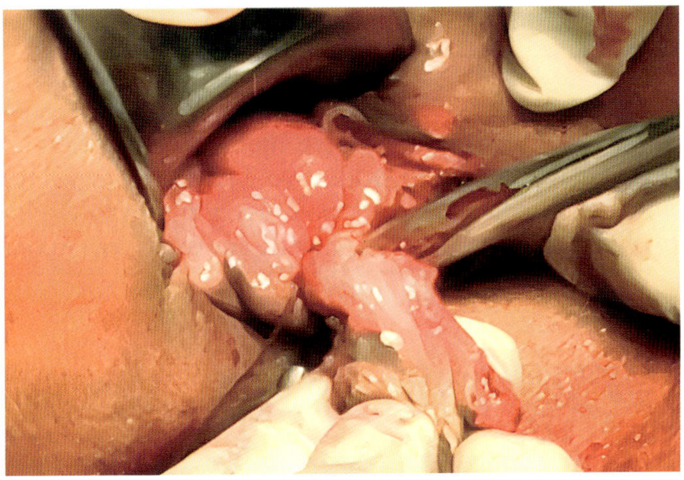

Fig. 3.3F: Milligan Morgan technique. F) Excision of the hemorrhoidal mass upto the anorectal ring.

Pitfalls of Milligan Morgan Hemorrhoidectomy

- Pain
- Mucosal or anal canal stenosis
- Bleeding (early and delayed)
- Prolonged healing time

FERGUSON'S CLOSED HEMORRHOIDECTOMY

Steps of Procedure

Steps I to 5: Same as in open hemorrhoidectomy (Fig. 3.3A to F).

Step 6: Once the hemorrhoidal tissue is excised, the margins are approximated from the anorectal ring upto the perianal skin by interrupted sutures, leaving a small margin at the end for draining the collection. The suture used is polyglactin 3-0 (Fig. 3.4A–C).

Advantages of Ferguson's over Milligan Morgan

In Milligan Morgan's excisional hemorrhoidectomy, large raw areas are created, causing pain and delayed healing. Scar retraction may result in anal stenosis.

Ferguson's technique outperforms Milligan Morgan's. The advantages are:

- Lesser bleeding
- Better wound healing
- Less post-operative pain
- Early mobilization

Conclusion

Excisional hemorrhoidectomy has a few pitfalls. These include post-operative pain, large raw areas, prolonged healing time, and a delayed return to work. Many novel strategies have developed over time to reduce morbidity. Due to smaller incisions, lesser pain, early return to work, and the preservation of anatomical integrity, minimally invasive procedures offer an advantage over conventional surgeries.

Scan QR Code for Video on
Ferguson's Hemorrhoidectomy

VIDEO 7

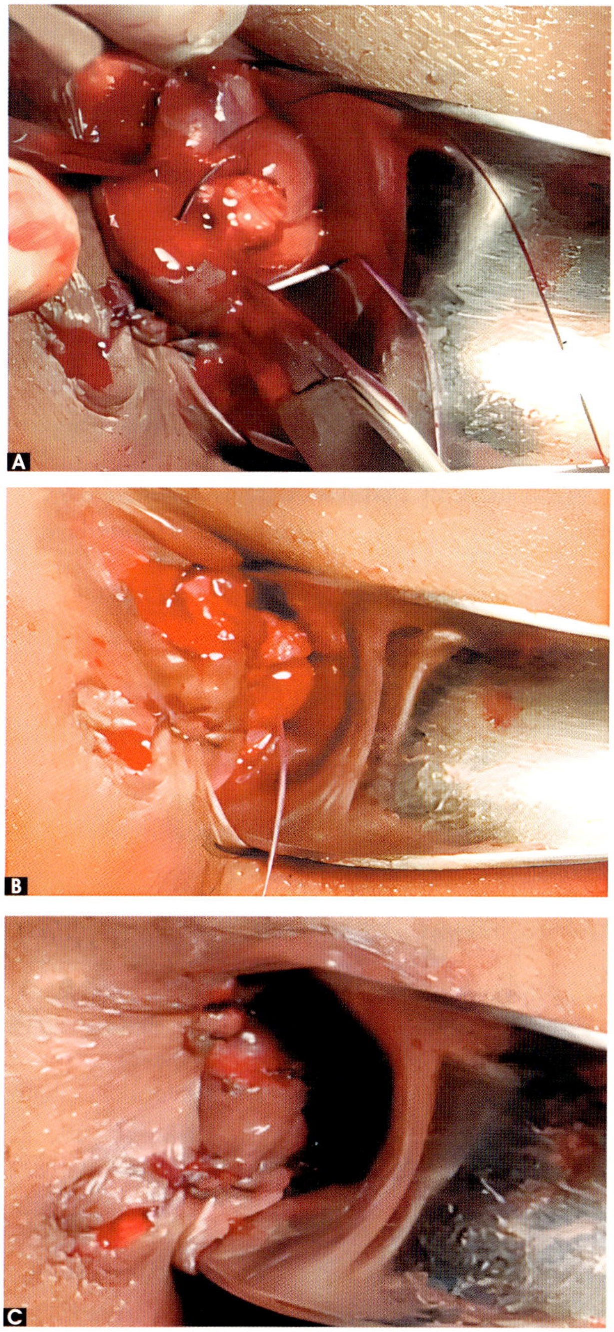

Fig. 3.4(A-C): A, B) Continuous suturing of the raw area leaving about 5 mm of open wound at the end for drainage purposes. C) Final wound as seen at the end of the procedure.

FURTHER READING

- Arbman G, Krook H, Haapaniemi S. Closed vs open hemorrhoidectomy—is there any difference? Dis Colon Rectum. 2000;43:31–4.
- Ayfan J. Complications of Milligan-Morgan hemorrhoidectomy. Dig Surg. 2001;18(2):131–3. https:// doi.org/10.1159/000050113.
- Bhatti MI, Sajid MS, Baig MK. Milligan-Morgan (open) versus Ferguson Hemorrhoidectomy (closed): a systematic review and meta-analysis of published randomized controlled trials. World J Surg. 2016;40(6):1509–19. https://doi.org/10.1007/s00268-016-3419-z.
- Borse H, Dhake S. A comparative study of open (Milligan-Morgan) versus closed (Ferguson) hemorrhoid-ectomy. MVP J Med Sci. 2016;3(1):7–10.
- Ferguson JA, Heaton JR. Closed hemorrhoidectomy. Dis Colon Rectum. 1959;2(2):176–9. https://doi. org/10.1007/BF02616713.
- Ferguson JA, Mazier WP, Ganchrow MI, Friend WG. The closed technique of hemorrhoidectomy. Surgery. 1971 Sep;70(3):480–4. PMID: 5568533.
- Hardy A, Chan CLH, Cohen CRG. The surgical management of hemorrhoids—a review. Dig Surg. 2005;22(1-2):26–33.
- Hosch SB, Knoefel WT, Pichlmeier U. Surgical treatment of piles: a prospective, randomized study of Parks vs. Milligan-Morgan hemorrhoidectomy. Dis Colon Rectum. 1998;41:159–64.
- Milligan ETC, Morgan CN, Jones L, Officer R. Surgical anatomy of the anal canal and the operative treatment of hemorrhoids. Lancet. 1937;230(5959): 1119–24.
- Pata F, Gallo G, Pellino G, Vigorita V, Podda M, Di Saverio S, D'Ambrosio G, Sammarco G. Evolution of surgical management of hemorrhoidal disease: an his- torical overview. Front Surg. 2021;8:727059. https:// doi.org/10.3389/fsurg.2021.727059.
- Pokharel N, Chhetri RK, Malla B, Joshi HN, Shrestha RK. Hemorrhoidectomy: Ferguson's (closed) vs. Milligan-Morgan's technique (open). Nepal Med Coll J. 2009;11(2):136–7.
- Shaikh AR, Dalwani AG, Soomro N. An evaluation of Milligan-Morgan and Ferguson procedures for hemorrhoidectomy at Liaquat University Hospital Jamshoro, Hyderabad, Pakistan. Pak J Med Sci. 2013;29(1):122–7. https://doi.org/10.12669/pjms.291.2858.
- Tomasicchio G, Martines G, Lantone G, Dibra R, Trigiante G, De Fazio M, Picciariello A, Alto- mare DF, Rinaldi M. Safety and effectiveness of tailored hemorrhoidectomy in outpatients setting. Front Surg. 2021;8:708051. https://doi.org/10.3389/fsurg.2021.708051.
- Watts JM, Bennett RC, Duthie HL, Goligher JC. Healing and pain after hemorrhoidectomy. Br J Surg. 1964;51:808–17. https:// doi.org/10.1002/ bjs.1800511104.
- Yeo D, Tan KY. Hemorrhoidectomy - making sense of the surgical options. World J Gastroenterol. 2014 Dec 7;20(45):16976–83. doi: 10.3748/wjg.v20.i45.16976. PMID: 25493010; PMCID: PMC4258566.

Chapter

4

Hemorrhoids Minimally Invasive Procedures

Minimally invasive techniques for managing hemorrhoids emerged in the late 20th and the early 21st centuries. These include

- Doppler Guided hemorrhoidal artery ligation
- Stapled hemorrhoidopexy (PPH)
- Laser hemorrhoidoplasty (LHP)
- Transanal suture hemorrhoidopexy
- Superior hemorrhoidal artery embolisation

DOPPLER GUIDED HEMORRHOIDAL ARTERY LIGATION

The technique was invented by a Japanese surgeon Kazumasa Morinaga in 1995.

Principle

- Locating and ligating the terminal branches of the superior hemorrhoidal artery using a proctoscope with a Doppler probe coupled with a Doppler transducer.
- The ligation is carried out 2–4 cm above the dentate line (Fig. 4.1).

Indications

- Grade II to IV hemorrhoids

Contraindications

- Circumferential prolapse of hemorrhoids
- Hemorrhoids with rectal prolapse
- Hemorrhoids with active proctitis
- Hemorrhoids associated with anorectal sepsis
- Grade IV necrotic hemorrhoids
- Post surgery scarring and fibrosis

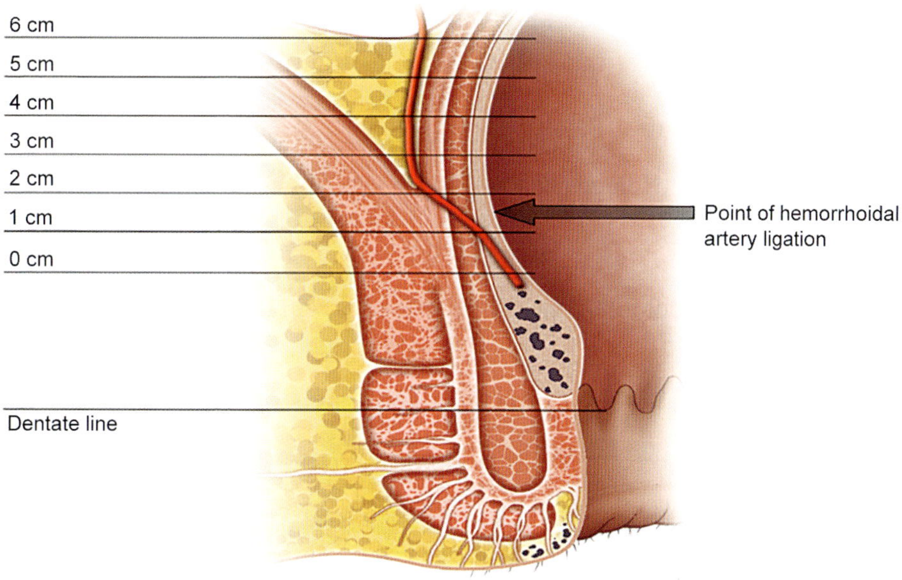

Fig. 4.1: Point of hemorrhoidal artery ligation.

Instrumentation

- Proctoscope with a built-in ultrasound transducer, light, and a special window for ligation (Fig. 4.2A).
- A Doppler machine that displays a graph (Fig. 4.2B)
- Special tipped needle holder.
- A strong atraumatic 27 mm 5/8 circle round body needle and 2/0 polyglactin suture (Fig. 4.2C, E).
- Forceps.
- Scissors.
- Knot pusher (Fig. 4.2D).
- A set of long jaw 9-inch thin artery forceps (Fig. 4.2D).
- Lubricant jelly.
- Trilogy probe (Fig. 4.2F).
- Recently a modified/wireless Bluetooth-enabled proctoscope with a Bluetooth speaker/echo sounder has been introduced.

Preoperative preparation: Two tablets of bisacodyl are given a night prior to the surgery.

Position of the patient: Lithotomy/Left lateral.

Type of anaesthesia: Spinal/General/Pudendal nerve block.

Principle of Doppler

- The disposable HAL proctoscope has a Doppler transducer on its tip. This proctoscope is connected to a Doppler instrument and generates acoustic signals. The influx of arterial blood in the internal hemorrhoidal plexus can be identified using acoustic signals, and the arteries can be selectively ligated.
- In the new doppler version, acoustic sounds can be heard through a Bluetooth-enabled smartphone. A trio probe replaced the earlier HAL proctoscope with a ligation window (Fig. 4.2F).

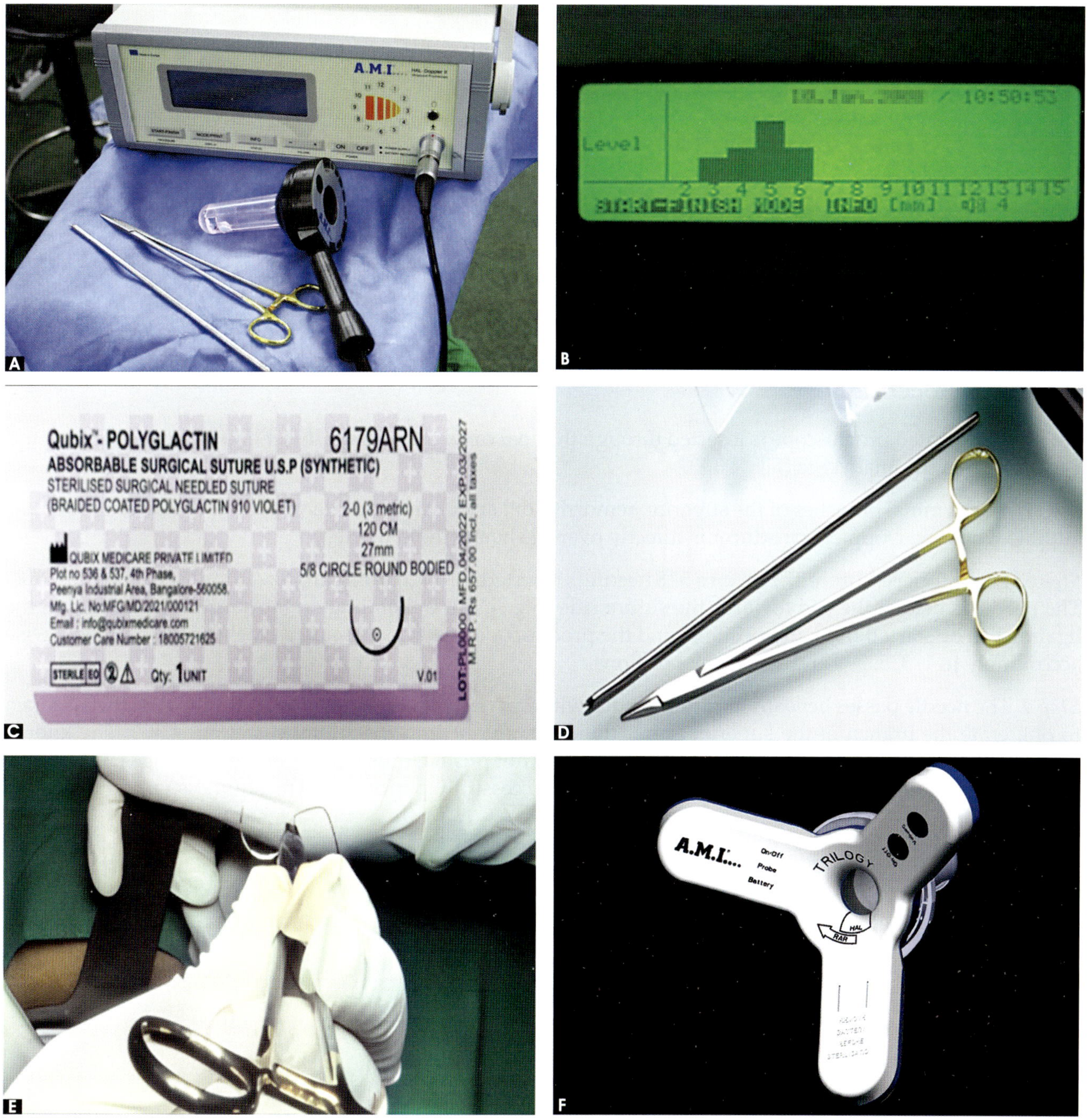

Fig. 4.2(A-F): Doppler equipment. A, B) Doppler proctoscope and monitor. C) Vicryl 2-0 suture. D) Needle holder and knot pusher. E) Needle on the needle holder. F)Trilogy probe.

Steps of the Procedure

Step 1: A lubricated proctoscope is inserted through the anal canal to reach the lower end of the rectum, around 5 to 7 cm from the anal verge (Fig. 4.3A).

Step 2: The terminal branches of the superior hemorrhoidal artery are accurately located. The arterial sound is audible when the Doppler transducer is directly over the hemorrhoidal artery.

Step 3: The 2/0 vicryl suture 27 mm on a 5/8 needle is inserted through the ligation window of the proctoscope. The needle is held at the end towards the suture side (Fig. 4.3B). Depending on the surgeon's preference, the ligation can be started from any position, and the proctoscope needs to be rotated clockwise or anti-clockwise accordingly to 1, 3, 5, 7, 9 and 11 o'clock positions.

Step 4: The needle passes beneath the artery and is withdrawn for safer reinsertion. A figure of 8 stitch is taken to obliterate the branch of the superior hemorrhoidal artery behind the submucosa (Fig. 4.3C). The knot is tied externally, pushed down into the mucosa with the knot pusher, thus ligating the artery (Fig. 4.3D, E). The Doppler sound disappears as soon as the ligation is successfully performed. The suture is cut with scissors (Fig. 4.3F, G).

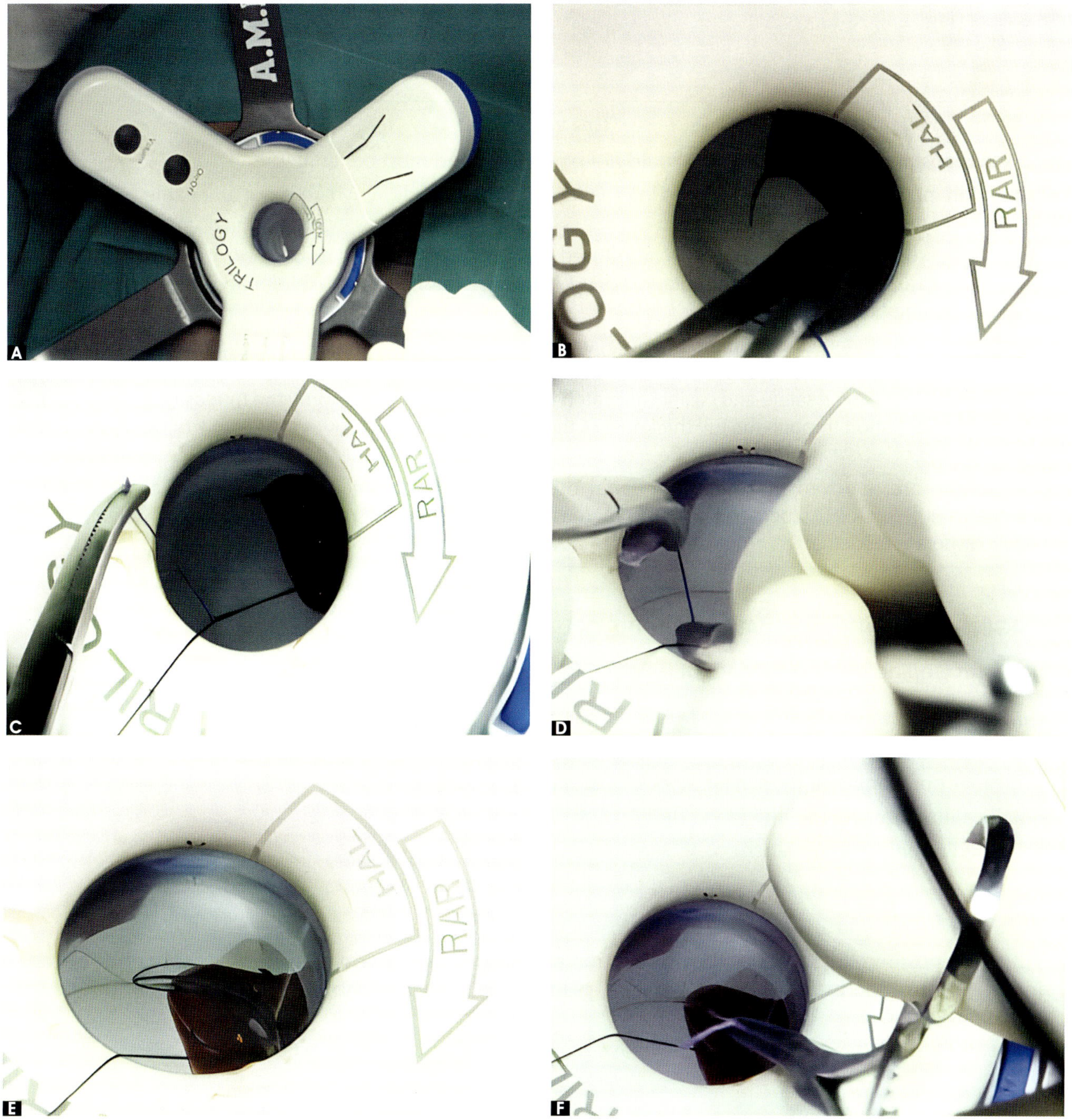

Fig. 4.3A to F: Technique of Doppler-guided hemorrhoidal artery ligation (DGHAL). A) Insertion of HAL proctoscope inside the anal canal. B) Insertion of the needle to ligate the branches of the superior hemorrhoidal artery. C) A Figure of 8 stitch taken to ligate the artery. D to E) Tying and pushing the knot with a knot pusher. F) Cutting of the suture.

All the branches are identified and ligated (Fig. 4.3H, I).

As a result of dearterialization, the shrinkage of the hemorrhoids starts immediately and continues over 6 to 8 weeks (Fig. 4.3J, K, L).

Tips and Tricks

- The prolapsing hemorrhoidal tissue should not be fibrosed and must be reducible.
- Attention must be paid to misdiagnosed internal rectal intussusception, which is not amenable to mucopexy used for hemorrhoidal prolapse.
- Blood pressure should be accurately monitored during surgery. A systolic blood pressure higher than 100–110 mmHg allows better auscultation of a Doppler signal necessary for identifying the hemorrhoidal arteries, making the procedure easier.
- There is a demarcated groove in the proximal end of the proctoscope in which the tip of the needle holder rotates to obliterate and ligate the vessels in a standard fashion. With this manoeuvre, the depth of the transfixed stitch can be safely and easily calibrated in a way that it includes only the mucosa and submucosa, to avoid penetration through the full thickness of the rectal wall, thereby lowering the risk of perirectal fistula and abscess.
- No tissues are removed from the anal canal other than hypertrophied papillae. External tags are not removed during DGHAL because doing so increases discomfort to the patient and may obscure the source of postoperative edema.

MANAGING CHALLENGING SITUATIONS ON THE OPERATING TABLE

Difficulty in Getting an Audio Signal at a Particular Point

Possibilities

- Improper lubrication of the sensor.
- Improper positioning of the sensor.
- Small calibre branch with low blood flow.
- Sclerosed or obliterated branch.

Solution

- Check for lubrication and reinsert the proctoscope.
- Tilt and reposition the sensor as the distribution patterns of the superior hemorrhoidal artery (bifurcation in 82%, trifurcation in 12%) and the entering points of its branches into the rectal wall musculature vary immensely.
- If the audio signal is absent after all the above manoeuvres, move to the next branch.

Scan QR Code for Video on

DGHAL

VIDEO 8

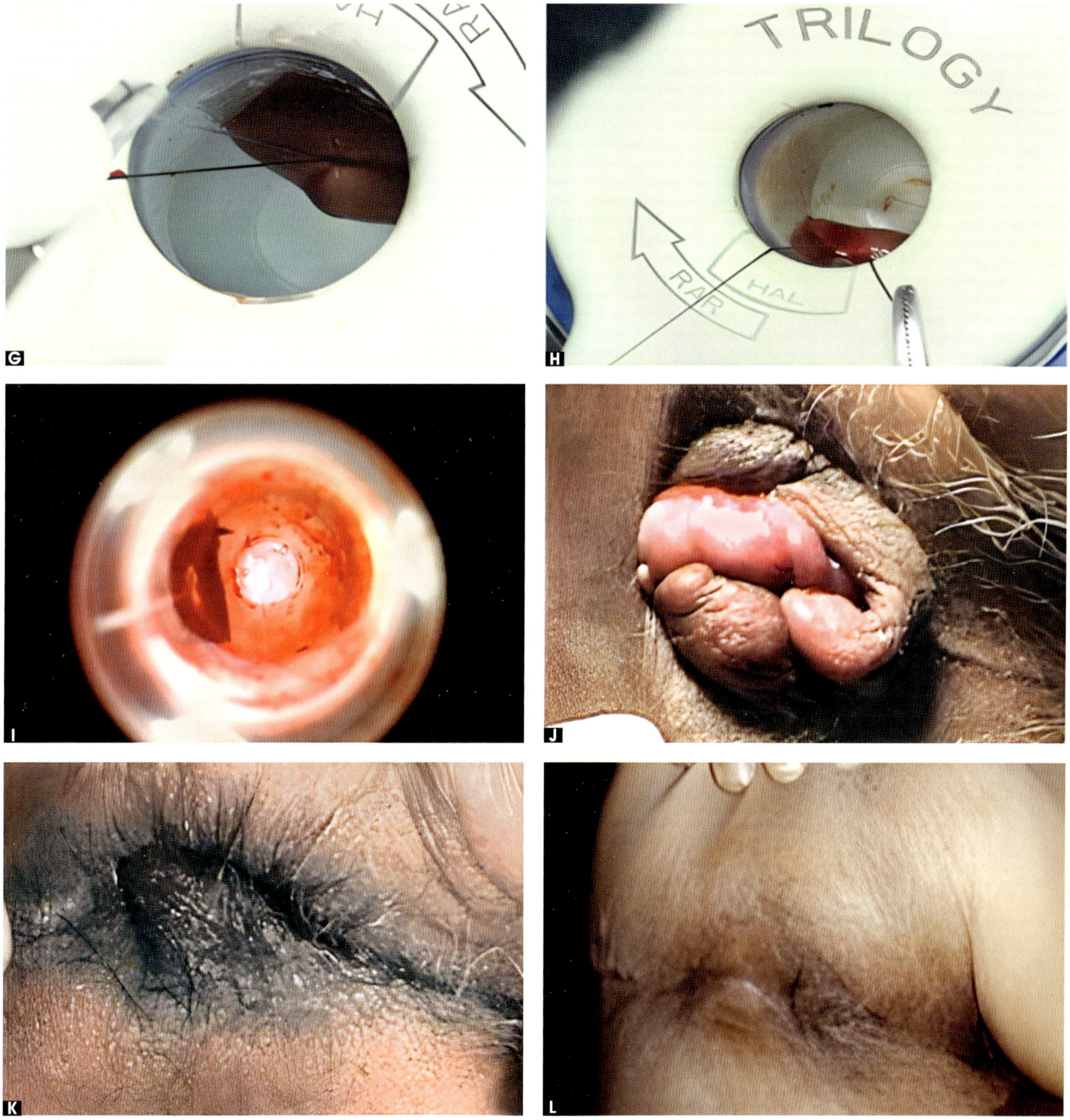

Fig. 4.3G to L: Technique of Doppler-guided hemorrhoidal artery ligation (DGHAL). G) Final picture seen through the proctoscope. H, I) Ligation at other positions. J, K) Preoperative and postoperative images. L) Post-operative image after 6 months. Procedure courtesy Dr. Ajit Kukerja.

The Audio Signal Persists Even After Ligation

Possibilities

- The vessel is not obliterated properly.
- Sounds are from adjoining small vessels after the primary branch is ligated.

Solution

- Take another ligature 1.5 to 2 cm proximal to the previous one. The sound usually disappears.
- Every time after passing the needle in the submucosa, pull the strings of the ligature. If the sound disappears, it is suggestive that the ligature is behind the vessel. If the sound persists, it is presumed to be from nearby small vessels (bifurcating or trifurcating branches).

RECTOANAL REPAIR (RAR)/MUCOPEXY

Indications

- Grade 3 and 4 hemorrhoids (Fig. 4.4A, B)

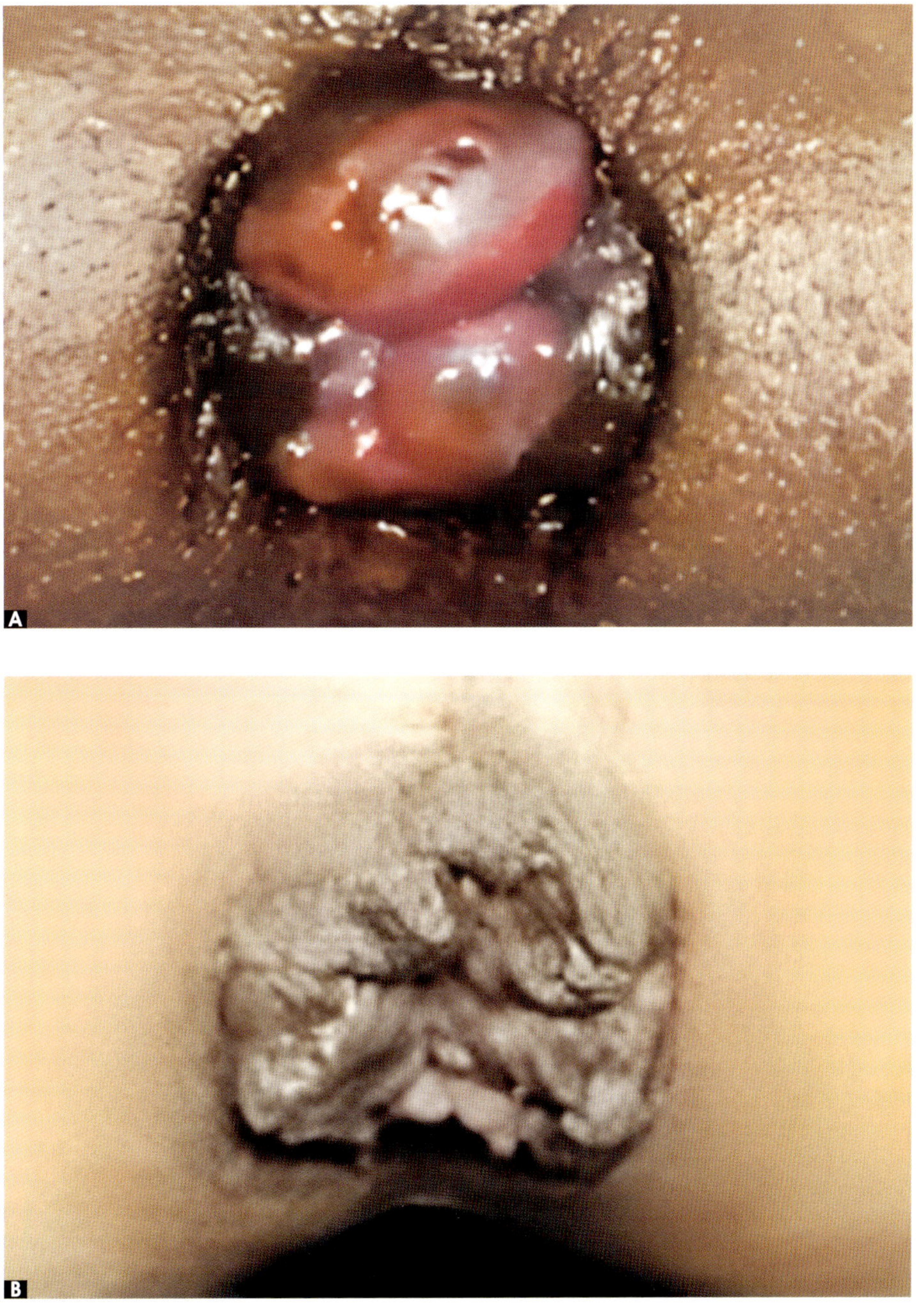

Fig. 4.4A, B: Grade 3 and 4 hemorrhoids.

Steps of the Procedure

Step 1: Continuing from the Doppler-guided dearterialization figure of 8 stitch, the sleeve is rotated to expose the mucosa.

Step 2: Longitudinal stitches spaced at 0.5 cm are started from the dearterialization stitch to the dentate line, and a kissing knot is gently tied to prevent a bowstring, which is moved in the proximal direction, to take its physiological position above the anal canal. Each stitch is taken at a depth of 2–3 mm.

Step 3: The last stitch is taken approximately 5mm above the dentate line. The sutures are always taken in a running fashion (Fig. 4.5A, B, C).

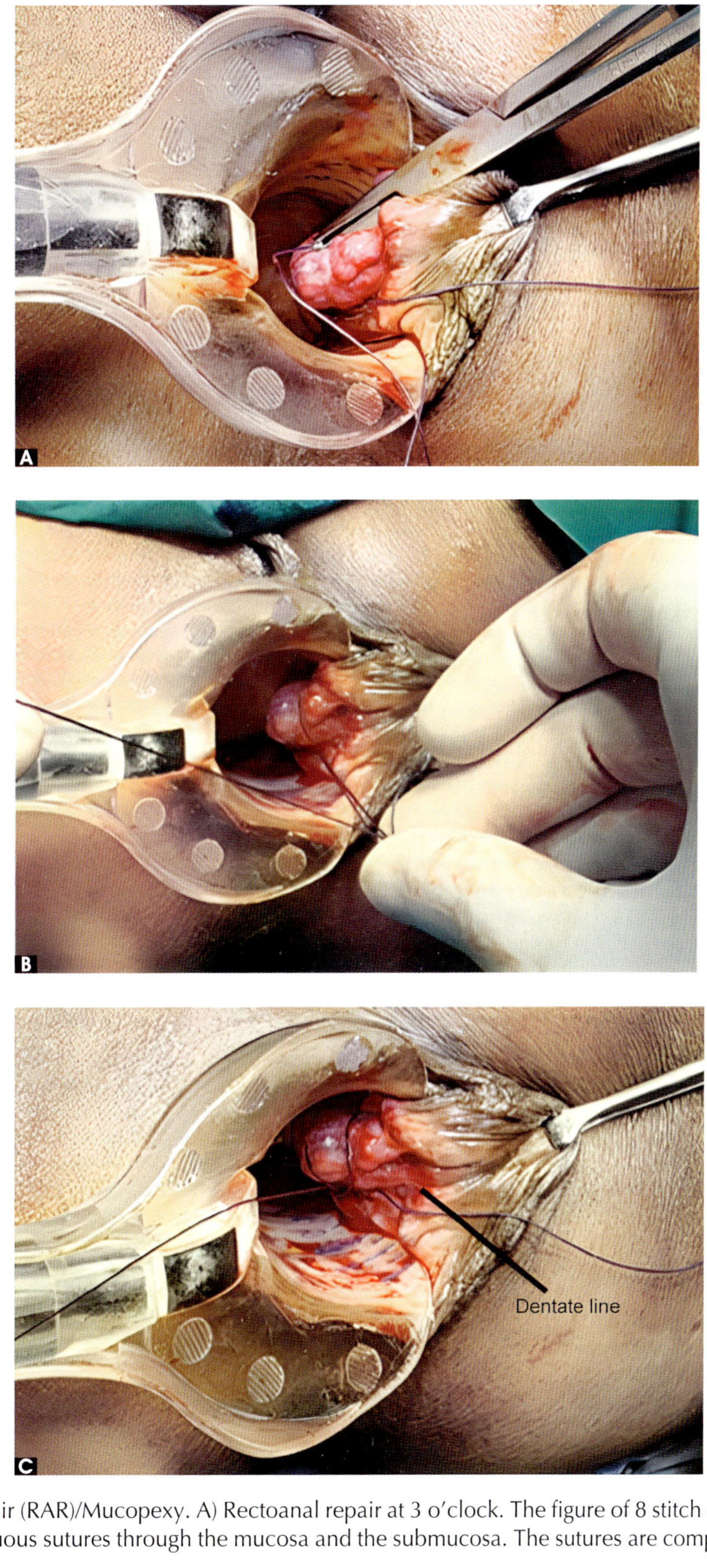

Fig. 4.5A–C: Rectoanal repair (RAR)/Mucopexy. A) Rectoanal repair at 3 o'clock. The figure of 8 stitch is taken at the apex of the pile mass. B, C) Showing continuous sutures through the mucosa and the submucosa. The sutures are completed above the dentate line.

Step 4: Once the stitching is over, both the ends of the thread are ligated at the apex, and the prolapsed tissue is pushed upwards towards the anal canal (Fig. 4.5D, E).

Tips and Tricks

- A short interval of suture stitches increases the risk of mucosal ischemia, whereas if the interval of suture stitches is long, "creeping" of the mucosa occurs.
- Adjacent vertical rows should be adequately spaced to ensure enough blood outflow from the hemorrhoids via the venous plexus.
- A relative contraindication to the procedure is circumferential prolapse, where circumferential repairs can lead to obliteration of the rectal tissue and obstruction of the blood and, consequently, an increased risk of postoperative thrombosis.

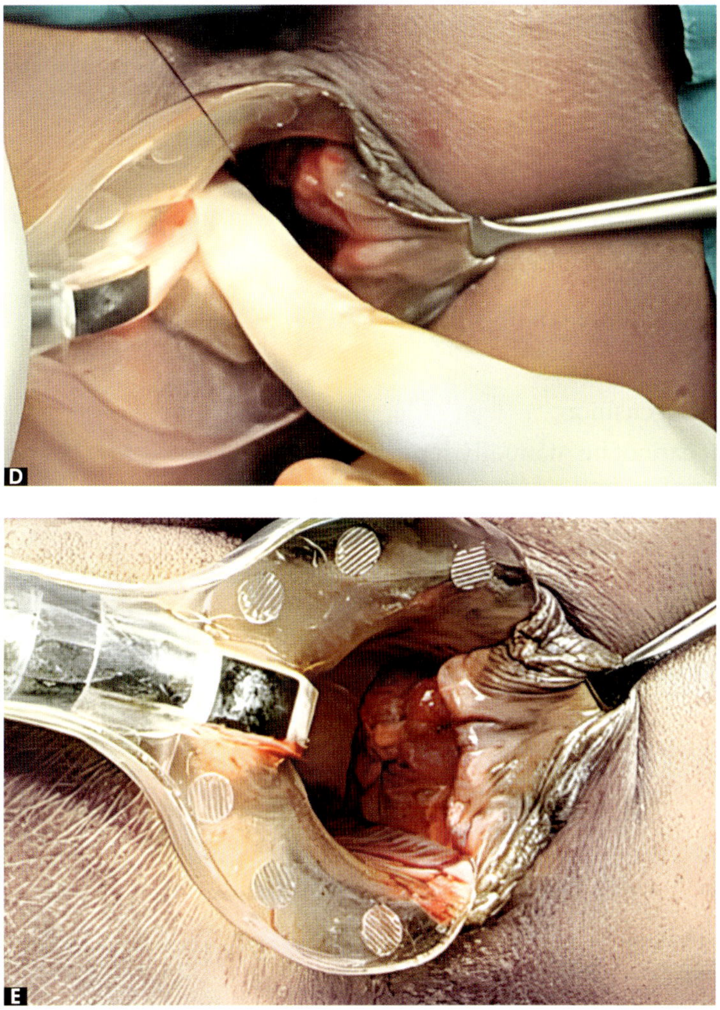

Fig. 4.5D-E: Rectoanal repair (RAR)/Mucopexy. D)The hemorrhoidal mass is pushed upwards towards the apex. E) Final picture of the interior of the anal canal at the end of the rectoanal repair.

STAPLED HEMORRHOIDOPEXY

Stapled hemorrhoidopexy was invented by Dr Longo from Italy in 1998. A circular device is used to reduce prolapsed hemorrhoidal mass.

Principle

- Excision of the rectal mucosa as a ring above the hemorrhoidal cushions with re-anastomosis of the mucosa.

Indications
- Grade 2 to 4 hemorrhoids (Circumferential)

Contra-indication
- Presence of a single prolapsed cushion.
- Fibrosed hemorrhoids that cannot be manually repositioned (Fig. 4.6).
- Inability to introduce circular anal dilator due to previous surgery causing scarring and fibrosis

Instrumentation (Fig. 4.7)

- A 33 mm stapler gun
- A detachable/non-detachable anvil
- A transparent anal dilator
- A purse-string crochet threader hook
- A purse-string speculum
- Prolene 2-0 (available with stapler equipment)

Preoperative preparation: The patient is prepared one night before the intervention by giving two bisacodyl tablets.

Position of the patient: Lithotomy

Type of anaesthesia: Spinal/General/Pudendal nerve block.

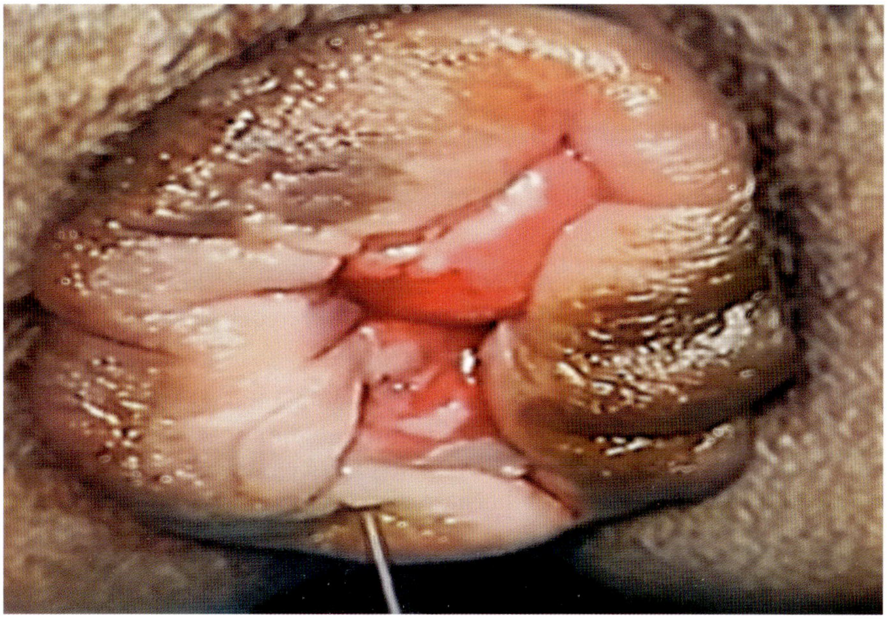

Fig. 4.6: Fibrosed circumferential hemorrhoids.

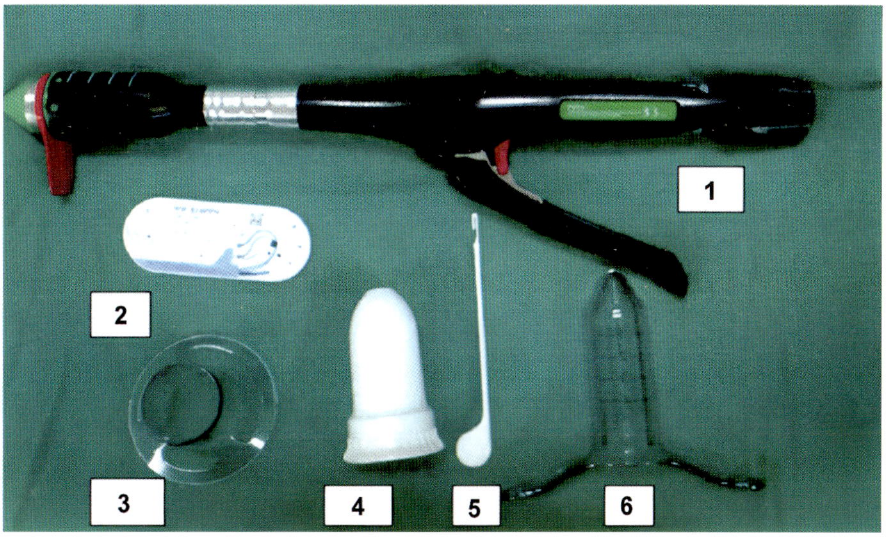

Fig. 4.7: Stapler equipment. 1) 33 mm stapler gun. 2) Prolene 2-0. 3) Transparent anal dilator. 4) Anal Dilator. 5) Purse-string crochet threader hook. 6) Transparent proctoscope.

Steps of the Procedure

Step 1: Reduce the prolapsed hemorrhoids in the head low position. Gentle anal dilatation is done either with lubricated fingers or the obturator to facilitate the introduction of the circular anal dilator (CAD) with an obturator in the anal canal (Fig. 4.8A).

Step 2: The obturator is removed, and the CAD is fixed to the perianal skin by stitching through the CAD window using a silk thread to secure it firmly. The dentate line is seen below the transparent body of the CAD. A half-cut anoscope is introduced through the dilator (Fig. 4.8B).

Step 3: The half-cut anoscope pushes the prolapsing mucosa against the rectal wall along a circumference of 270 degrees. The mucosa and the submucosa that protrude through the anoscope window are held with the help of a stitch using prolene 2-0 (Fig. 4.8C). The first stitch is taken 3-4 cm above the dentate line and proximal to the hemorrhoidal apex, starting from 3 o'clock. Alternatively, one can start the purse-string suture at 9 o'clock.

Step 4: The half-cut proctoscope is withdrawn after each stitch and reintroduced after slight clockwise rotation for the next stitch. This ensures that the purse string stitches are at the same level along the entire circumference.

The anoscope is gently rotated through the rectal circumference to complete a "purse-string" suture (Fig. 4.8D). A counter stitch opposite to the starting point is taken with the length kept long.

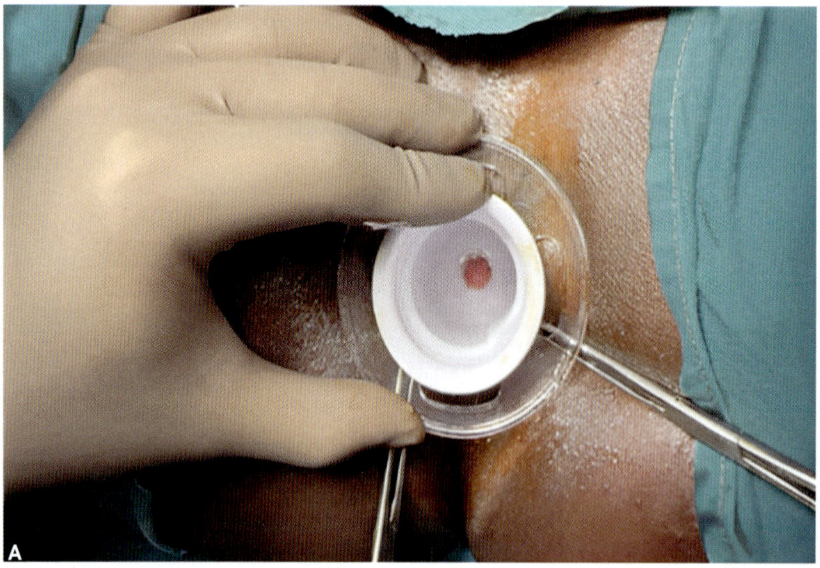

Fig. 4.8A: Stapler technique for hemorrhoids. A) Insertion and fixation of circular anal dilator followed by insertion of anoscope.

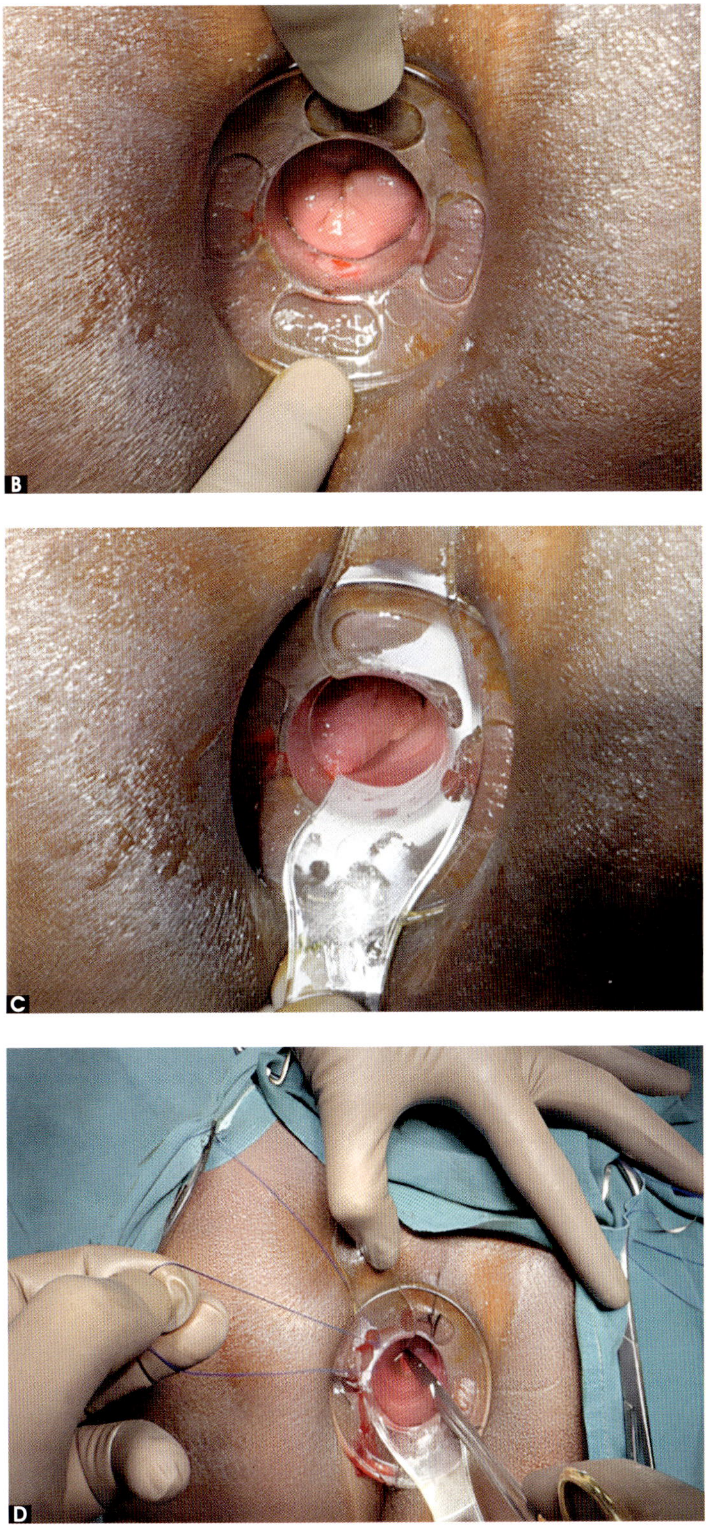

Fig. 4.8B-D: Stapler technique for hemorrhoids. B, C) Removal of the obturator to visualize the prolapsing mucosa against the rectal wall. D) Rotation of anoscope and starting of the purse string suture.

Step 5: The stapler is then unfolded to its maximum limit and introduced with the opened stapler head placed beyond the purse string suture. The purse string is tied over the stapler shaft with one throw knot. Both suture ends are externally tied or clamped with a forceps (Fig. 4.8E).

Step 6: Along the anal canal axis, the stapler is aligned and closed, keeping a normal amount of tension on the string (Fig. 4.8F). After the stapler is closed, it is held for a minute to reduce interstitial oedema. A finger is passed into the vagina in a female patient to check the posterior vaginal wall and to ensure this is not incorporated into the purse string.

Step 7: The stapler is fired, releasing a row of double-staggered titanium staples through the tissue. The tissue comprising of the mucosa and the submucosa is excised circumferentially by the circular stapler knife. The stapler device is removed by opening the head partially with half rotation on either side.

The doughnut is checked. It should contain a 2 cm wide rectal mucosal strip (Fig. 4.8G).

Scan QR Code for Video on
Stapled Hemorrhoidopexy Procedure for Prolapsed Hemorrhoids
VIDEO 9

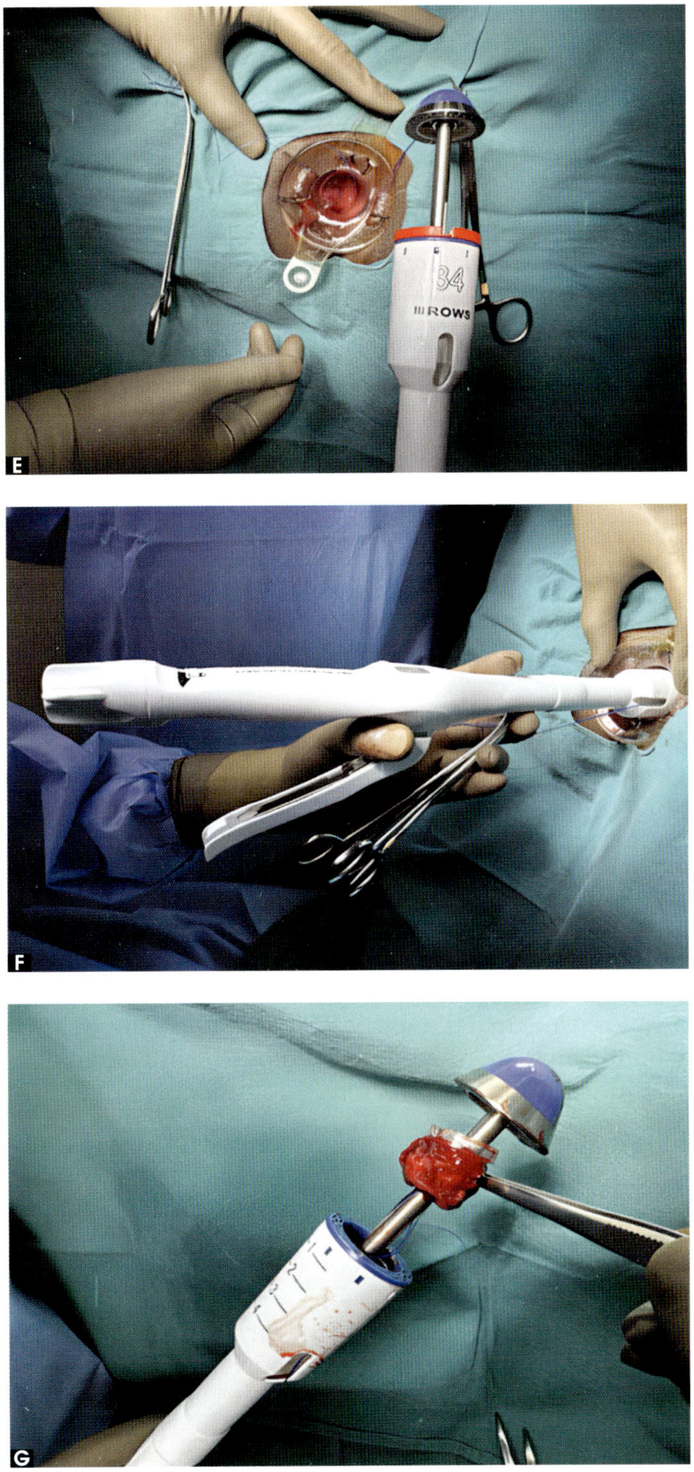

Fig. 4.8E-G: Stapler technique for hemorrhoids. E) Tying of the purse string with one throw knot. F) Insertion of stapler device. G) Donut as seen after releasing the staplers. (Procedure, video and images courtesy Dr. Nitish Jhawar, Mumbai).

TROUBLE SHOOTING IN PPH

Bowel preparation: Laxative should be given a night prior to the procedure. Handling a solid stool on the table is better than a liquid one. The liquid stool particles may get entrapped in the staple line, leading to a rectal pocket syndrome.

Position: Extended lithotomy position is preferred over the conventional one for the proper fixation of the circular anal dilator and to facilitate the procedure.

Park's manoeuvre: It is done to reproduce the prolapse on the table and for deciding the level of purse string suturing. It can be done by putting a dry gauze inside the anus and pulling it out using Allis forceps.

Anal dilation: Two-finger-controlled anal dilatation is recommended to facilitate smooth passage and positioning of the obturator and the circular anal dilator. This would prevent any drag while pushing the anoscope inside, and a staggered or skewed staple line can be avoided. If there is a drag, the dentate line may get pushed inside, and the final staple line will come close to the dentate line, causing excruciating pain.

Narrow pelvis with close ischial tuberosities: In some cases, the distance between the two tuberosities is narrow, and it will not allow passage of the obturator or circular anal dilator. In such a case, a size 32 can be used in place of 34, which is routine.

Heavy buttocks preventing fixation of the circular anal dilator: In case of heavy butt cheeks causing difficulty in fixing the circular anal dilator, the flanges may be cut, or a circular anal dilator which has two prongs can be used.

Fixing the CAD: The fixing of CAD is of utmost importance. If it changes its position during the surgery, the staple line may be skewed, leading to an incomplete procedure, along with post-operative pain and bleeding. Proper fixation can be achieved by taking sutures through the windows provided and the assistant holding it in position throughout the surgery.

Purse string suture: The suturing is done using the stapler device and the monofilament sutures provided by the vendor. For a right-handed surgeon, it's advisable to start suturing at 9 o'clock so that the difficult part is initially covered. The distance from the dentate line should be around 4 to 5 cm, and the depth should be up to the level of the submucosa. To ensure that the suture is not too shallow, one should not be able to see the suture through the mucosa. Similarly, to ensure that the suture is not too deep, there should be a tenting of the suture line when we lift the suture off the mucosa. If the suture is too deep, it will take the internal anal sphincter in the donut, which can affect continence and cause massive post-operative pain.

Belt loop suture: To ensure the donut is uniform and complete, the belt loop suture can be taken opposite the starting point of the purse string suture. Usually, we prefer taking it at 3 o'clock to give a uniform donut.

Stapling device: The anvil of the stapler should be completely opened and then inserted beyond the purse string suture so that both the purse string and the belt loop suture can be pulled out from the window provided on the sides of the stapler head.

The direction of the stapling device should be towards the sacral hollow and in the midline. Once the stapler is closed, the traction should be applied on the sutures in a bowstring manner so that the tissue will not slip out of the housing of the stapler. It is recommended to wait for 30 to 60 seconds before the staple is fired so that the excess fluid can be pushed out of the tissue and the staple is secure and haemostatic.

Firing zone: It is important to look for the indicator in the firing zone and fire only when it has come on to the line, as indicated on the anvil. The stapling gun should be fired only once. If fired twice, it will cut twice, but staple only once, which can lead to profuse bleeding.

Avoiding the vagina in female patients: It should be a routine practice to ensure that the posterior wall of the vagina is not taken in the stapling device. After closing the stapler, one should examine the vaginal wall for any puckering. The same can be ensured by lifting the posterior vaginal wall off the floor. Any vaginal packing is to be avoided.

Firing: Firing of the stapler should be aimed only once, with full force and in a standing position to get maximum mechanical advantage. Immediately after firing, the lock should be placed back in position to avoid repeat firing.

Opening the stapler: After firing, the stapler is opened by rotating the knob anticlockwise by 270°. The stapler is then rotated on both the sides by 90° and removed by fishtailing.

Examining the donut: After firing, and once the stapler is opened fully and removed, the donut should be examined without changing its orientation. Any discontinuity in the donut should be corrected by taking a figure of eight suture using Vicryl 2-0 in the corresponding area.

Stuck Stapler: Sometimes, when we try to remove the stapler, it may not come out easily, in such cases, we can cut the sutures holding the CAD in place and remove the entire assembly in one go.

Misfiring: There have been incidences in which the stapler was fired, but it only cut and did not staple, leaving a 360° raw area with profuse bleeding. In such cases, four quadrant stitches using Vicryl 2-0 are taken using a purse string anoscope to visualise the individual quadrants. Once this is achieved, a continuous double-locking suture can be taken all around, bringing the cut ends together. Using time-tested products from good companies can prevent this problem.

Bleeding: After firing the stapler, examine the suture line for any bleed. In case there is bleeding, take a figure of eight stitch using Vicryl 2-0 or 3-0. Taking the first bite above the staple line and the second bite below the staple line can control the bleeding effectively.

Skin tags: If there are skin tags associated with internal hemorrhoids, the patient should be explained that the staplers are not going to cure the tags. Removing the skin tags can cause pain, but if not removed, they may become turgid in the post-operative period and cause discomfort to the patient. It is a good practice to remove large skin tags.

Post-operative pain: This complication can be avoided by taking purse string sutures all around, 4 to 5 cm above the dentate line. If there is pain in the immediate postoperative period, local block using xylocaine or methylene blue can be used for prolonged pain relief. If the patient complains of severe pain 4 to 5 days post-surgery, the possibility of infective complications like a rectal pocket syndrome (submucosal abscess) should be considered and treated accordingly.

Stricture: It is a good practice to carry out a DRE in the postoperative period. If one finds a soft stricture developing, the patient can be given an anal dilator for regular use, to prevent stricture formation. If the patient comes back with a history of passing a narrow calibre stool, one should suspect the possibility of a stricture formation. If the stricture is mature, hard and very tight, then stricturoplasty or Aggraphectomy can be done. This complication of stricture formation can be avoided by taking the sutures up to the submucosa and refraining from taking the sphincter in the stapler.

Recurrence: In cases where the donut is incomplete or the suture line is improper, the patient may develop recurrent hemorrhoidal disease, which can be treated by repeat stapling, rubber band ligation, sclerotherapy, excision or DGHAL.

Transanal Suture Hemorrhoidopexy

The technique was introduced by Dr.Chivate from India in 2012.

Principle

The principle is based on dearterialization, achieved by blocking the vessels at two sites, 2 cm and 4 cm proximal to the dentate line. This prevents the formation of collaterals and subsequent recurrence.

Instrumentation (Fig. 4.9)

- Self-illuminating proctoscope with a ligation window
- Half-cut proctoscope
- Three Allis forceps
- Two Needle holders
- Scissors
- One forceps
- HAL suture
- Light source

Position of the patient: Lithotomy

Type of anaesthesia: Spinal/General/Pudendal nerve block.

Preoperative preparation: The patient is prepared one night before the intervention by giving two bisacodyl tablets.

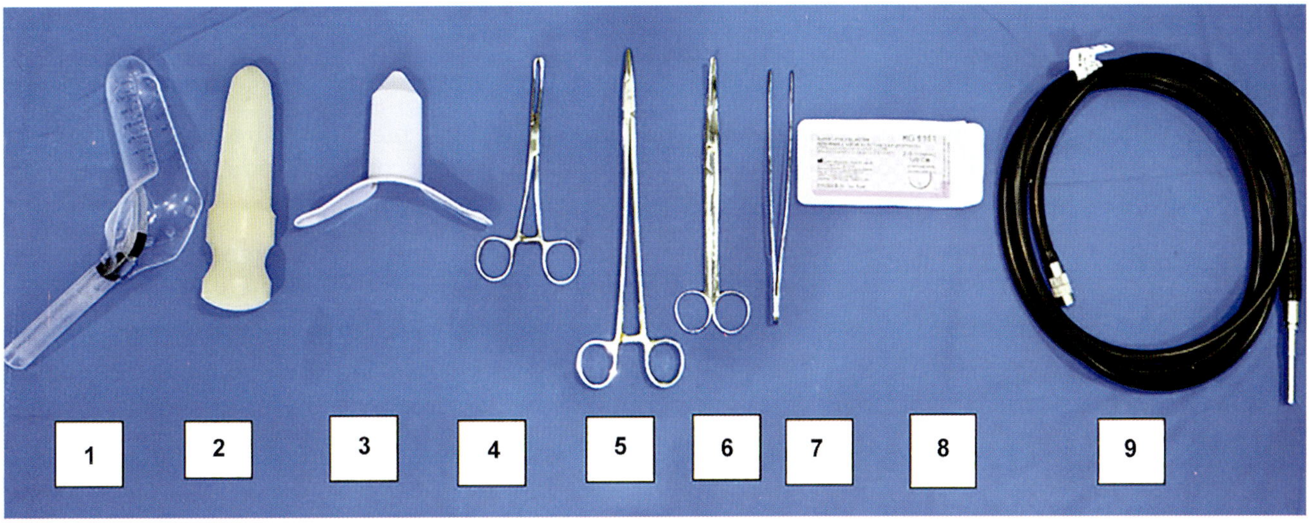

Fig. 4.9: 1. Self-illuminating proctoscope. 2. Half-cut proctoscope. 3. Three Allis forceps. 4. Needle holders. 5. Scissors. 6. Forceps. 7. HAL suture. 8. A light source. 9. Laser fibre.

Steps of the Procedure

Step 1: The patient is placed in a lithotomy position, and three rolled gauge pieces are introduced to assess the degree of the hemorrhoids (Fig. 4.10A, B). A well-lubricated half-cut proctoscope is introduced to evaluate the position of the pile masses.

Step 2: Once the position and degree of the pile masses are assessed, a specially designed, self-illuminated sliding valve proctoscope with a slit is inserted. The engorged mucosa and the dentate line are visualized (Fig. 4.10C, D).

Step 3: The sutures are started at 3 o'clock, 4 cm proximal to the dentate line and are passed through the mucosa, submucosa, and the internal sphincter to fix the laxed submucosa and the mucosa. A 27 mm atraumatic 5/8 circle needle with 2-0 polyglactin (Vicryl) is used for the stitch. The pile masses are milked to reduce engorgement before the knot is tied (Fig. 4.10 E, F, G). Some surgeons prefer 2-0 polyglactin 30 mm ½ circle needle.

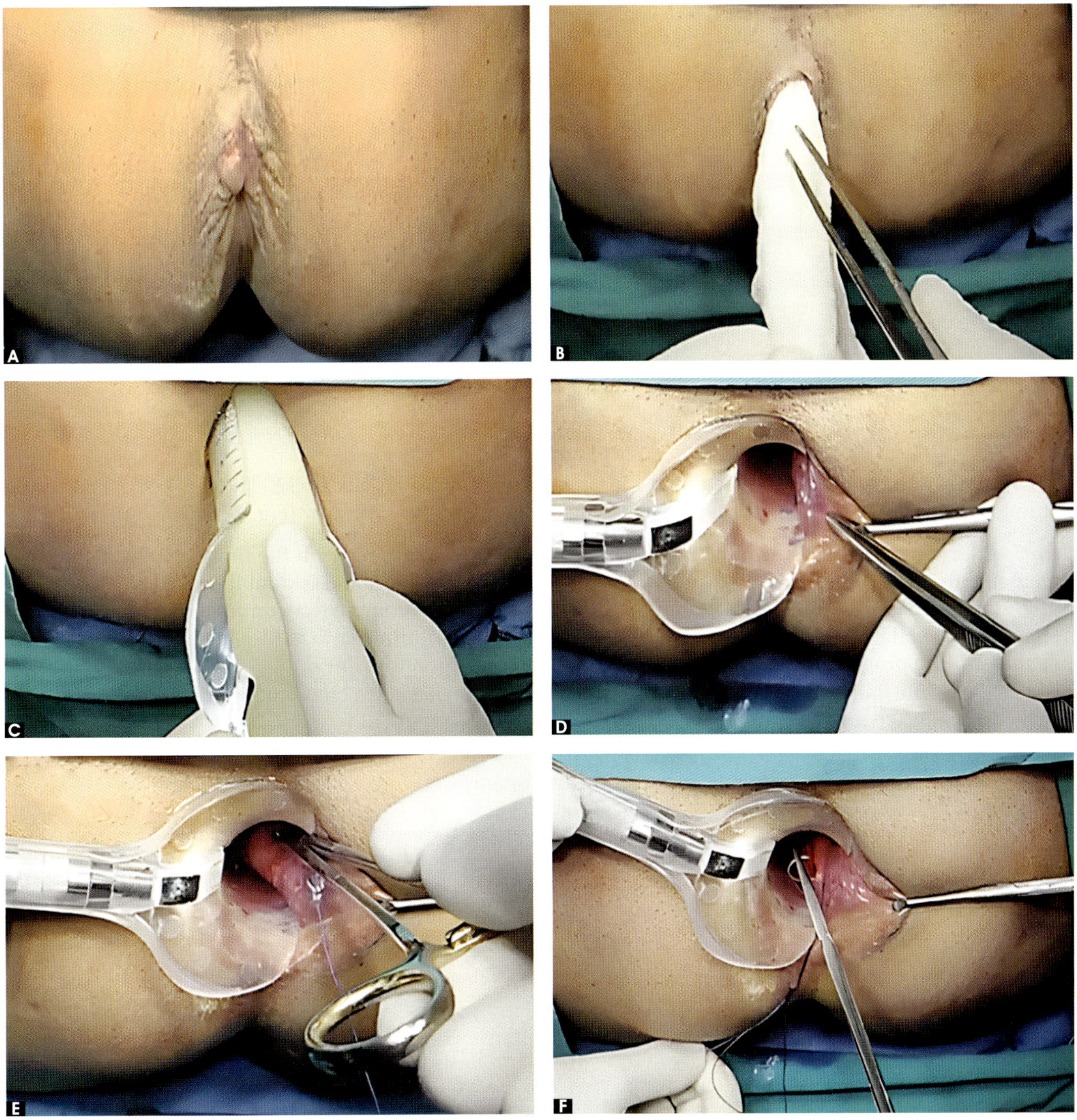

Fig. 4.10A–F: Transanal suture hemorrhoidopexy. A, B) Placement of patient in the lithotomy position and assessment of hemorrhoids. C, D) Introducing self-illuminated proctoscope to visualize the dentate line. E, F) Taking the sutures through the mucosa, submucosa, and the internal anal sphincter muscle starting at 3 o'clock, 4 cm proximal to the dentate line.

Step 4: The obturator is reintroduced, and the proctoscope is rotated clockwise. The reintroduction of the obturator helps prevent the pile mass from entering the proctoscope's window (Fig. 4.10H).

Step 5: After tying the first stitch, the next stitch is taken by overlapping with the first stitch by 1–2 mm to occlude all the branches of SHA. Each suture is taken 0.5 to 1 cm apart and is double-locked to prevent the purse-string effect (Fig. 4.10I, J, K). The sutures are taken around the complete circumference of the rectal wall at the same level. Each time a suture is taken, the obturator is reintroduced to reduce the engorgement of the pile masses. The proctoscope is rotated clockwise to complete the suture line.

Once the suture line is completed, both ends of the suture are tied at 3 o'clock, the site of starting of the first stitch.

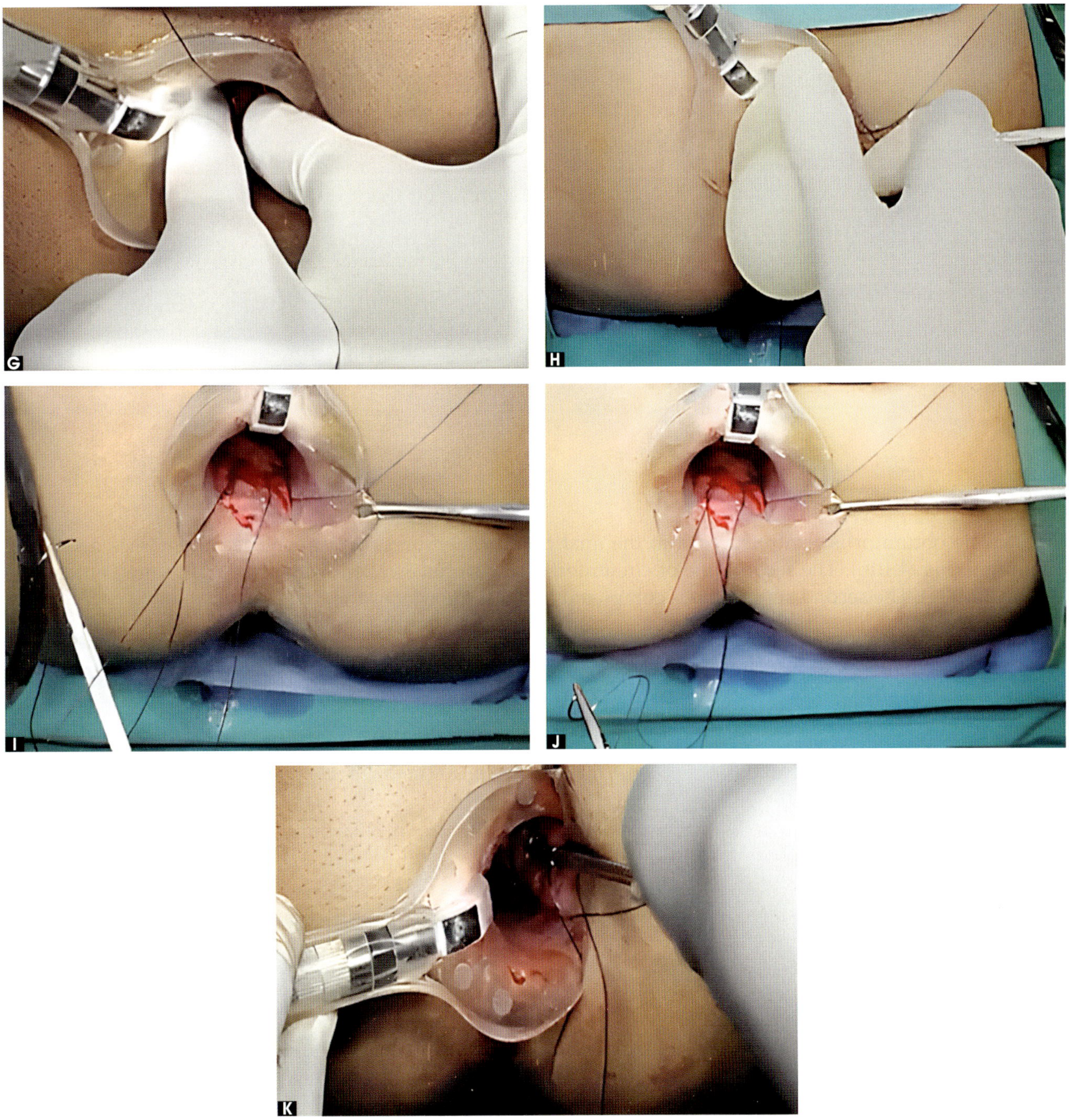

Fig. 4.10G-K: Transanal suture hemorrhoidopexy. G) Taking the sutures through the mucosa, submucosa, and the internal anal sphincter muscle starting at 3 o'clock, 4 cm proximal to the dentate line. H) Introducing the obturator into the anal canal to compress and reduce the pile masses projecting into the window of the proctoscope. I, J, K) Completion of the first line of suturing.

Step 6: The obturator is reintroduced into the anal canal to compress and push the pile masses inside the anal canal (Fig. 4.10L). The second line of circumferential sutures is taken 2 cm proximal to the dentate line (Fig. 4.10M, N). The second suture line is completed in the same way as the first.

Step 7: After completion of the procedure, the pudendal nerve block is given (Fig. 4.10O, P). The final wound picture is shown in Fig. 4.10Q.

Scan QR Code for Video on
Transanal Suture Hemorrhoidopexy

VIDEO 10

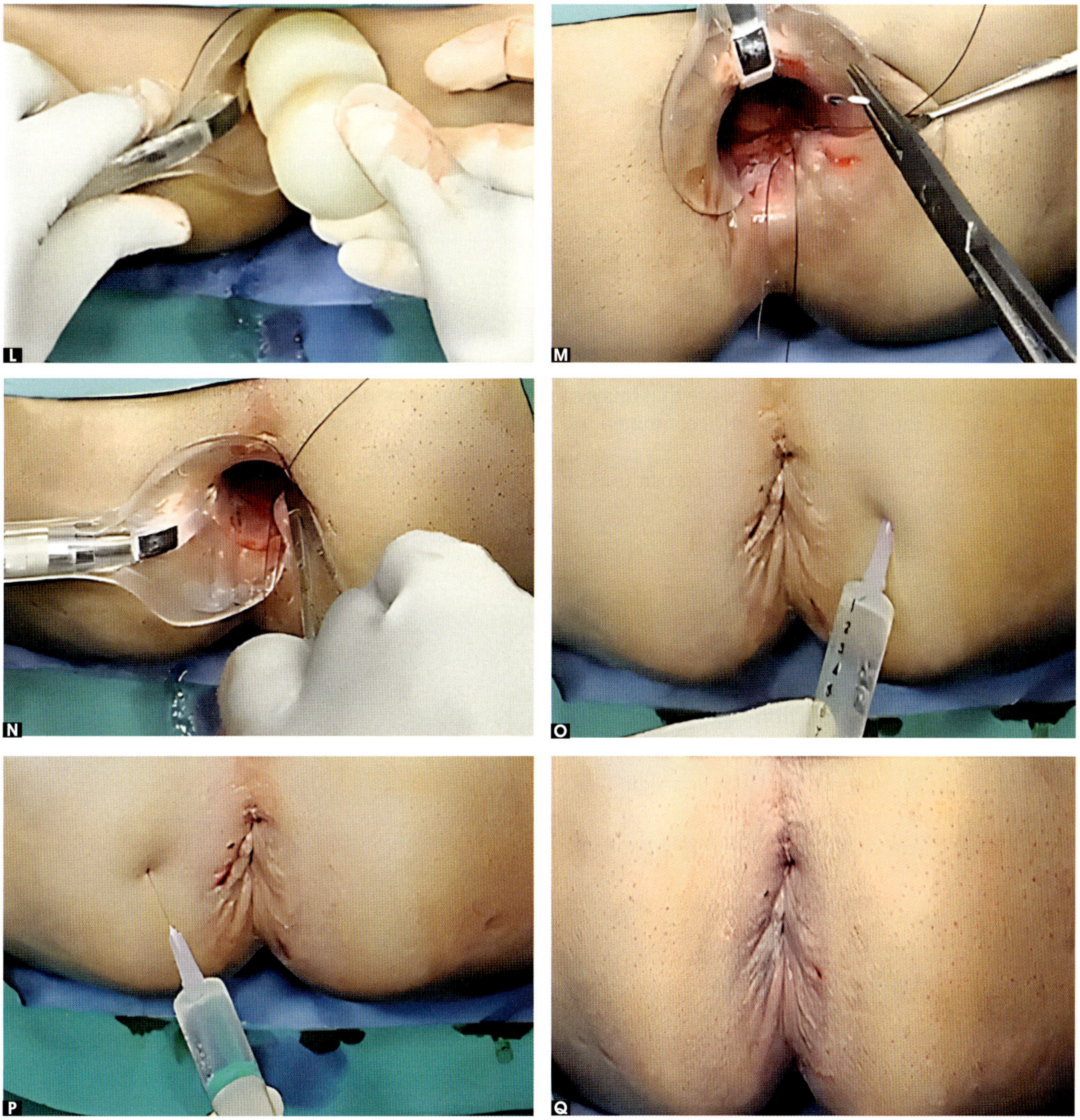

Fig. 4.10M-Q: Transanal suture hemorrhoidopexy. L) Reintroduction of the obturator into the anal canal to compress and reduce the pile masses projecting into the window of the proctoscope. M, N) Second line of circumferential sutures 2 cm proximal to the dentate line. O, P) Pudendal nerve block. Q) Final picture as seen after the completion of the procedure.

Laser Hemorrhoidoplasty (LHP)

Laser hemorrhoidoplasty is a procedure that takes care of both the vascular and the non-vascular components of the anal cushions. The procedure is combined with Finger-guided hemorrhoidal artery ligation (FGHAL), and is called a "Hybrid procedure."

Since with DGHAL or FGHAL, the transmural or intramural branches cannot be ligated, the results of the hybrid technique are better.

Instrumentation (Fig. 4.11)

- Scissors
- Two-needle holders 9″ each
- Allis forceps
- Fine-tip artery forceps
- Half-cut proctoscope 33.5 mm
- Anal dilator
- Vicryl 2-0 5/8 round body on 27 mm needle
- Laser equipment 1470 nm (Fig. 4.12)

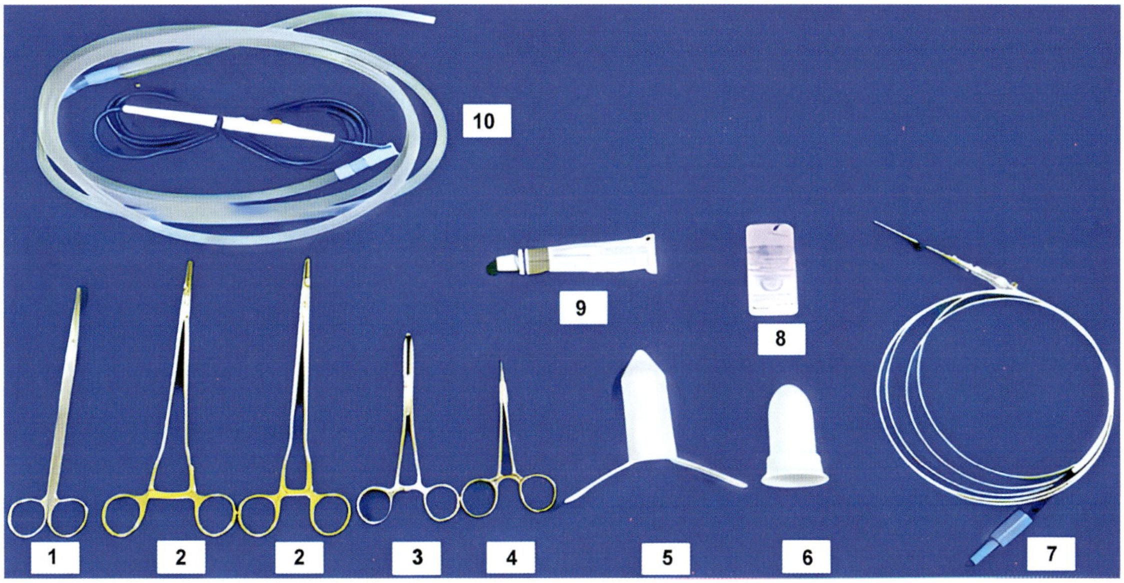

Fig. 4.11: Equipment for FGHAL and LHP. 1) Scissors. 2) Needle holders. 3) Allis. 4) Mosquito. 5) Half - cut proctoscope. 6) Anal dilator. 7) Laser fibre. 8) Vicryl 2-0. 9) Lidocaine jelly. 10) Suction tip and cautery lead.

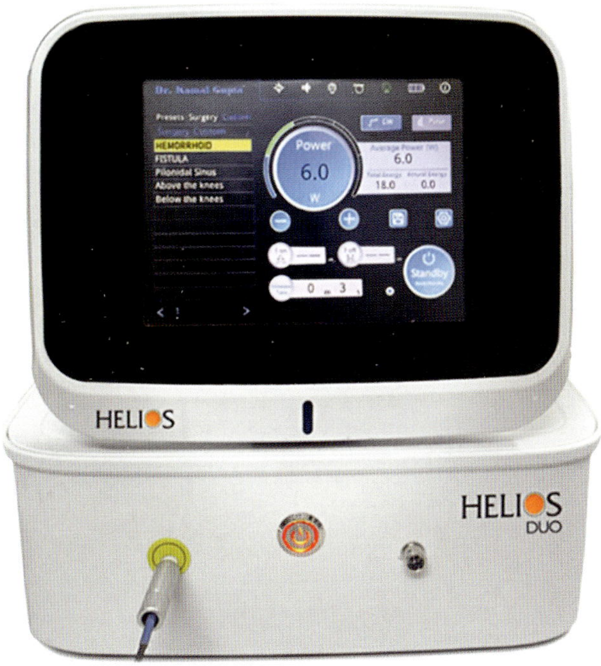

Fig. 4.12: Laser equipment 1470.

- Eye protection glasses (Fig. 4.13)
- Conical laser fibre with handle (Fig. 4.14A, B)
- Suction tip
- Electrosurgical cautery
- Lidocaine jelly

Position of the patient: Lithotomy

Anaesthesia: Spinal/General.

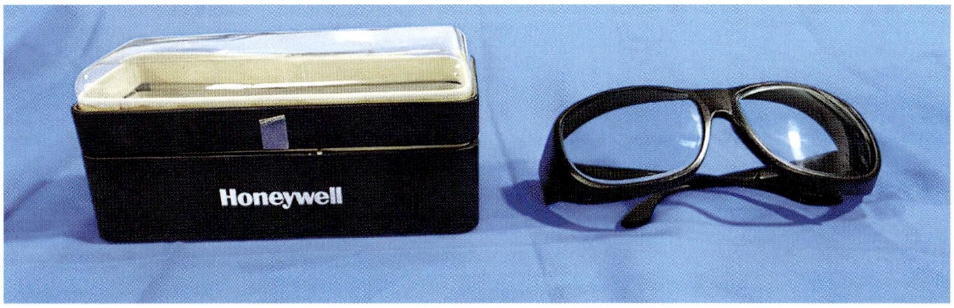

Fig. 4.13: Eye protection glasses.

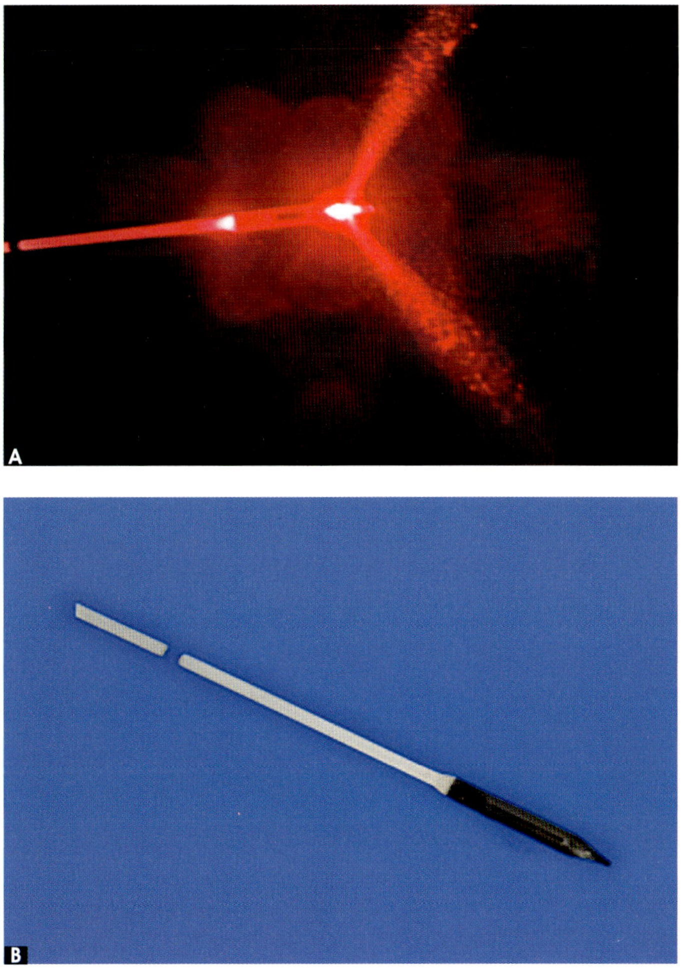

Fig. 4.14A,B: Special conical sharp glass tip fibre for hemorrhoid puncture.

Steps of Procedure (Finger-Guided Hemorrhoidal Artery Ligation)

Step 1: After positioning the patient under spinal anaesthesia, the head side of the operating table is lowered by 15 degrees (Fig. 4.15A).

Step 2: Three pieces of rolled gauze are inserted inside the anal canal and gently pulled out to determine the degree of hemorrhoids (Fig. 4.15B).

Step 3: After lubricating with lignocaine hydrochloride jelly, a half-cut proctoscope is introduced into the anal canal (Fig. 4.15C). The Allis forceps is applied at the anal verge at 3 o'clock, and the hemorrhoidal tissue is slowly pulled outwards. The dentate line is identified, and the left-hand index finger is inserted into the anal canal up to the apex of the hemorrhoidal mass. The SHA branch is palpated at 3 o'clock.

Step 4: Once the vessel has been palpated, ligation is done using Vicryl 2-0, 27 mm 5/8 round body needle by taking a figure of 8 stitch (Fig. 4.15D). The threaded end of the needle is held with the tip of the needle holder just at the edge of the needle holder (Fig. 4.15E, F).

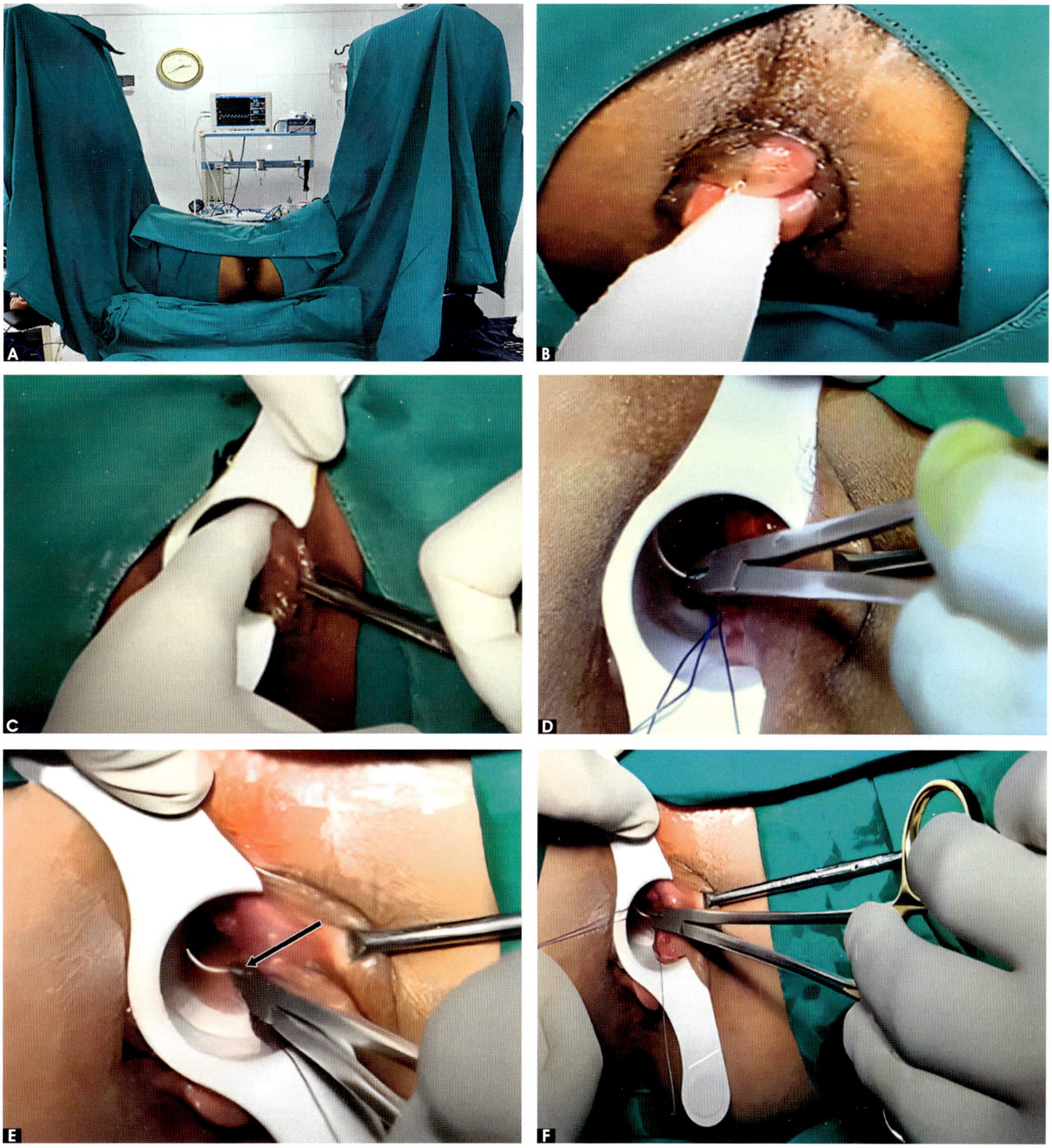

Fig. 4.15(A–F): Technique of Finger guided hemorrhoidal artery ligation. A) Positioning of the patient. B) Insertion of three gauze pieces to assess the degree of hemorrhoids. C) Insertion of half-cut proctoscope inside the anal canal and palpation of the vessels at 3 o'clock. D) Figure of 8 stitch with Vicryl. E, F) Position to hold the needle with the needle holder.

The stitch is taken deep enough to include a few fibres of the internal anal sphincter. The wrist should move freely with both supine and prone movements for inserting and withdrawing the needle smoothly (Fig. 4.15G, H). One should be careful not to puncture the vessel. Before taking the knot, the assistant is asked to milk the hemorrhoidal tissue to reduce the engorgement (Fig. 4.15I). Once the knot is tied, the vessel is palpated again to ensure proper ligation.

Step 5: After the ligation at 3 o'clock, the half-cut proctoscope is rotated clockwise by 360 degrees. All the branches are palpated and ligated (Fig. 4.15J). Preferably, it should be possible to ligate 4–6 branches.

Step 6: The proctoscope is removed, and three rolled-up gauze pieces are inserted into the anal canal to assess the size of the pile masses. A reduction in the size of the hemorrhoids can be seen on the operating table in grade 3 and 4 hemorrhoids (Fig. 4.15K).

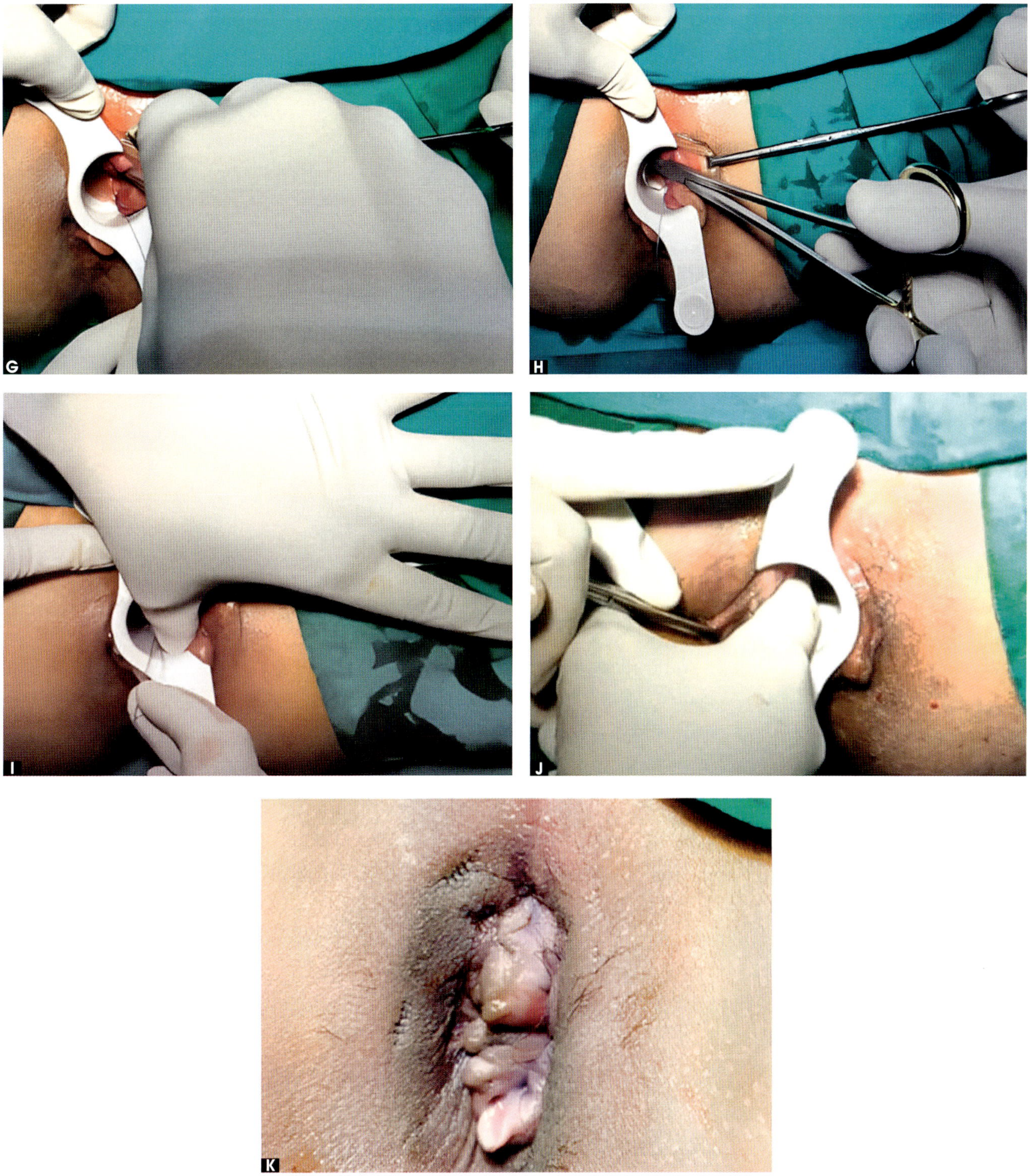

Fig. 4.15(G-K): Technique of Finger guided hemorrhoidal artery ligation. G, H) Pronation and supination movements of the wrist while taking a stitch. I) Milking of the hemorrhoidal mass. J) Ligation of the remaining branches. K) Reduction in size of the pile masses after HAL.

Technique of Laser Hemorrhoidoplasty

After the completion of the hemorrhoidal artery ligation, laser hemorrhoidoplasty is done.

Fibre/Dosage/Energy/Mode

Fibre: Sharp tip conical. However, bare-tip fibre can also be used.

Dosage

- At the time of fibre insertion: 6 Watts, 1-second pulse
- At the time of fibre activation: 6 Watts, 3-second pulse

  The dosage is calculated as follows:

  Watt × time in second = Joule (1 Watt × 1 Sec = 1 Joule per second (J/s).

Energy

The energy is calculated in joules. The overall dose should not exceed 150 to 200 Joules per hemorrhoidal mass.

Mode: Pulse mode

Point of Entry of Fibre

The mucocutaneous junction (white line of Hilton) is the entry point for the laser fibre (Fig. 4.16).

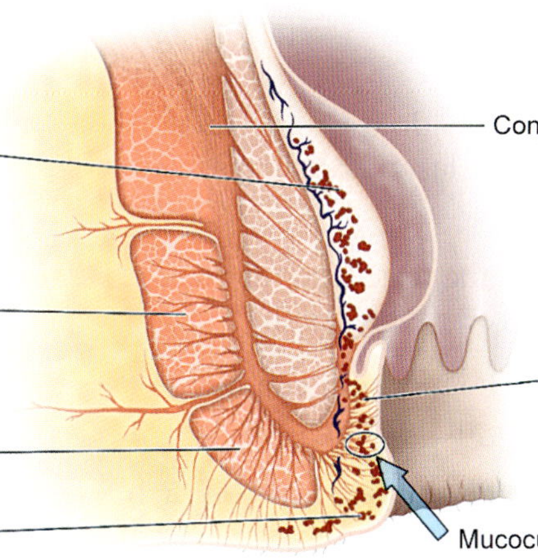

Fig. 4.16: Mucocutaneous junction (point of entry of fibre).

Steps of Laser Hemorrhoidoplasty

Step 1: A half-cut proctoscope is inserted inside the anal canal. An Allis forceps is applied at the anal verge at 3 o'clock. It is pulled outwards, and the laser fibre is inserted from the mucocutaneous junction into the submucosal space (Fig. 4.17A).

Step 2: Once inside the submucosal space, the fibre stops at the distal end, where the HAL was performed. The energy dose at the fibre entry point is 6 watts × 1 second.

Step 3: Check the red light of the fibre. The red light can be seen inside the submucosa of the anal cushions (Fig. 4.17B). Ensure the light is neither bright nor dim (Fig. 4.17C).

Step 4: The fibre is activated once inside the submucosal hemorrhoidal tissue. The energy dosage is 6 watts × 3 seconds pulse (Fig. 4.17D). Crackling sounds are heard due to the release of hydrogen ions.

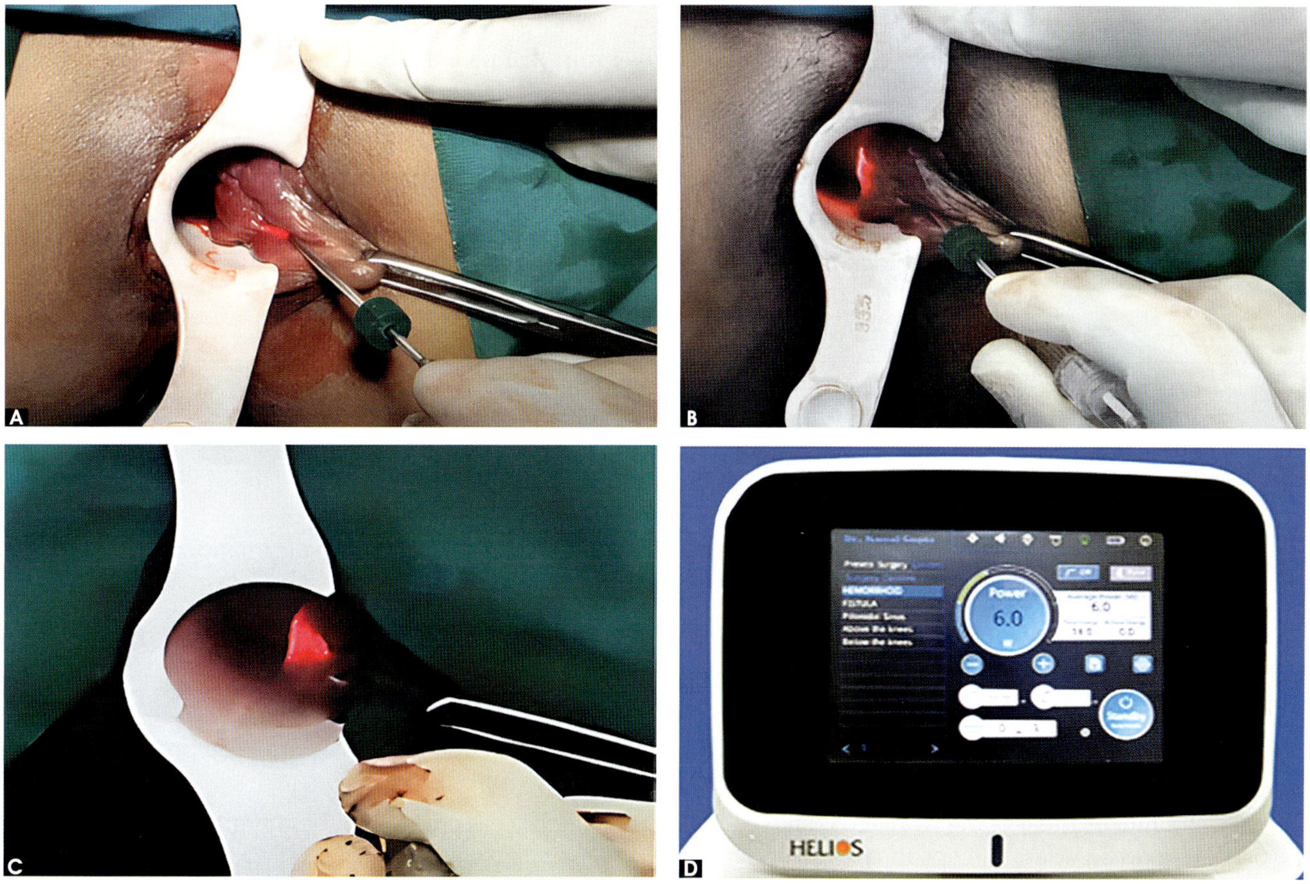

Fig. 4.17A-D: Technique of Laser hemorrhoidoplasty. A) Insertion of laser fibre through the mucocutaneous junction at 3 o'clock. B) Illumination with red light after insertion of fibre in the submucosal space. C) Bright light is seen when the fibre tip is too close to the mucosa. D) Settings of laser energy as seen on the equipment.

Step 5: Slowly rotate the fibre during activation to prevent it from sticking to the tissue. Keep withdrawing the fibre every 5 mm because the fibre covers approximately 4 mm distance in one activation.

Step 6: After the hemorrhoidal mass is managed at 3 o'clock, the same procedure is repeated at 7 and 11 o'clock (Fig. 4.17E, F). If an accessory hemorrhoid is present at 6 o'clock, it is treated in the same way. At the end of the procedure, an ice finger is inserted inside the anal canal for 8 to 10 minutes to reduce postoperative edema (Fig. 4.17G).

Step 7: Finally, a pudendal nerve block is given to reduce postoperative pain.

Tips and Tricks—Hemorrhoidal artery ligation

- The depth of the needle while doing FGHAL is roughly 5 mm.
- The figure of 8 stitch taken during the procedure is not for ligation of the vessel per se. It compresses the surrounding tissue to squeeze the vessel, leading to dearterialization.
- While ligating, if the needle pierces the vessel, and there is bleeding or hematoma formation:
  - o Do not withdraw the needle.
  - o Complete the ligature and press the area with gauze for 2 minutes. If the bleeding persists or the hematoma increases, ligate 1.5 to 2 cm proximally.
- The needle cuts through the mucosa:
  - o Chances are the local area is inflamed; avoid another ligature. Look for normal mucosa proximally and distally; if convinced, ligate under Doppler guidance.
  - o If the mucosa tear is big or bleeds, take a small loose stitch to approximate the margins and press with gauze on an artery forceps to arrest bleeding.
- The needle breaks or gets lost in the submucous plane before the tip comes out.
  - o Please do not panic. Remove the scope, not the suture. Take adequate jelly on the finger, gently palpate the needle and gradually milk it out until the tip is visible and can be held by the artery forceps. As shown in the videos, another needle holder can be used to pull out the needle from the mucosa.

Scan QR Code for Video on
Finger Guided Hemorrhoidal Artery Ligation with Laser Hemorrhoidoplasty
VIDEO 11

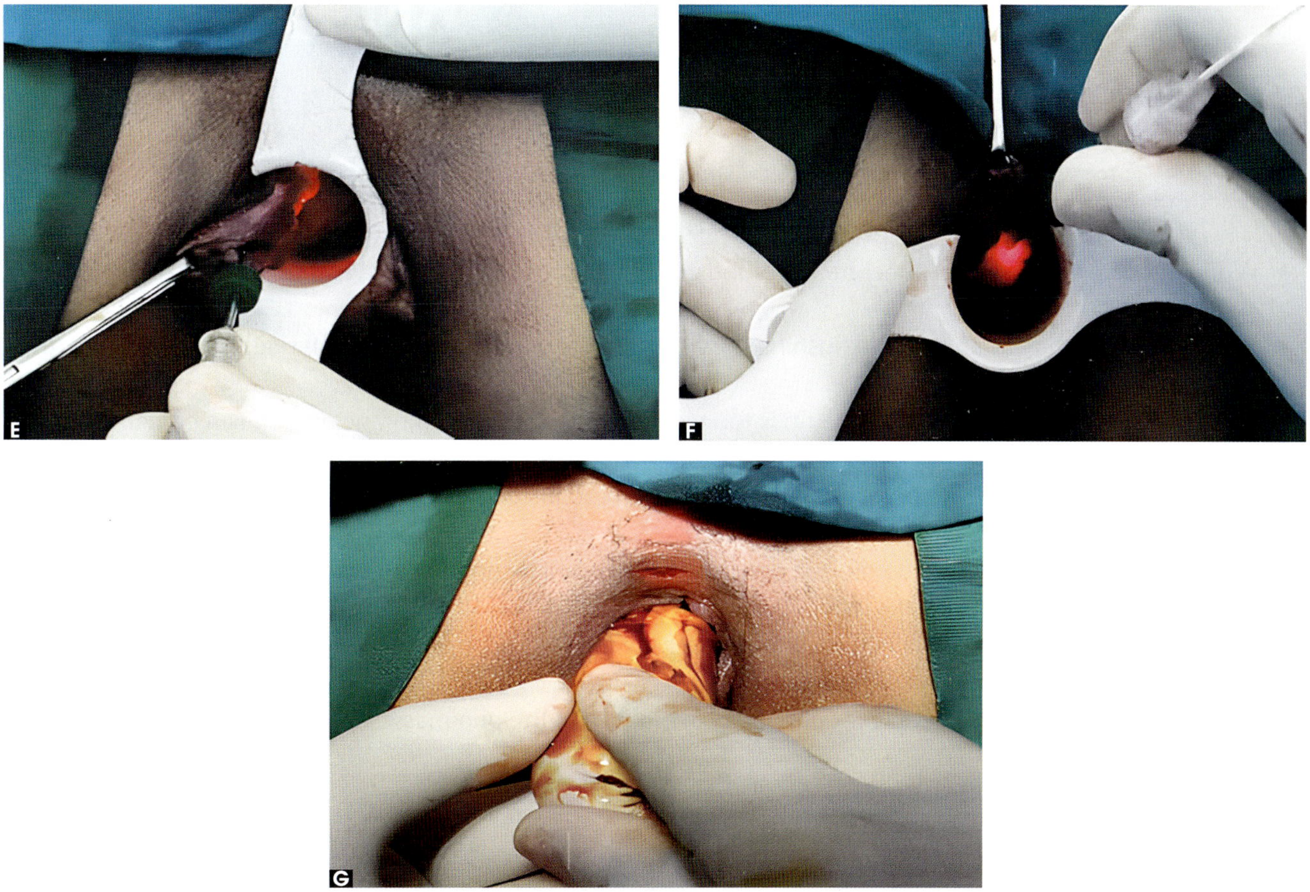

Fig. 4.17E-G: Technique of laser hemorrhoidoplasty. E, F) Insertion of laser fibre at 7 and 11 o'clock. G) Insertion of ice finger.

Tips and Tricks—Laser Hemorrhoidoplasty

- While ligating, ensure not to puncture the blood vessel with the needle. If the vessel is pierced, a hematoma appears immediately.
- Ensure there is no resistance while pushing the fibre into the submucosal space. If one feels resistance, the fibre is in the wrong plane.
- Too bright light indicates that the fibre tip is too close to the mucous membrane, which can be damaged by thermal energy.
- A dim light indicates that the tip of the fibre lies somewhere inside the internal sphincter, which may cause damage to the sphincters with subsequent fibrosis.
- In grade 3 and grade 4 hemorrhoids, one can use a fan-shaped technique to release more energy (Fig. 4.18). However, the total energy for each pile mass should not exceed 200J.
- With repeated use of the laser fibre, the power intensity tends to decrease. It is better to increase the dosage to 8w × 3-sec pulse.
- Educate the patient. It takes 6 to 8 weeks for the shrinkage of the pile masses.

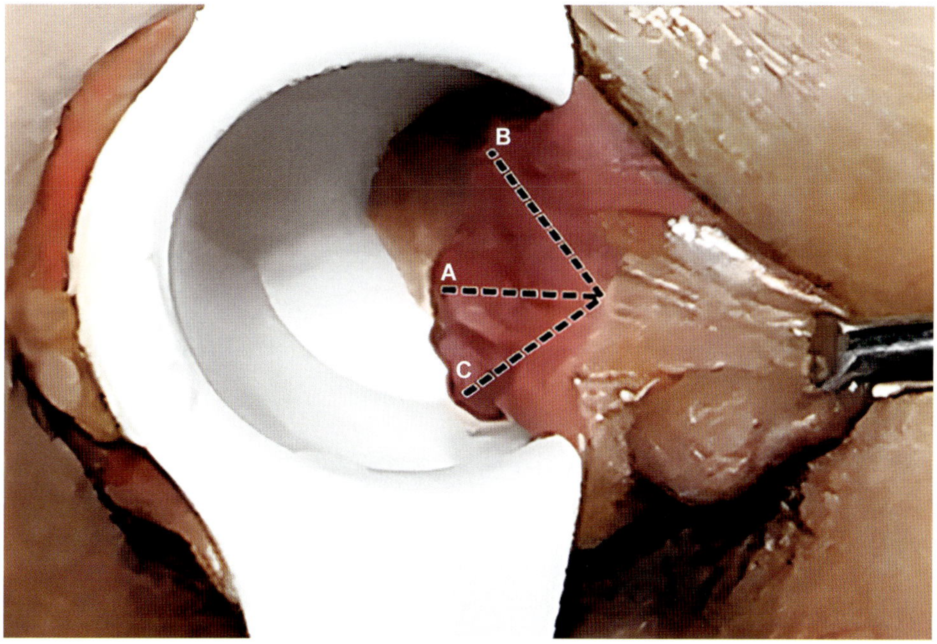

Fig. 4.18: Fan shape technique for release of laser energy in large pile masses.

Laser Hemorrhoidoplasty in Thrombosed Hemorrhoids

After doing FGHAL, clot evacuation can be done in thrombosed internal haemorrhoids, followed by laser hemorrhoidoplasty (Fig. 4.19A to D).

Scan QR Code for Video on
Thrombosed Hemorrhoids

VIDEO 12

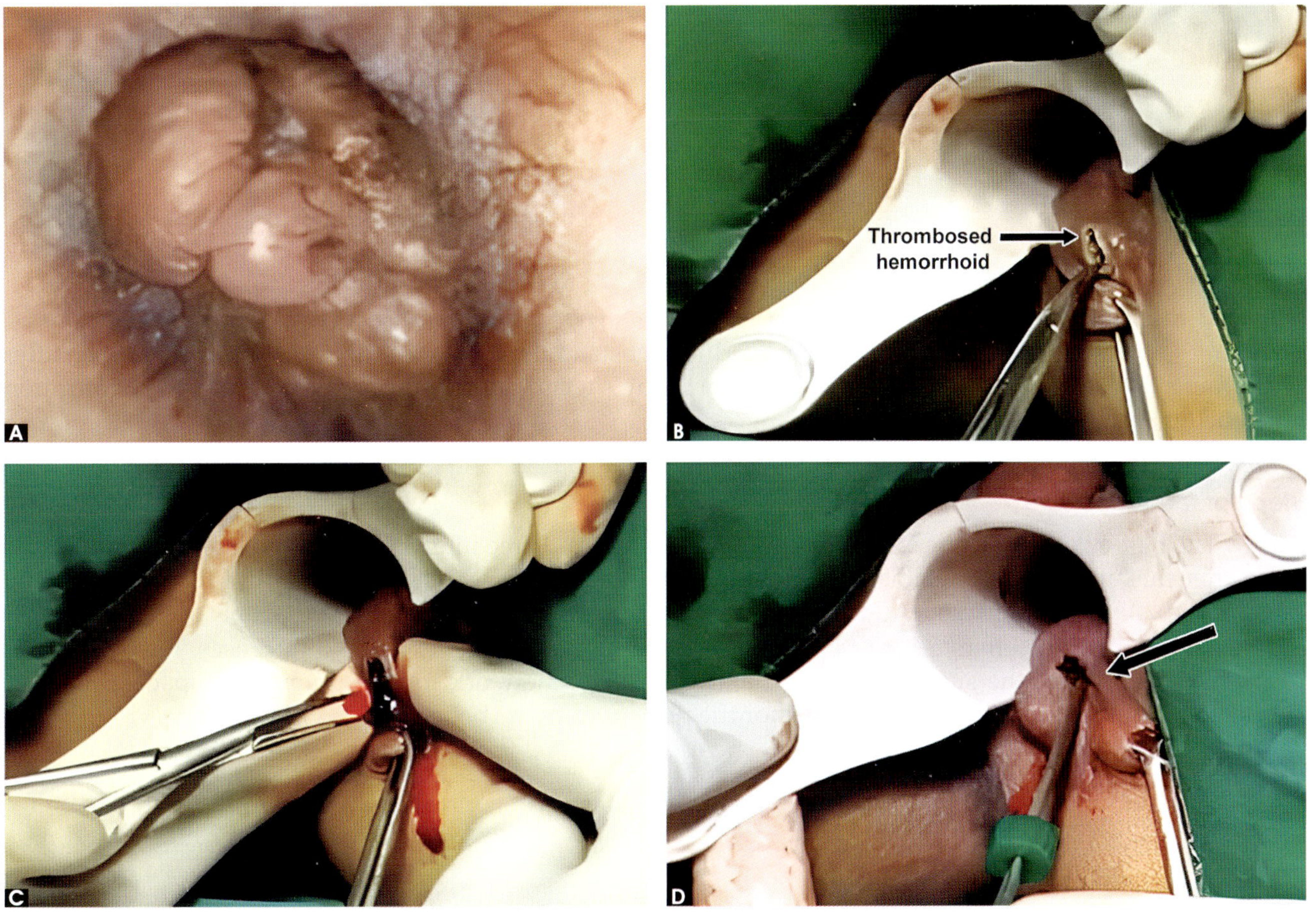

Fig. 4.19(A-D): Managing thrombosed hemorrhoids. A) Thrombosed hemorrhoids. B) Incision given over the clot. C) Clot evacuation being done. D) Point of entry of laser fibre at the site of clot evacuation.

TOP-UPS

Blaisdell Technique -For better dearterialization and management of prolapse in grade 3 and 4 hemorrhoids

Sometimes, the hemorrhoidal tissue does not reduce substantially in grade 3 and 4 hemorrhoids, even after performing HAL and LHP. Performing Blaisdell or Farag's technique of mucopexy leads to dearterialization and a better cosmetic effect.

Steps of the Procedure

Step 1: The half-cut proctoscope is inserted into the anal canal. Three interrupted sutures are taken at the pile mass after pushing it inside the anal canal. The first suture is taken just below the apex of the hemorrhoidal mass (Fig. 4.20A, B). The suture encloses mucosa, submucosa, and fibres of the internal anal sphincter.

Blaisdell's technique offers a better outcome than simple RAR as it serves two purposes. Firstly, there is dearterialization since the suture encloses the arteriovenous network in the submucosal space. Secondly, deepening the suture into the IAS helps anchor the prolapsed tissue better.

Scan QR Code for Video on
Blaisdell's Technique

VIDEO 13

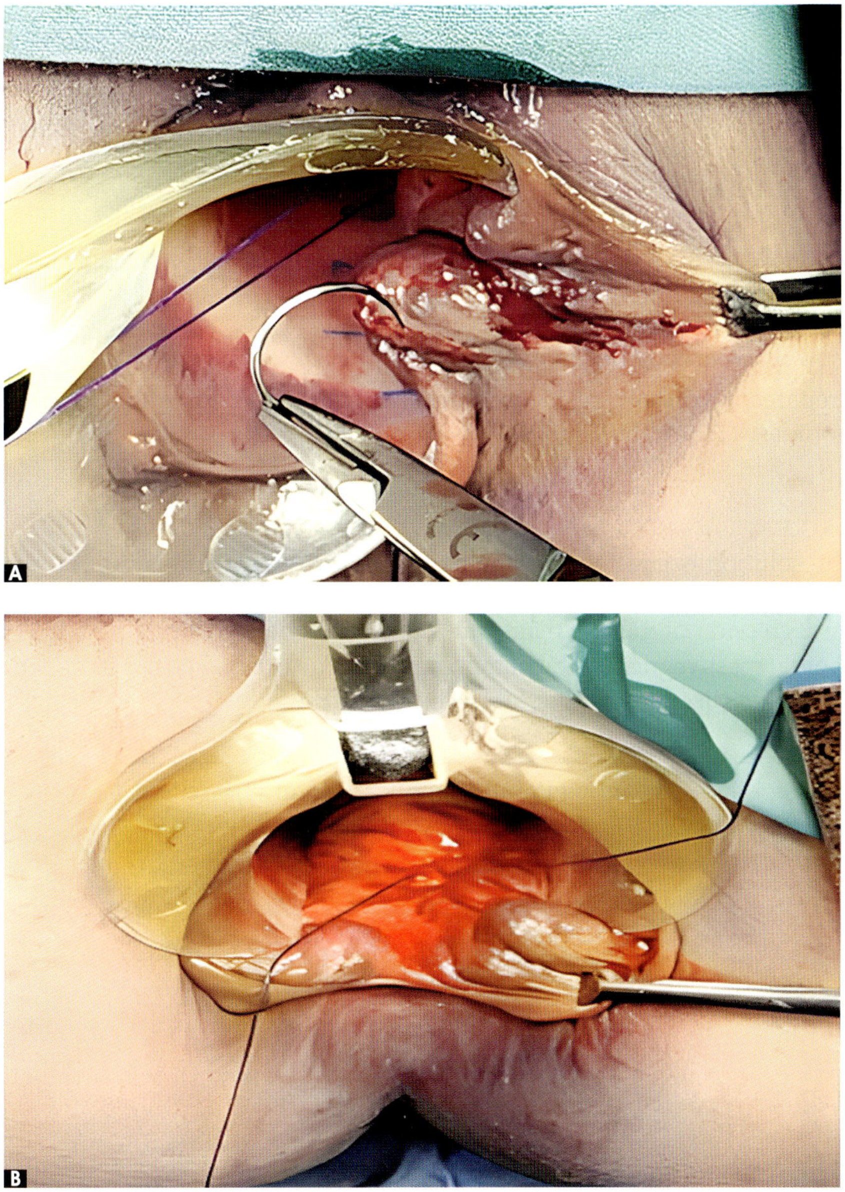

Fig. 4.20A, B: Mucopexy by taking three interrupted sutures by Blaisdell technique.

Role of Injection Hylase

Indication

Grade 4 hemorrhoids with substantial edema.

Principle

Increases tissue permeability leading to a decrease in edema.

Point of injection

Injection hylase (Hyaluronidase) can be injected into the submucosa of the hemorrhoids.

Preparation of solution

- Injection hylase is available in powder form.
- The solution is prepared by dissolving the powder in 1 ml of distilled water or saline. Each ml contains 1500 IU of hyaluronidase (Fig. 4.21).

Technique

After preparation, the solution is injected into the hemorrhoidal tissue. The syringe's piston is pulled out to ensure the needle is not inside a blood vessel. 1–2 ml of hylase is injected into each hemorrhoidal mass (Fig. 4.22A, B). Immediate regression of the pile mass can be observed on the operating table (Fig. 4.22C).

Once the hemorrhoidal mass regresses, the hemorrhoids can be pushed back into the lumen. The remaining steps of the procedure are as discussed under FGHAL and LHP.

Learning Point: Complications of Hylase

Allergic reactions reported in 0.05 to 0.69 per cent of cases are:

- Erythema
- Itching and pain
- Urticaria and angioedema

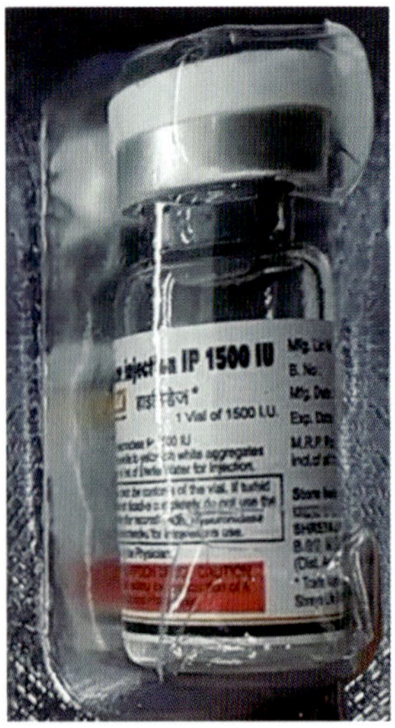

Fig. 4.21: Injection hylase.

Scan QR Code for Video on

Grade 4 Hemorrhoids with Injection Hylase

VIDEO 14

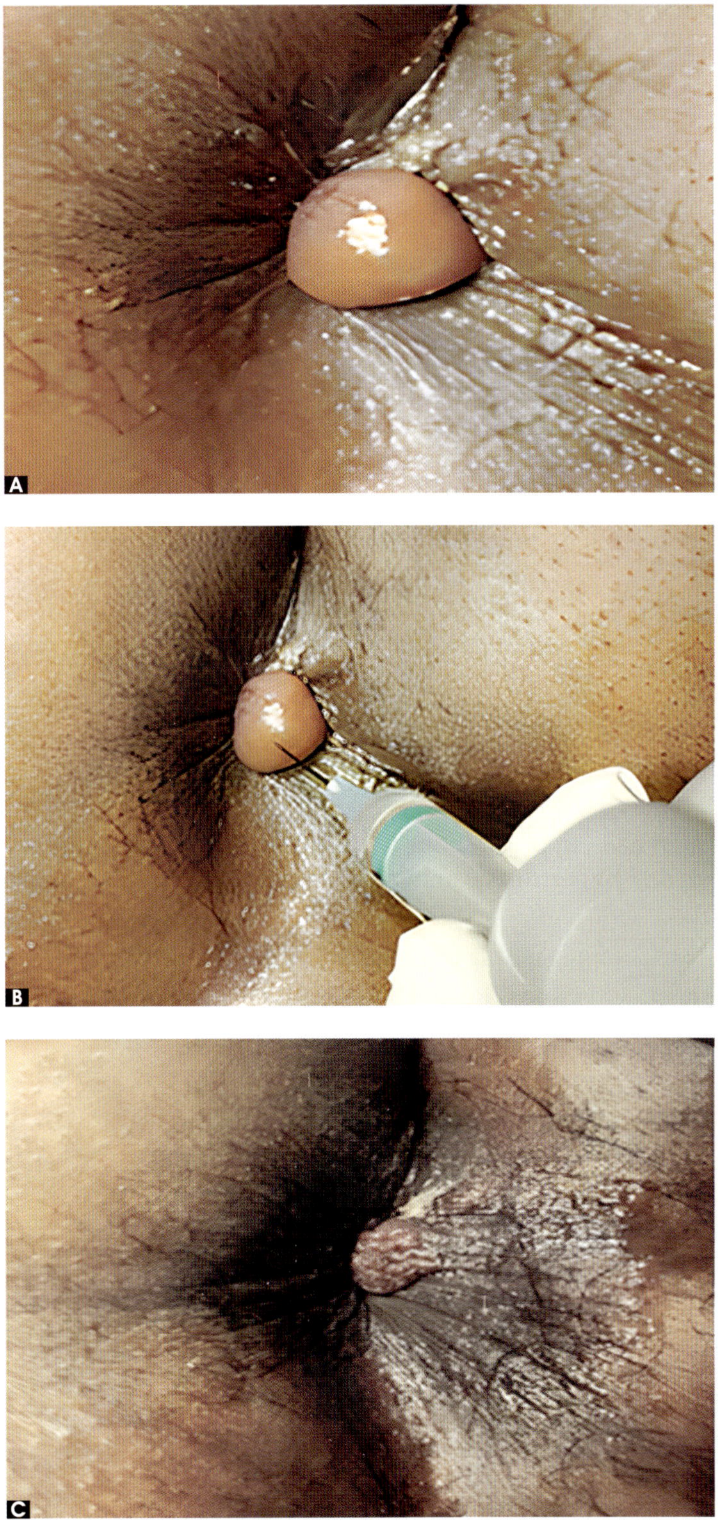

Fig. 4.22A-C: Injection hylase. A) Edematous hemorrhoidal mass. B) Injecting 1 ml of hylase solution into the pile mass. C) Regression of the pile mass.

Excision of Skin Tags and Fibrous Anal Polyp

Anal skin tags are painless skin growths located around the anus. They cause irritation and difficulty during defecation. A fibrous anal polyp is a pedunculated fibrous tissue in the anal cushions.

Management

Position of the patient: Lithotomy position

Anaesthesia: Spinal/Pudendal nerve block.

Technique

Step 1: Insert a well-lubricated half-cut proctoscope into the anal canal. Rotate the proctoscope gently to assess the canal for fibrous polyps and hypertrophic anal papillae. Look for anterior and posterior tags around the anal orifice (Fig. 4.23A, B).

Step 2: Hold the anterior skin tag with Allis forceps over the proctoscope (Fig. 4.23C). Gently cut the tag radially in a circular motion over the proctoscope (Fig. 4.23D, E). Radial incisions always have a good cosmetic effect. One can use bare fibre for cutting and coagulation, but cautery is good enough. Once the excision is complete, a fine circular cut can be made.

Step 3: Now rotate the proctoscope to excise the posterior skin tag in a similar way as the anterior tag (Fig. 4.23F).

Scan QR Code for Video on
Excision of Skin Tags

VIDEO 15

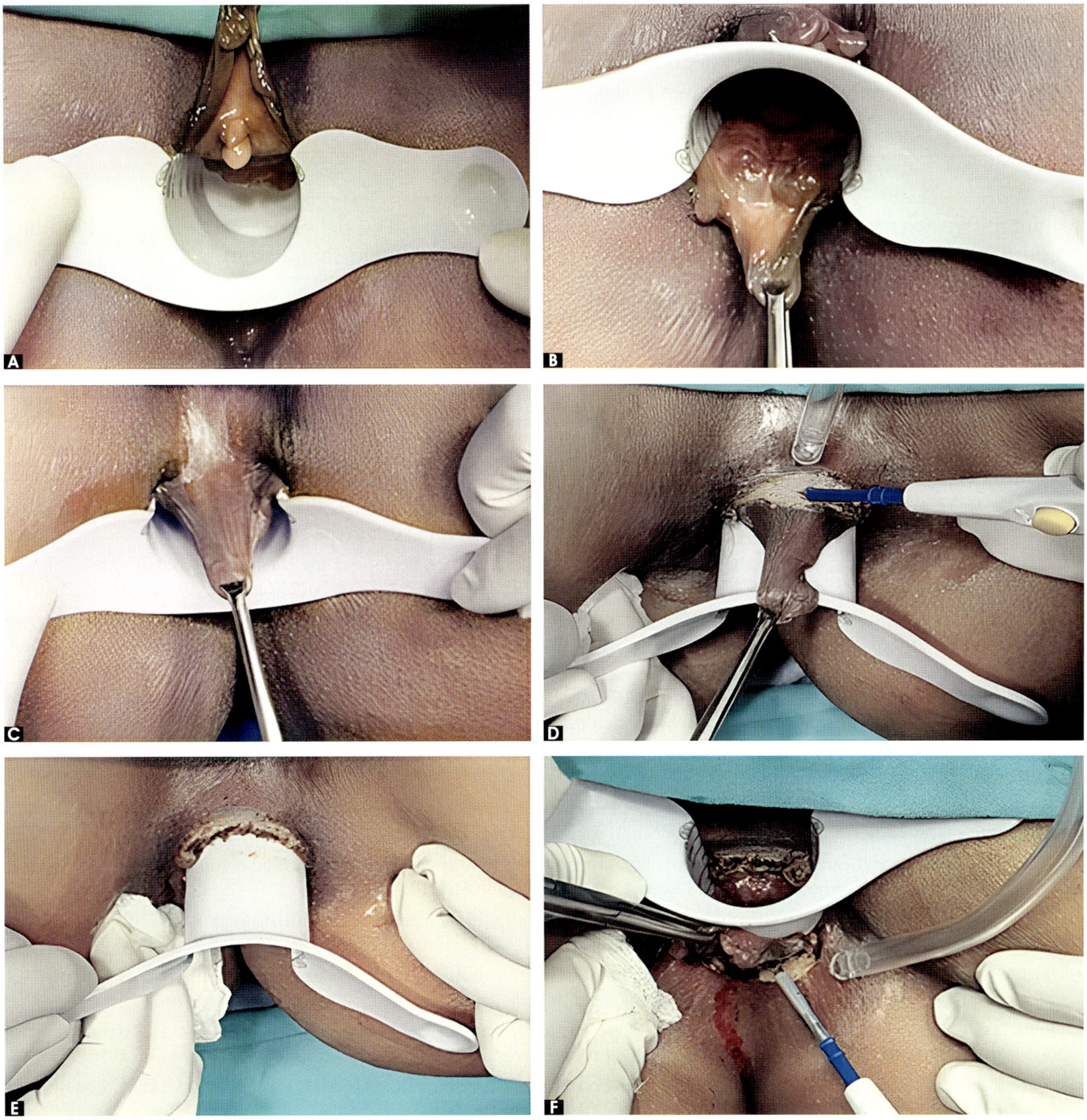

Fig. 4.23A–F: Excision of skin tags. A, B) Presence of large skin tags anteriorly and posteriorly. C, D, E) Excision of the anterior skin tags radially after inverting the half-cut proctoscope. F) Excision of the posterior skin tag.

Step 4: Once the excision of the tags is complete, look for fibrous polyps and hypertrophic anal papillae. Hold the papillae with an Allis forceps and excise them using cautery (Fig. 4.23G).

Step 5: After the procedure, the pudendal nerve block is given along with bupivacaine infiltration in the perianal area to block the perineal branch of the pudendal nerve (Fig. 4.23H, I, J).

The final postoperative picture is shown in Fig. 4.23K.

Conclusion

Minimally invasive procedures are associated with less morbidity. The patient can return to work at the earliest. The VAS score is much less as compared to an excisional hemorrhoidectomy.

FURTHER READING

- Aigner F, Bodner G, Conrad F, Mbaka G, Kreczy A, Fritsch H. The superior rectal artery and its branching pattern with regard to its clinical influence on ligation techniques for internal hemorrhoids. Am J Surg. 2004;187:102–8. https://doi.org/10.1016/j.amjsurg.2002.11.003.
- Blaisdell PC. Office ligation of internal hemorrhoids. Am J Surg. 1958;96:401–4.
- Chia YW, Darzi A, Speakman CT, Hill AD, Jameson JS, Henry MM. CO2 laser hemorrhoidectomy— does it alter the anorectal function or decrease pain compared to conventional hemorrhoidectomy? Int J Colorectal Dis. 1995;10(1):22–4.
- Chivate SD, Ladukar L, Ayyar M, Mahajan V, Kavathe S. Transanal Suture Rectopexy for Haemorrhoids: Chivate's Painless Cure for Piles. Indian J Surg. 2012 Oct;74(5):412–7. doi: 10.1007/s12262-012-0461-4. Epub 2012 Mar 22. PMID: 24082598; PMCID: PMC3477406
- De A, Roy P. Hybrid digitally guided hemorrhoidal artery ligation with laser hemorrhoidoplasty: our experience with a new approach to hemorrhoidal dis- ease. Int Surg J. 2021;8(10):2968–73.
- Figueiredo MN, Campos FG. Doppler-guided hemorrhoidal dearterialization/transanal hemorrhoidal dearterialization: technical evolution and outcomes after 20 years. World J Gastrointest Surg. 2016;8(3):232–7. https://doi.org/10.4240/wjgs.v8.i3.232.
- Giamundo P. Advantages and limits of hemorrhoidal dearterialization in the treatment of symptomatic hemorrhoids. World J Gastrointest Surg. 2016;8(1):1–4.
- Gupta K, Agarwal N, Mital K. Clinical outcomes in patients with hemorrhoids treated by finger-guided hemorrhoidal artery ligation with laser hemorrhoidoplasty: a retrospective cohort study. J Adv Med. 2021;33(18):143–52.
- Gupta K, Mital K, Kant R. Surgical management of hemorrhoids – a new approach finger- guided hemorrhoidal artery ligation (FGHAL) with laser hemorrhoidoplasty. Int J Recent Sci Res. 2019;10(05):32186–7.
- Gupta PJ. Hypertrophied anal papillae and fibrous anal polyps, should they be removed during anal fissure surgery? World J Gastroenterol. 2004 Aug 15;10(16):2412-4. doi: 10.3748/wjg.v10.i16.2412. PMID: 15285031; PMCID: PMC4576300.
- Hardy A, Chan CL, Cohen CR. The surgical management of haemorrhoids—a review. Dig Surg. 2005; 22(1–2):26–33. https://doi.org/10.1159/000085343.
- Hoyuela C, Carvajal F, Juvany M, et al. HAL-RAR (Doppler-guided haemorrhoid artery ligation with recto-anal repair) is a safe and effective procedure for hemorrhoids. Results of a prospective study after a two-year follow-up. Int J Surg. 2016;28:39–44.
- Jongen J, Bach S, Stübinger SH, et al. Excision of Thrombosed External Hemorrhoid Under Local Anesthesia. Dis Colon Rectum 46, 1226–1231 (2003). https://doi.org/10.1007/s10350-004-6719-6.
- Jung H. Hyaluronidase: An overview of its properties, applications, and side effects. Arch Plast Surg. 2020 Jul;47(4):297-300. doi: 10.5999/aps.2020.00752. Epub 2020 Jul 15. PMID: 32718106; PMCID: PMC7398804.
- Kumkumsingh, Kamal Gupta, Ajit Naniksingh Kukreja, Tamonas Chaudhry, Shalu Gupta. Hemorrhoids Practice Guidelines 2021. Association Colon & Rectal Surgeons of India, Nov 30 2021

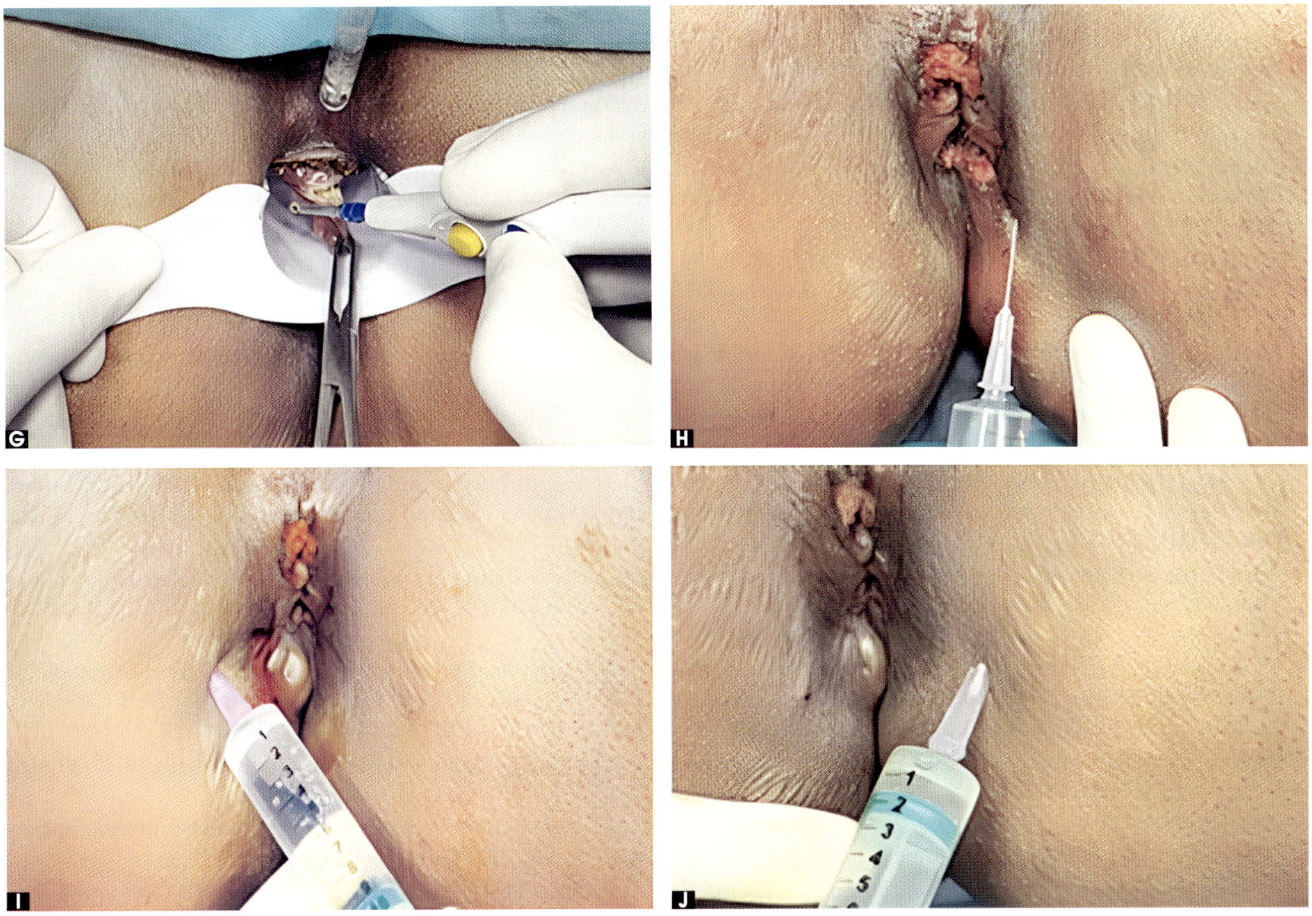

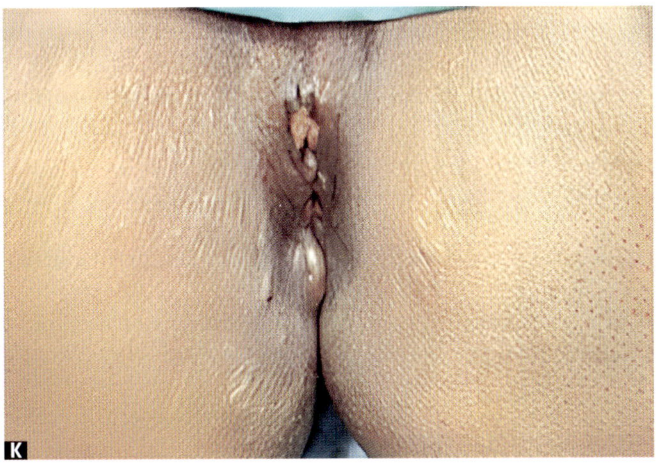

Scan QR Code for Video on
2nd Degree Hemorrhoids with Fistula
VIDEO 16

Scan QR Code for Video on
2nd Degree Hemorrhoids with Fissure
VIDEO 17

Fig. 4.23G–K: Excision of skin tags. G) Excision of hypertrophic anal papilla at 12 o'clock. H) Local infiltration of bupivacaine. I, J) Pudendal nerve block at 3 and 11 o'clock. K) Final picture at the end of the procedure.

- Laughlan K, Jayne DG, Jackson D, Rupprecht F, Ribaric G. Stapled haemorrhoidopexy compared to Milligan-Morgan and Ferguson haemorrhoidectomy: a systematic review. Int J Color Dis. 2009;24(3):335– 44. https://doi.org/10.1007/s00384-008-0611-0.
- Lienert M. Literature review on dearterialization of hemorrhoids and mucopexy. In: Ratto C, Parello A, Litta F, editors. Hemorrhoids, Coloproctology, vol. 2. Cham: Springer; 2018. https://doi. org/10.1007/978-3-319-53357-5_41.
- Longo A. Treatment of hemorrhoids disease by reduction of mucosa and hemorrhoidal prolapse with a circular-suturing device: a new procedure. Proceedings of the Sixth World Congress of Endoscopic Surgery, Rome, Italy; 1998. p. 777.
- Maloku H, Gashi Z, Lazovic R, Islami H, Juniku- Shkololli A. Laser hemorrhoidoplasty procedure vs open surgical hemorrhoidectomy: a trial comparing 2 treatments for hemorrhoids of the third and fourth degree. Acta Inform Med. 2014;22(6):365–7.
- Markaryan D, Tulina I, Garmanova T, Bredikhin M, Alikperzade A, Tsarkov P. Hemorrhoidal artery ligation with Doppler guidance vs digital guidance for grade II–III hemorrhoidal disease treatment: study protocol clinical trial (SPIRIT Compliant). Medicine (Baltimore). 2020;99(15):e19424.
- Morinaga K, Hasuda K, Ikeda T. A novel therapy for internal hemorrhoids: ligation of the hemorrhoidal artery with a newly devised instrument (Moricorn) in conjunction with a Doppler flowmeter. Am J Gastroenterol. 1995;90(4):610–3.
- Morinaga K, Hasuda K, Ikeda T. A novel therapy for internal hemorrhoids: ligation of the hemorrhoidal artery with a newly devised instrument (Moricorn) in conjunction with a Doppler flowmeter. Am J Gastroenterol 1995; 90:610–3.
- Murray G, Convery C, Walker L, Davies E. Guideline for the Safe Use of Hyaluronidase in Aesthetic Medicine, Including Modified High-dose Protocol. J Clin Aesthet Dermatol. 2021 Aug;14(8):E69-E75. Epub 2021 Aug 1. PMID: 34840662; PMCID: PMC8570661.
- Ortiz H, Marzo J, Armendáriz P, De Miguel M. Stapled hemorrhoidopexy vs diathermy excision for fourth-degree hemorrhoids: a randomized, clinical trial and review of the literature. Dis Colon Rectum. 2005;48(4):809–15. https://doi.org/10.1007/ s10350-004-0861-z.
- Papadopoulos IN, Danias N, Zoumpouli CK. Fibroepithelial polyp in an anal fistulous track: a sign of chronic pathology. BMJ Case Rep. 2010;2010:bcr08.2009.2169. doi: 10.1136/bcr.08.2009.2169. Epub 2010 Jan 13. Erratum in: BMJ Case Rep. 2010;2010:doi/10.1136/bcr.08.2009.2169corr1. Zoumpouli, Christine K [added]. PMID: 22242043; PMCID: PMC3027388.
- Plapler H. A new method for hemorrhoid surgery: an experimental model of diode laser application in monkeys. Photomed Laser Surg. 2008;26:143–6.
- Poskus T, Danys D, Makunaite G, et al. Results of the double-blind, randomized controlled trial comparing laser hemorrhoidoplasty with sutured mucopexy and excisional hemorrhoidectomy. Int J Color Dis. 2020;35(3):481–90.
- Practice parameters for the treatment of hemor- rhoids. The Standards Task Force American Society of Colon and Rectal Surgeons. Dis Colon Rectum. 1993;36(12):1118–20.
- Ratto C, Giordano P, Donisi L, Parello A, Litta F, Doglietto GB (2011) Transanal haemorrhoidal dearterialization (THD) for selected fourth-degree hemorrhoids. Tech Coloproctol 15:191–197. https://doi.org/10.1007/s10151-011-0689-1.
- Ratto C, Parello A, Veronese E, et al. Doppler-guided transanal haemorrhoidal dearterialization for haemorrhoids: results from a multicenter trial. Colonrectal Dis 2015;17(1):O10–O19.
- RJ J (1956). The management of hemorrhoidal thrombosis. GP, 14(1), 82–86.
- Scheyer M, Antonietti E, Rollinger G, Mall H, Arnold S. Doppler-guided hemorrhoidal artery ligation. Am J Surg. 2006;191(1):89–93. https://doi.org/10.1016/j. amjsurg.2005.10.007.
- Schuurman JP, Go PM, Bleys RL. Anatomical branches of the superior rectal artery in the distal rectum. Color Dis. 2009;11(9):967–71. https://doi. org/10.1111/j.1463-1318.2008.01729.x.
- Wałega P, Scheyer M, Kenig J, Herman RM, Arnold S, Nowak M, et al. Two-centre experience in the treatment of hemorrhoidal disease using Doppler-guided hemorrhoidal artery ligation: functional results after 1-year follow-up. Surg Endosc. 2008;22(11):2379–83.
- Wilkerson PM, Strbac M, Reece-Smith H, Middleton SB. Doppler-guided haemorrhoidal artery ligation: long-term outcome and patient satisfaction. Colour Dis. 2009;11(4):394–400. https://doi. org/10.1111/j.1463-1318.2008.01602.x.
- Yilmaz İ, Sücüllü İ, Karaka DÖ, Özdemir Y, Yücel E, Akin ML. Doppler-guided hemorrhoidal artery ligation: experience with 2 years follow-up. Am Surg. 2012;78(3):344–8.
- Zhai M, Zhang YA, Wang ZY, Sun JH, Wen J, Zhang Q, Li JD, Wu YZ, Zhou F, Xu HL. A randomized controlled trial comparing suture-fixation mucopexy and Doppler-guided hemorrhoidal artery ligation in patients with grade III hemorrhoids. Gastroenterol Res Pract. 2016;2016:8143703. https://doi.org/10.1155/2016/8143703.

Chapter

5

Surgical Management of Anorectal Abscess

Anorectal abscess is a common clinical condition in surgical practice. As there is no role of antibiotics, the abscess must be drained at the earliest. The abscess may often be associated with a communicating fistula, where a primary fistulotomy can be carried out with abscess drainage.

The surgeon must be familiar with two surgical techniques for managing an anorectal abscess with a communicating fistula.

Park's Technique

In Park's technique, an oval incision is given 0.5 cm above the internal opening. The mucosa, submucosa, and surrounding tissue are excised, and the fibres of the internal anal sphincter are incised to reach the deep intersphincteric space. The space is curetted, and the necrotic material is removed.

Since this procedure is performed through an intra-anal approach, all the extensions can easily be identified and explored.

Eisenhammer's Technique

Eisenhammer recommended laying the fistula tract open from the external to the internal opening, followed by curetting.

Either of the above techniques can be used to manage an abscess with a communicating fistula tract.

Instrumentation: Figure 5.1A–D.

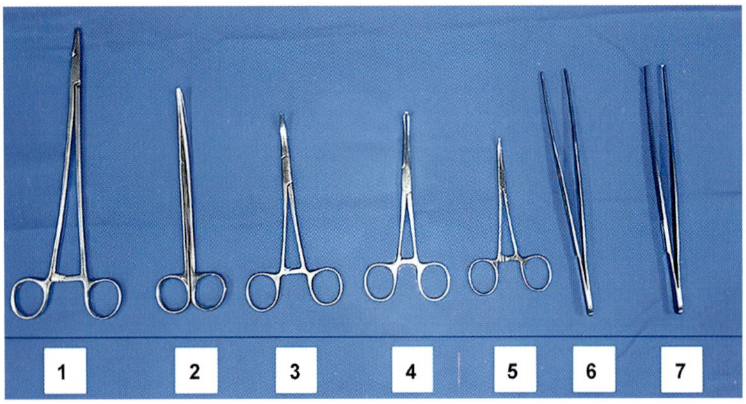

Fig. 5.1A: 1) Needle holder. 2) Scissors. 3) Blunt artery forceps. 4) Allis forceps. 5) Mosquito forceps. 6) Plain forceps. 7) Tooth forceps

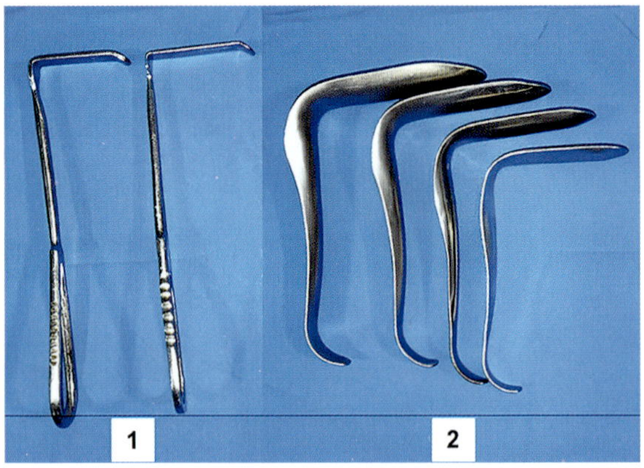

Fig. 5.1B: 1) A pair of right-angle retractors. 2) Sim's speculum

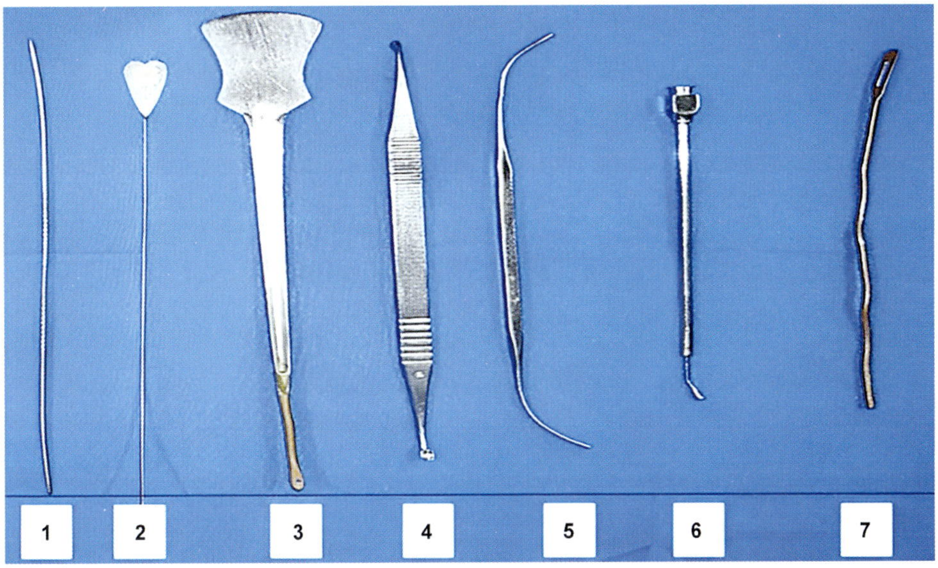

Fig. 5.1C: 1) Hager's dilator 3 mm. 2) Lockhart mummery probe. 3) Eye probe for seton placement. 4) Currette. 5) Curved probe. 6) Irrigation cannula. 7) Malleable metal probe

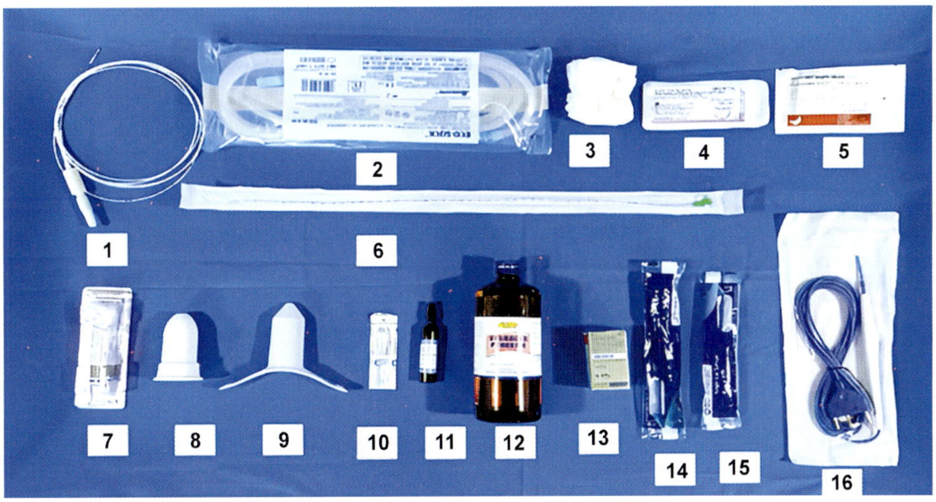

Fig. 5.1D: 1) Laser fibre 360 degrees radial. 2) Suction tip. 3) Gauze pieces. 4) Vicryl 2-0. 5) Cautery tip cleaner. 6) Infant feeding tube. 7) Xylocaine jelly. 5) Circular anal dilator. 9) Half-cut proctoscope. 10) Surgical blade 11 number. 11) Methylene blue ampule. 12) Hydrogen peroxide. 13) Injection bupivacaine 0.5%. 14) Disposable syringe 10 ml. 15) Disposable syringe 5 ml. 16) Cautery pencil

PERIANAL ABSCESS

A perianal abscess appears as a swelling in the perianal space. It is formed due to downward extension of infection from the intersphincteric space. A perianal abscess may or may not be associated with a communicating fistula tract (Fig. 5.2A, B).

Surgical Management of Perianal Abscess

Instrumentation: Figure 5.1A-D.

Type of anaesthesia: Spinal/General

Position of the patient: Lithotomy

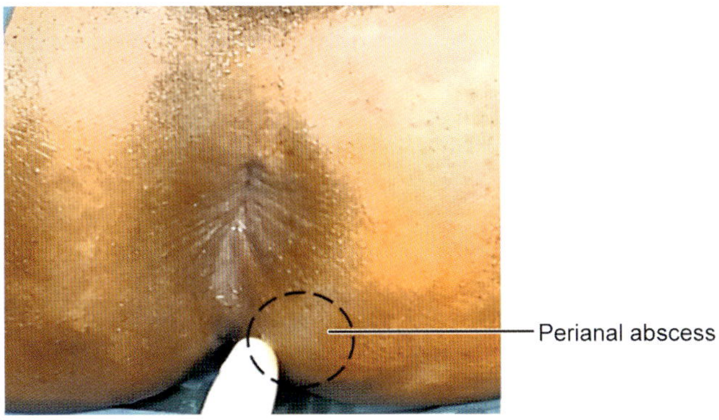

Fig. 5.2A: Perianal abscess

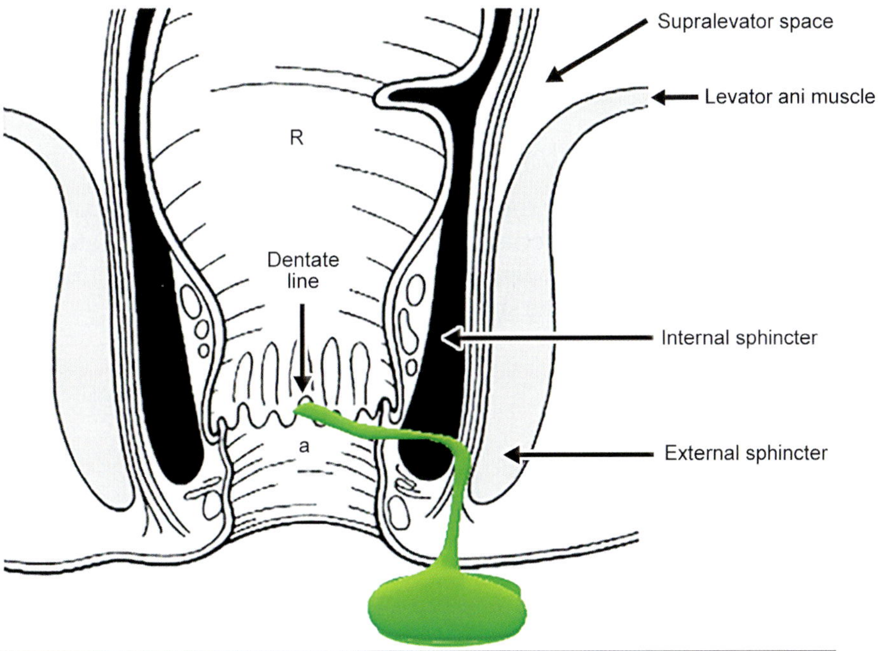

Fig. 5.2B: Diagrammatic representation of MRI of perianal abscess

MANAGING PERIANAL ABSCESS WITH A COMMUNICATING INTERSPHINCTERIC FISTULA

Steps of the Procedure

Step 1: The abscess is palpated, the outline is demarcated, and needle aspiration is done from the most medial part of the abscess. Methylene blue and hydrogen peroxide are injected through the abscess to identify any communicating fistula tract. If the bubbles are seen coming out of the anal canal, it indicates a communicating fistula, usually the inter-sphincteric tract (Fig. 5.3A).

Step 2: A stab incision is given over the most medial part of the abscess as close to the anal verge as possible using 11 number blade, and the pus is drained (Fig. 5.3B). A blunt artery forceps is inserted through the incision, and the blades of the artery forceps are opened using modified Hilton's technique to drain the pus.

Step 3: A probe is inserted through the external opening and brought out through the internal opening (Fig. 5.3C).

Step 4: An incision is given over the probe or the artery forceps using electrosurgical cautery, and the fistula tract is laid open (Fig. 5.3D). The tract is curetted and irrigated. Methylene blue stained granulation tissue indicates one is in the right tract, and no iatrogenic opening has been created (Fig. 5.3E). Park's technique to excise the internal opening can also be used, as shown in Fig. 5.3F and G.

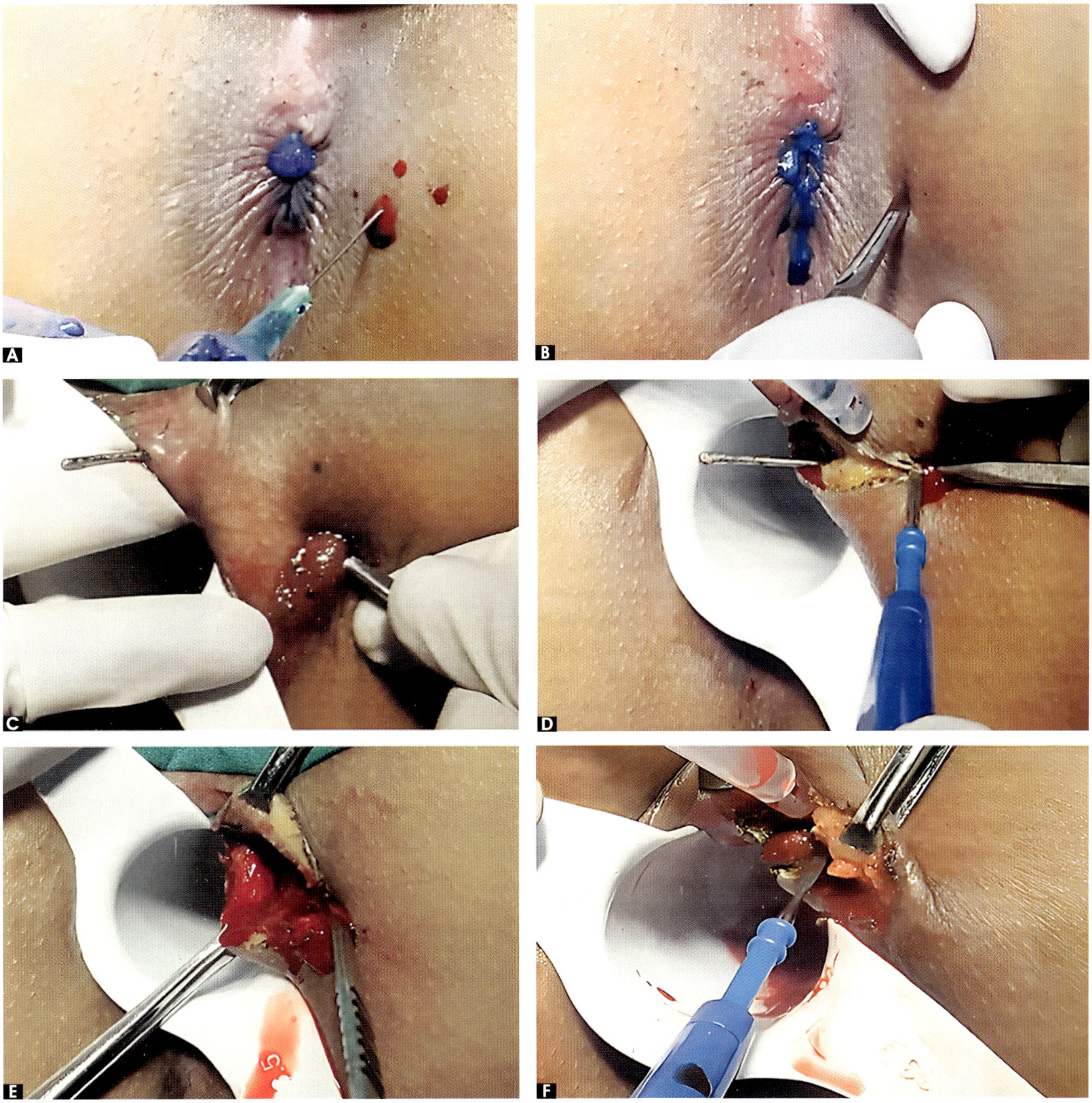

Fig. 5.3A–F: Managing perianal abscess with a communicating intersphincteric fistula. A) Injecting methylene blue and hydrogen peroxide into the abscess cavity. Bubbles can be seen coming out of the internal opening. B) An incision is given towards the most medial part of the abscess, and the pus is drained. C) Insertion of the probe from the site of drainage of the abscess. The probe is brought out of the internal opening. D) Primary fistulotomy being carried out over the probe. E) Curetting and irrigation of the fistulotomy wound. F). Internal opening excision using Park's technique

Step 5: After the fistulotomy, marsupialization of the margins is carried out (Fig. 5.3H). The margins of the fistulotomy wound are stitched with the margins of the skin, taking interrupted sutures using polyglactin 2-0 or 3-0 on 27 mm on a 5/5 round body needle. The final picture at the end of the procedure is shown in Fig. 5.3I.

Scan QR Code for Video on
Perianal Abscess with Communicating Fistula

VIDEO 18

Tips and Tricks

- Sometimes due to the presence of a stricture, fibrosis, an hourglass deformity or necrotic material in the tract, bubbles may not appear at the site of the internal opening, on injecting hydrogen peroxide into the abscess cavity. If on DRE, the internal opening is palpable; one can try to inject hydrogen peroxide through it using an infant feeding tube to rule out a communicating tract. An increase in the size of the abscess indicates communication.
- If one is planning to do a primary fistulotomy in a communicating tract, taking blunt artery forceps from the drained abscess site towards the internal opening is always better. Due to inflammation, an iatrogenic opening may be created if a probe is inserted from the outside.If one plans to do a primary fistulotomy from the inside out, inserting a probe from the internal opening and bringing it out through the abscess drainage site is advisable.
- In Park's technique, a few fibres of the internal anal sphincter are incised to reach the deep intersphincteric space. One can identify the fibres of the internal anal sphincter as they are white and run transversely. The internal anal sphincter is a smooth muscle and on applying cautery, there is no twitching sensation. If one sees the twitching sensation, the external anal sphincter is being cut as it comprises of type 1 and 2 skeletal muscles and forms the lateral boundary of the deep intersphincteric space.
- Local infiltration of bupivacaine 0.5% at the wound site and a pudendal nerve block help decrease postoperative pain.

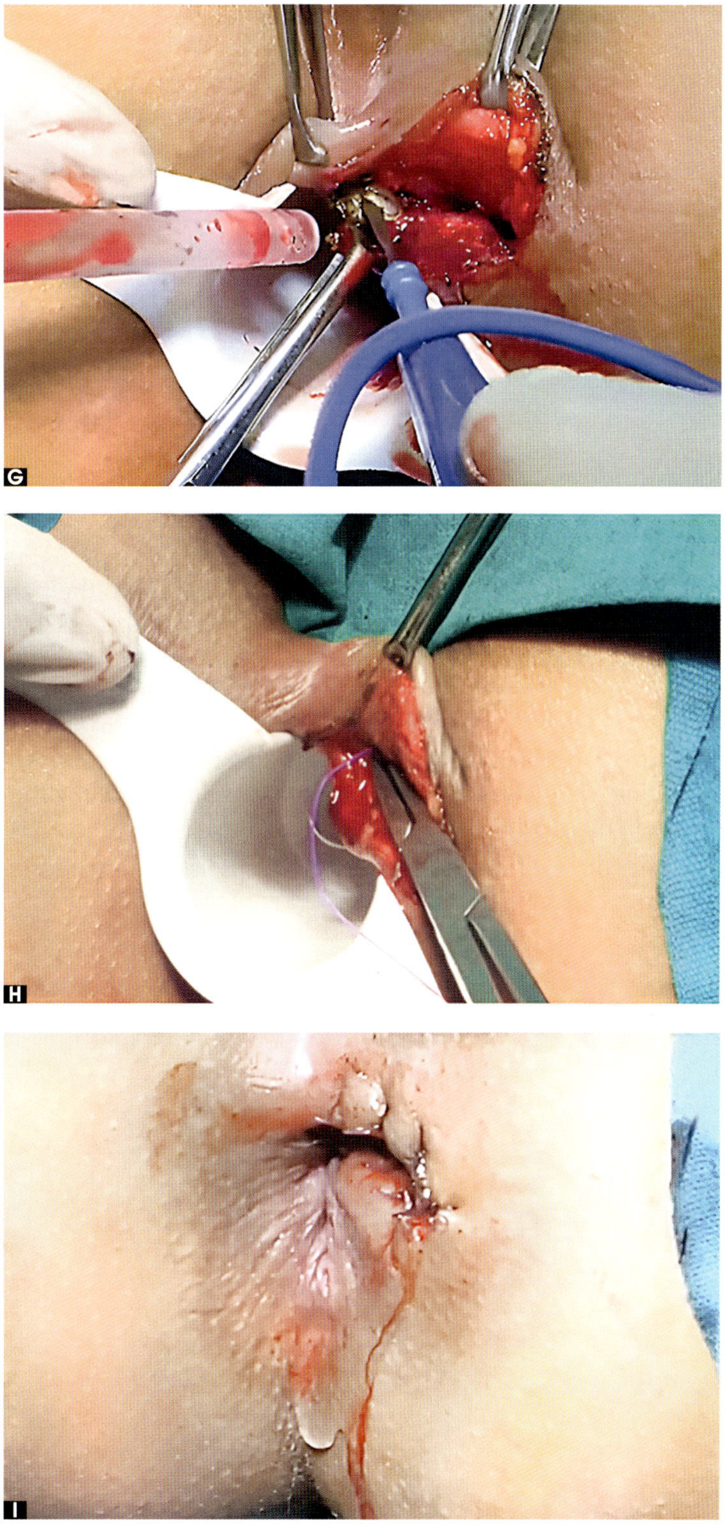

Fig. 5.3G and I: Managing perianal abscess with a communicating intersphincteric fistula. G). Internal opening excision using Park's technique. H) Marsupialization of the margins of the fistulotomy wound. I). Final wound as seen after completion of the procedure

MANAGING PERIANAL ABSCESS WITHOUT A COMMUNICATING FISTULA

If no bubbles are seen in the anal canal on injecting hydrogen peroxide into the perianal abscess, it indicates the absence of a communicating fistula (Fig. 5.4). Simple drainage of the abscess is sufficient in such cases.

Learning Points

- Always insert the proctoscope after the bubbles appear in the anal canal. Otherwise, one may wrongly assume that it is a non-communicating tract. Inserting the proctoscope before injecting the hydrogen peroxide may lead to stretching of the tract and closure of the internal opening.
- Always drain the abscess near the anal verge so that subsequent fistula formation, if any, is small.

ISCHIORECTAL ABSCESS

An ischiorectal abscess is a significant, edematous, brawny induration or tender mass in the ischiorectal space (Fig. 5.5 and 5.6).

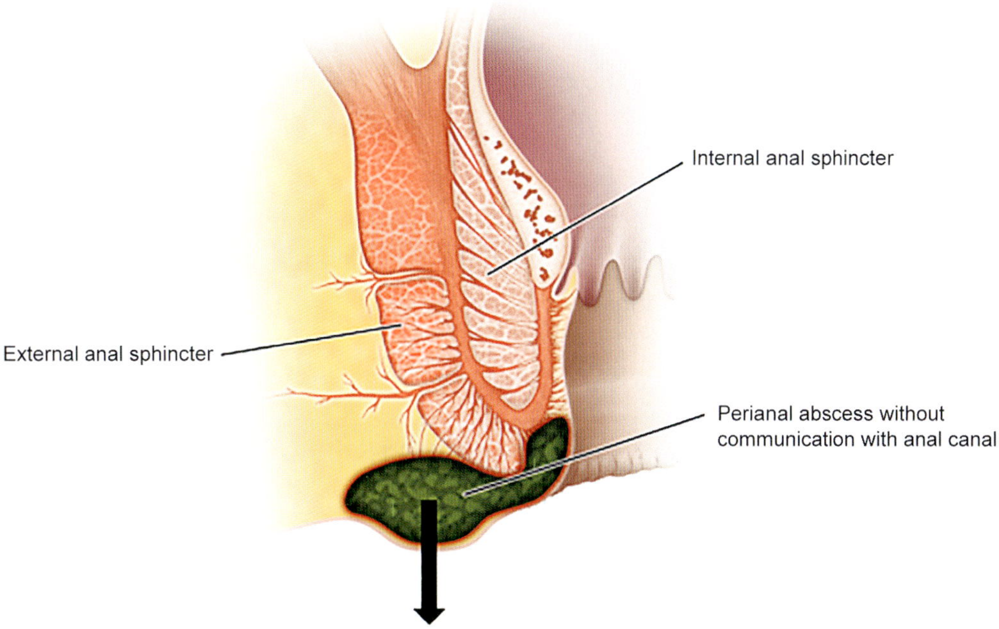

Fig. 5.4: Managing perianal abscess without a communicating fistula. The abscess is drained as close to the anal orifice as possible

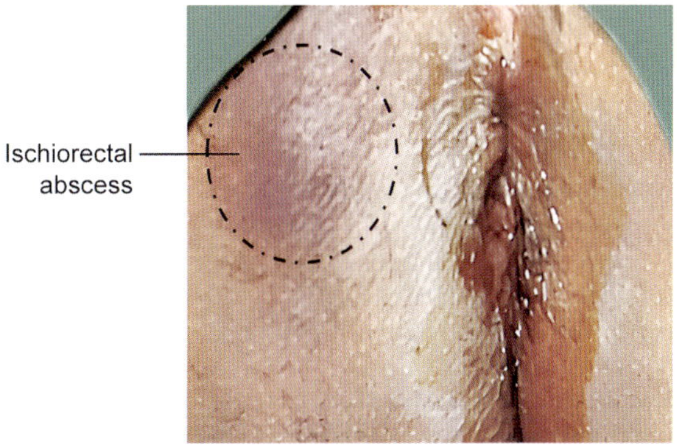

Fig. 5.5: Ischiorectal abscess

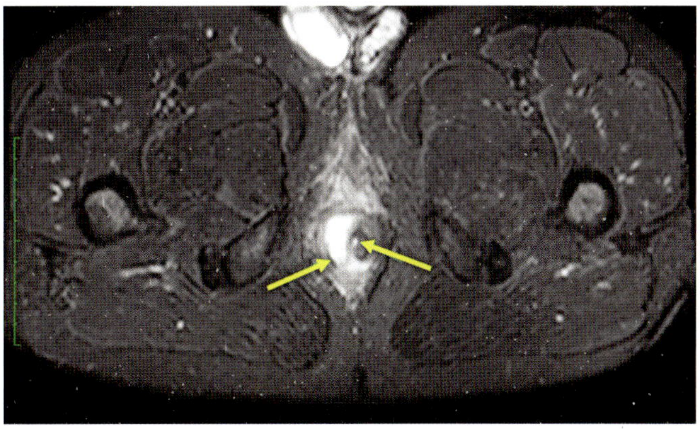

Fig. 5.6: MRI of the ischiorectal abscess

Surgical Management of an Ischiorectal Abscess

Instrumentation: Same as shown in Fig. 5.2A-D

Type of anaesthesia: Spinal/General/Regional

Position of the patient: Lithotomy

MANAGING ISCHIORECTAL ABSCESS WITH A COMMUNICATING FISTULA

The fistula associated with an ischiorectal abscess is trans-sphincteric. In such cases, primary fistulotomy with abscess drainage is sometimes challenging.

Steps of the Procedure

Step 1: Under anaesthesia, the patient is placed in the lithotomy position and cleaned and draped. The abscess is palpated, which is usually felt as a hard swelling. The extent of the abscess is demarcated (Fig. 5.7A).

Step 2: Needle aspiration of the abscess is done from the most medial part, as close to the anal verge as possible. Hydrogen peroxide and methylene blue are injected through the abscess to identify any communicating fistula tract. If the bubbles are seen coming out of the anal canal, it indicates a communicating fistula (Fig. 5.7B, C). Alternatively, after injecting hydrogen peroxide and methylene blue through the internal opening, if the size of the abscess increases, it indicates a communicating fistula tract.

Step 3: A well-lubricated half-cut proctoscope or a Sim's speculum is inserted into the anal canal, and the internal opening is identified. One can easily make out a blue-stained internal opening, usually at the dentate line.

Step 4: At the site of needle aspiration, a small radial incision about 3 mm wide is given (Fig. 5.7D). A blunt artery forceps is inserted, and the abscess is drained by modified Hilton's method (Fig. 5.7E). The margins of the abscess cavity are pressed for complete evacuation of pus and necrotic material. Thorough curetting and irrigation of the abscess cavity are done with a copious amount of normal saline. The pus is sent for culture sensitivity, and the necrotic material is sent for a histopathology examination. The incision can be widened up to 10 mm. Some surgeons prefer to give a cruciate incision.

Step 5: The communicating fistula tract can also be assessed by injecting hydrogen peroxide and methylene blue from the internal opening using a 6F infant feeding tube. The presence of bubbles at the drained abscess site confirms the presence of a communicating fistula tract (Fig. 5.7F)

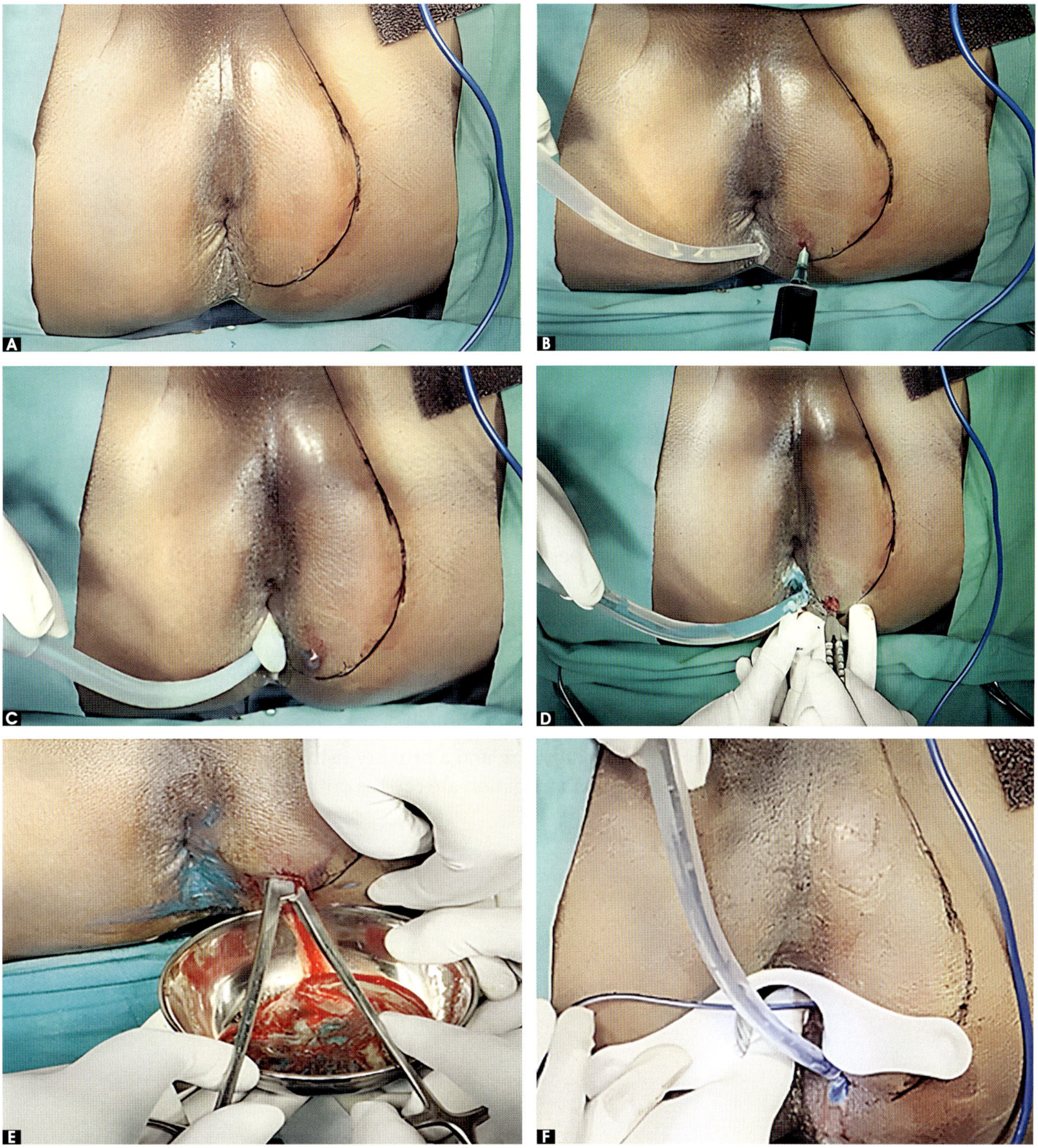

Fig. 5.7(A-F): Managing ischiorectal abscess with a communicating trans-sphincteric fistula. A) Demarcation of Ischiorectal abscess. B) Insertion of hydrogen peroxide and methylene blue through the abscess cavity. C) Bubbles are seen coming out of the internal opening at 6 o'clock. D) Incision given over the most medial part of the abscess. E) Pus drained from the abscess cavity by modified Hilton's technique, followed by thorough irrigation of the tract. F). Methylene blue is inserted through the internal opening. Bubbles seen coming out of the external opening indicate a communicating trans-sphincteric fistula

Step 6: The internal opening is excised along with mucosa, submucosa and a few fibres of the internal anal sphincter to reach the deep intersphincteric space (Fig. 5.7G, H).

Step 7: Sometimes, after opening the deep intersphincteric space, a methylene blue-stained extension can be seen going towards the intersphincteric space. The extension is laid open upto the anorectal ring, followed by a thorough curetting to remove the necrotic material (Fig. 5.7I, J).

Step 8: In an ischiorectal abscess with a communicating fistula, it is imperative to know the extent of the external anal sphincter involved. If more than 50% of the external sphincter is involved or the anatomy of the external sphincter is not precise due to the presence of inflammation, primary fistulotomy is not recommended.

Once the external sphincter is thoroughly assessed, one can proceed with primary fistulotomy. A blunt artery forceps is inserted through the incision site of the drained abscess and brought out of the excised internal opening site. An incision is given over the artery forceps, and a primary fistulotomy is carried out (Fig. 5.7K).

Once the fistula tract is laid open, curetting and irrigation are carried out (Fig. 5.7L).

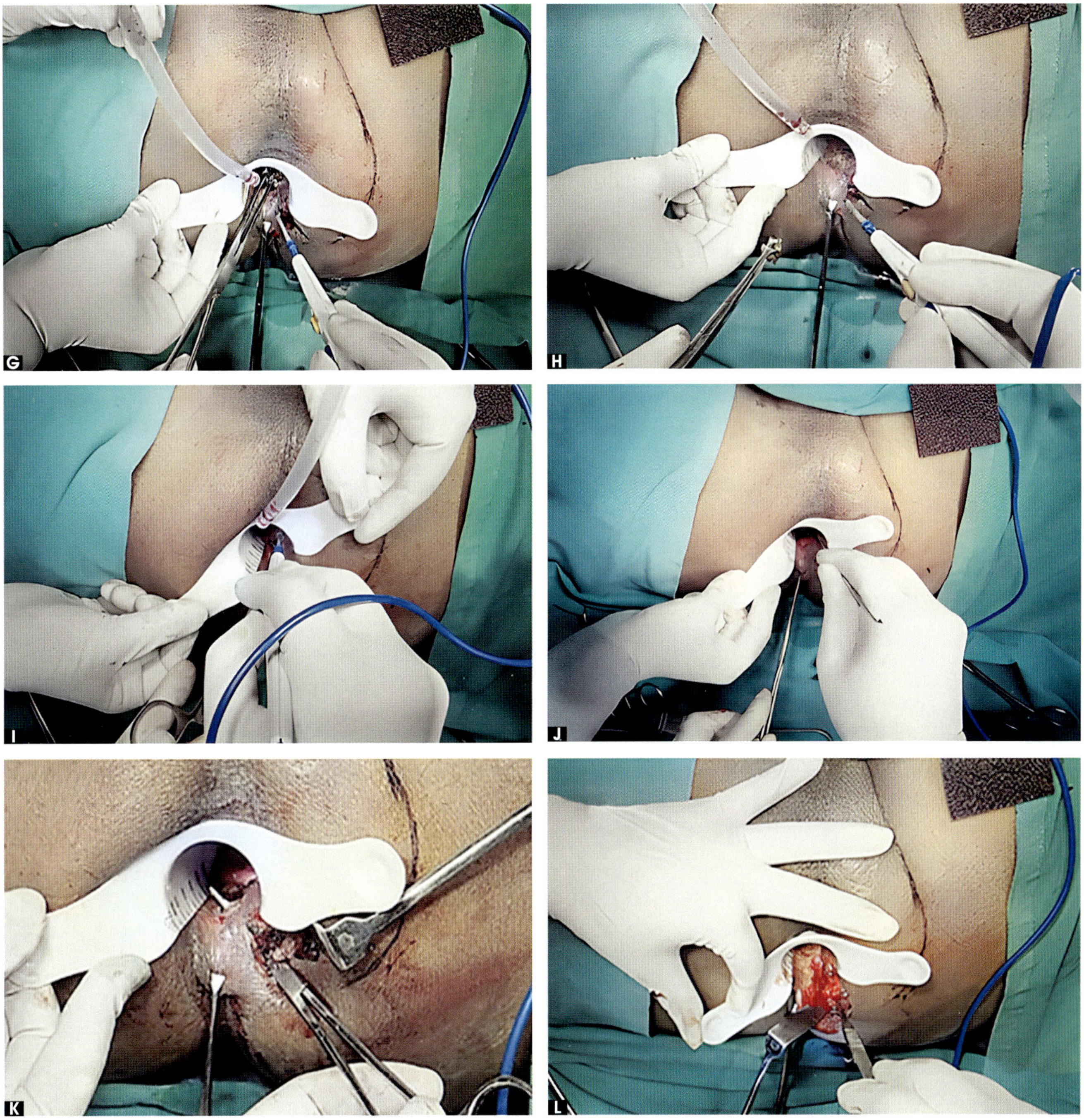

Fig. 5.7(G-L): Managing ischiorectal abscess with a communicating trans-sphincteric fistula. G) Excision of internal opening along with mucosa and submucosa. A few fibres of the internal anal sphincter are cut to reach the deep intersphincteric space. H) Primary fistulotomy done. I) Intersphincteric extension seen going upwards. The tract laid open up to the anorectal ring. J) Curetting of the upward extension. K) Primary fistulotomy done for trans-sphincteric fistula tract. L) Curetting of the tract after fistulotomy

Step 9: The blunt artery is inserted through the fistulotomy wound and extended anteriorly towards the upper extent of the abscess. An incision is given at the tip, and a draining seton is placed to prevent collection (Fig. 5. 7M, N).

Step 10: Primary sphincter repair using PDS 2-0 is done if the external anal sphincter is cut upto 50% (Fig. 5.7O). It helps to prevent postoperative anal incontinence.

Step 11: Marsupialization of the fistulotomy wound is done by taking interrupted sutures using polyglactin 2-0 or 3-0 on 27 mm on a 5/5 round body needle (Fig. 5.7P).

Step 12: Finally, a pudendal nerve block is given using 0.5% bupivacaine (Fig. 5.7Q, R).

Figure 5.7 S shows the wound at the end of the procedure.

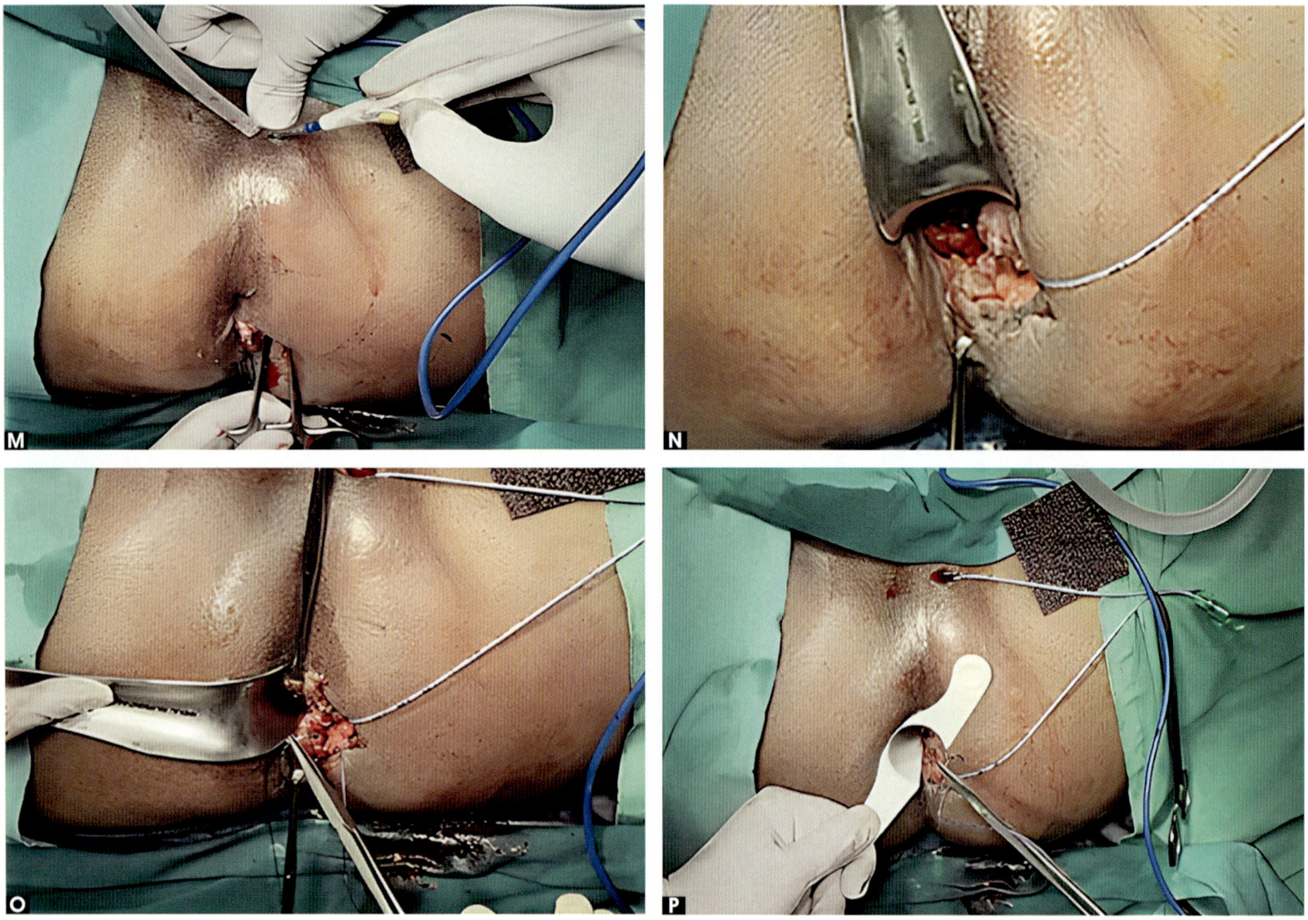

Fig. 5.7(M-N): Managing ischiorectal abscess with a communicating trans-sphincteric fistula. M) Insertion of a blunt artery forceps in the abscess cavity. N) Insertion of a draining seton. O) Primary sphincter repair using PDS 2-0. P) Marsupialization of the margins using Vicryl 3-0.

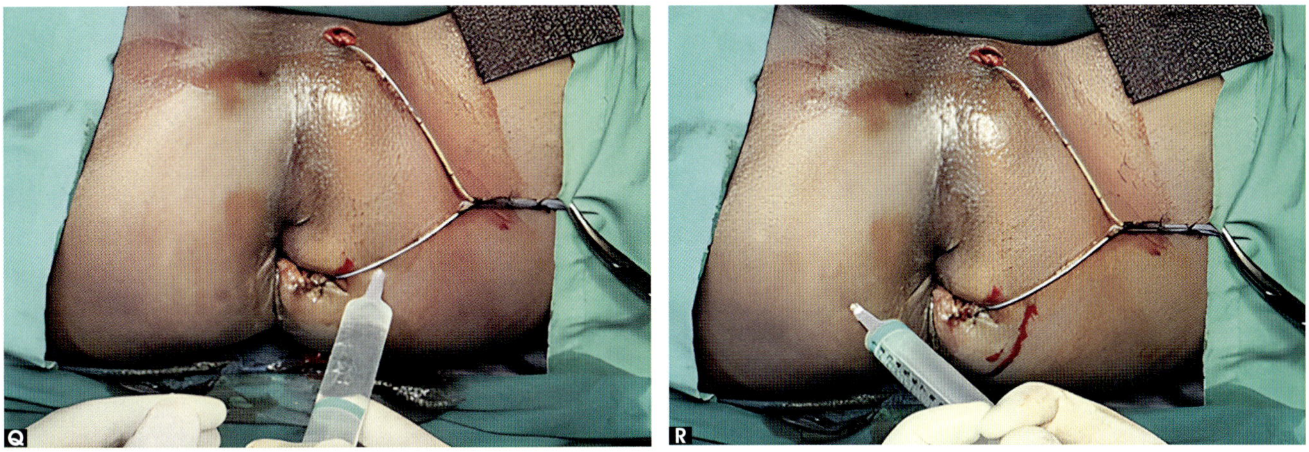

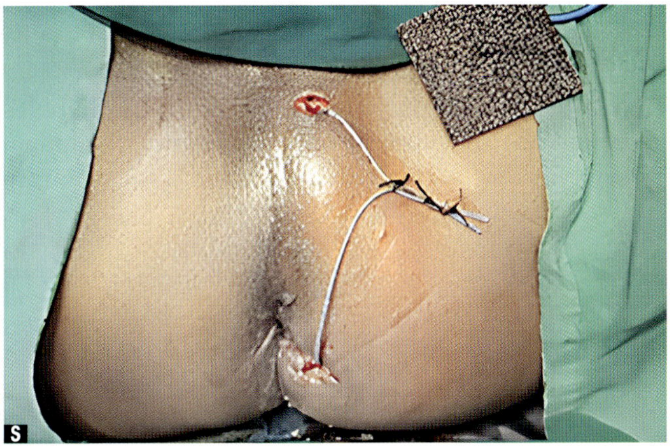

Scan QR Code for Video on
Managing Ischiorectal Abscess with Communicating Fistula
VIDEO 19

Fig. 5.7(O-S): Managing ischiorectal abscess with a communicating trans-sphincteric fistula. Q and R) Bilateral pudendal nerve block given. S) Final picture at the end of the procedure

Tips and Tricks

- While operating on an ischiorectal abscess, one should refrain from inserting a finger into the abscess cavity to break the loculi, as the loculi are never present. One can damage the fibres of the inferior rectal nerve branches and the branches of the pudendal vessels supplying the ischiorectal region. This can lead to postoperative paraesthesia of the skin over the ischiorectal region. Moreover, profuse bleeding may occur during the surgery due to injury to the pudendal vessels or the underlying muscles.
- While carrying out a primary fistulotomy, it is advisable not to insert a probe from the incision site of the drained abscess. Since there is inflammation, even a gentle insertion of a probe can lead to an iatrogenic opening. Insertion of blunt artery forceps is always a better option.
- A critical consideration during fistulotomy is to assess the extent of the external sphincter involved. If the anatomy of the external anal sphincter is not precise, a seton can be placed for drainage, followed by a second surgery for the fistula after three months. Cutting the external sphincter without proper assessment can lead to incontinence.

MANAGING ISCHIORECTAL ABSCESS WITH A NON-COMMUNICATING FISTULA TRACT

Once hydrogen peroxide and methylene blue are injected into the ischiorectal abscess, the absence of bubbles in the anal canal indicate a non-communicating fistula. In such a case, the pus is drained by a radial incision on the most medial part of the abscess (Fig. 5.8). The abscess cavity is thoroughly curetted and irrigated. A drain is placed for 72 hours for drainage and irrigation.

Learning Points

- Since the fistula tract associated with ischiorectal abscess is trans-sphincteric, assessing the extent of the external sphincter involved is essential. Primary fistulotomy should be performed with utmost care to avoid incontinence.
- A seton can also be placed in a communicating fistula if one is uncomfortable in carrying out a primary fistulotomy. A definitive procedure can be performed after three months when the inflammation subsides and the fistula tract matures.

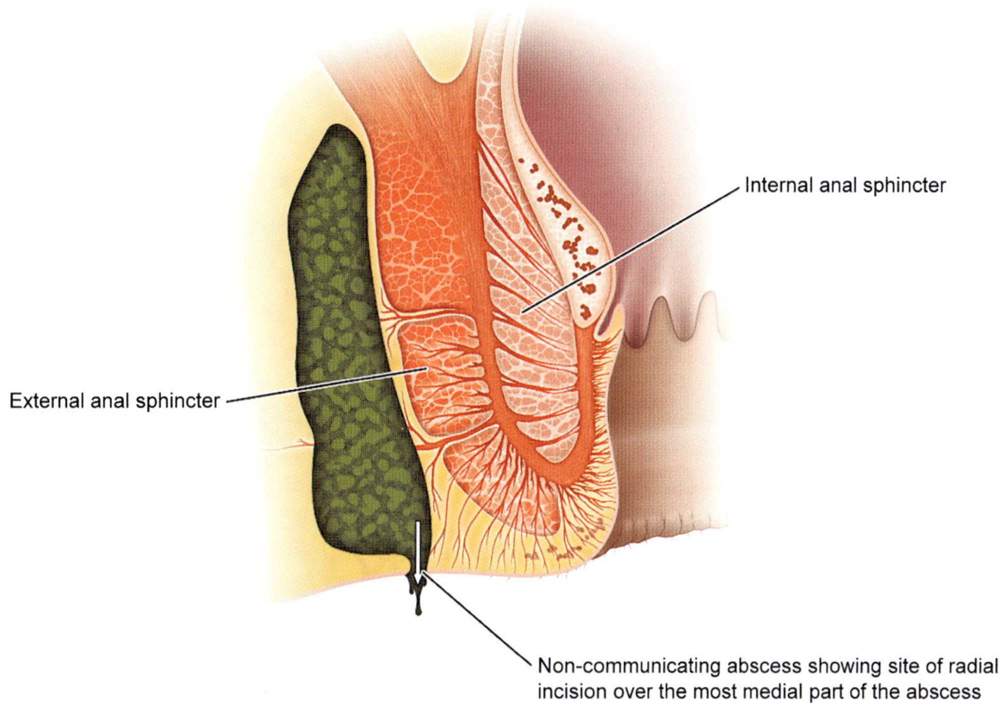

Fig. 5.8: Drainage of ischiorectal abscess in a non-communicating fistula tract. Drainage of pus from the most medial part of the ischiorectal abscess with a radial incision

INTERSPHINCTERIC ABSCESS

The intersphincteric abscess is formed in the intersphincteric space. It may extend downwards to form a perianal abscess or upwards to form a supralevator abscess.

MANAGING INTERSPHINCTERIC ABSCESS (ASSOCIATED WITH A4 TYPE OF FISTULA TRACT)

Instrumentation: As shown in Fig. 5.2A-D

Type of anaesthesia: Spinal/General

Position of the patient: Lithotomy

Steps of the Procedure

Step 1: Since no external opening is present, it is crucial to identify the internal opening from where the pus is oozing. A well-lubricated half-cut proctoscope is introduced into the anal canal to identify the internal opening (Fig. 5.9A). A blunt artery forceps can be inserted through the internal opening to demonstrate the deep intersphincteric space (Fig. 5.9B).

Step 2: Methylene blue is injected through the internal opening to stain the unhealthy granulation tissue and the intersphincteric space (Fig. 5.9C). The internal opening is excised by Park's technique. The fibres of the internal anal sphincter are incised to enter the intersphincteric and the deep intersphincteric space (Fig. 5.9D, E).

Step 3: A probe is inserted into the intersphincteric space, which is opened upto the anorectal ring (Fig. 5.9F).

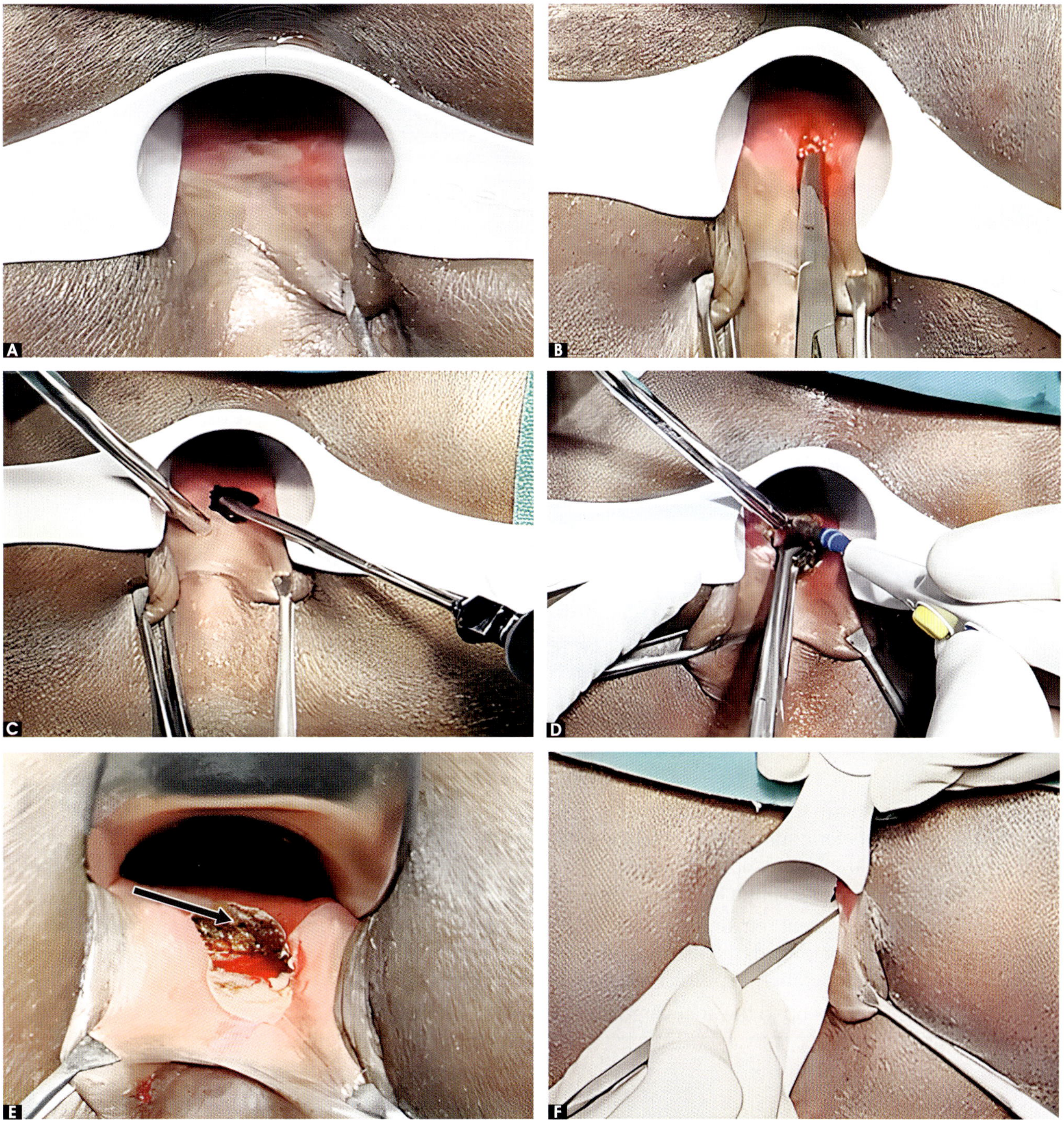

Fig. 5.9A-F: Management of intersphincteric abscess. A) Internal opening as seen after insertion of a half-cut proctoscope. B) Blunt artery is inserted through the internal opening to demonstrate the deep intersphincteric space. C) Methylene blue is injected to demarcate the internal opening and stain the unhealthy granulation tissue. D, E) Excision of the internal opening along with mucosa, submucosa, surrounding tissue and fibres of the internal anal sphincter (Park's technique). The deep intersphincteric space is opened. F) Insertion of the probe into the intersphincteric space. The space is opened over the probe

Methylene blue stained granulation tissue in the space indicates the abscess cavity. The pus is drained, and curetting is done to remove the necrotic material (Fig. 5.9G). If the abscess extends towards the levators, the supralevator space is also curetted. After curetting, the space is irrigated with normal saline (Fig. 5.9H). An alternative to the opening of intersphincteric space is laser ablation (Fig. 5.9I).

Step 4: A low-end fistulotomy may be carried out from the site of excised internal opening and extending upto the anal verge to facilitate drainage, followed by marsupialization of the margins (Fig. 5.9J).

Step 5: Bupivacaine 0.5% is infiltrated locally at the operated site, and a pudendal nerve block is given to reduce postoperative pain.

The final picture at the end of the procedure is shown in Fig. 5.9K.

Scan QR Code for Video on
Management of Intersphincteric Abscess
VIDEO 20

Tips and Tricks

- Removing the primary source of infection, i.e., the internal opening, opening of deep intersphincteric space and the intersphincteric space is essential for managing the intersphincteric abscess. Some authors feel that cutting the internal sphincter up to the anorectal ring can lead to anal incontinence. The technique described above for managing intersphincteric abscesses is Park's technique.
- The surgical management remains the same, whether one is dealing with intersphincteric abscess or intersphincteric extension towards the levators (supralevator space). The primary objective remains the drainage of an abscess. The operative steps for Type A 4 fistula also remain the same.
- A low-end fistulotomy up to the anal verge is necessary for proper drainage.

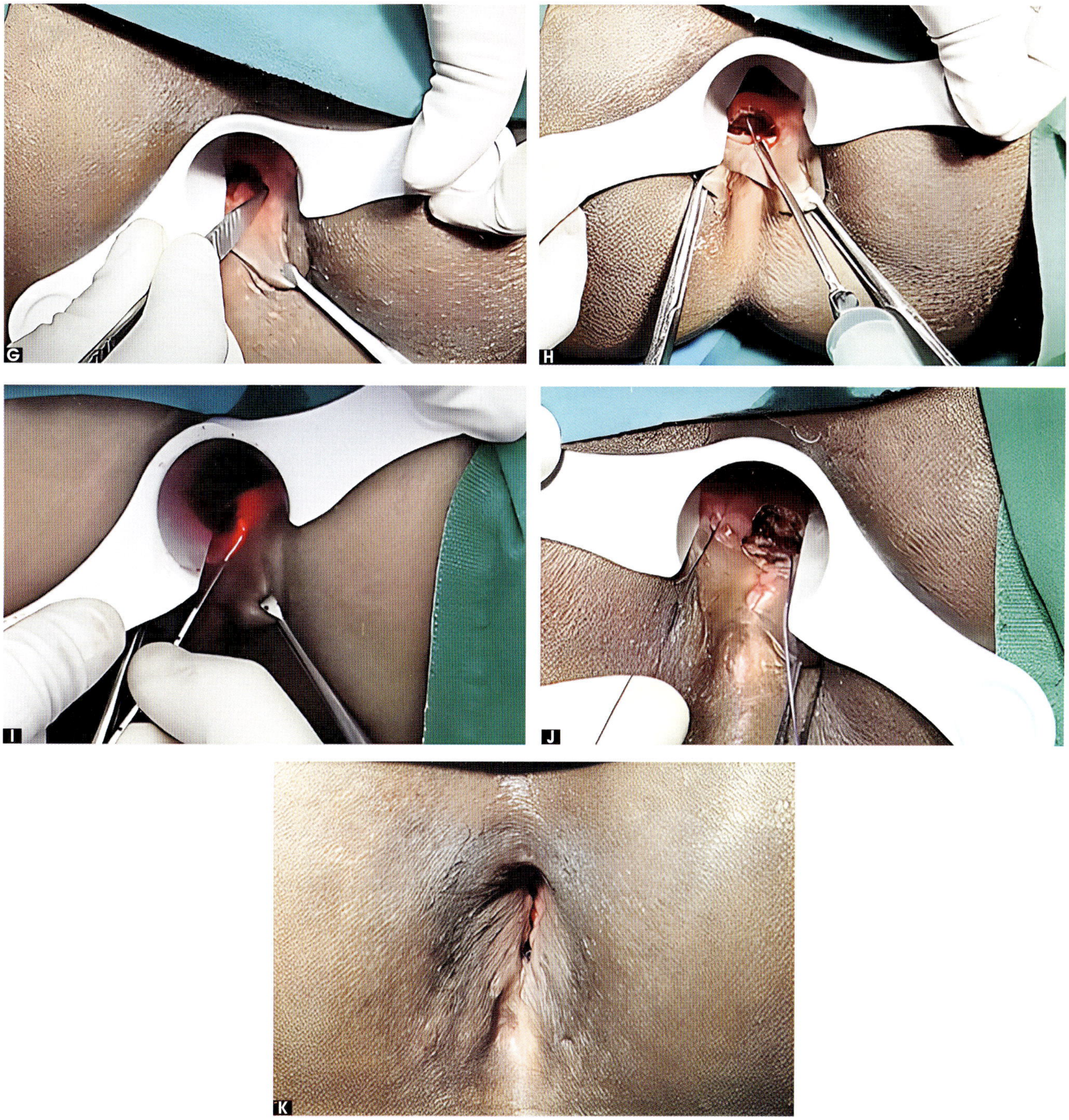

Fig. 5.9G-K: Management of intersphincteric abscess. G) Curretting and irrigation of the intersphincteric space. H) Irrigation of intersphincteric space. I) Laser ablation of intersphincteric space as an alternative to the opening of the space. J)Proximal fistulotomy and marsupialization of the margins. K) Final wound at the end of the procedure

SUPRALEVATOR ABSCESS

A supralevator abscess (Fig. 5.10A–C) can arise from:

- Upwards extension of an intersphincteric abscess
- Downward extension from pelvic disease
- Upwards extension of an ischiorectal abscess

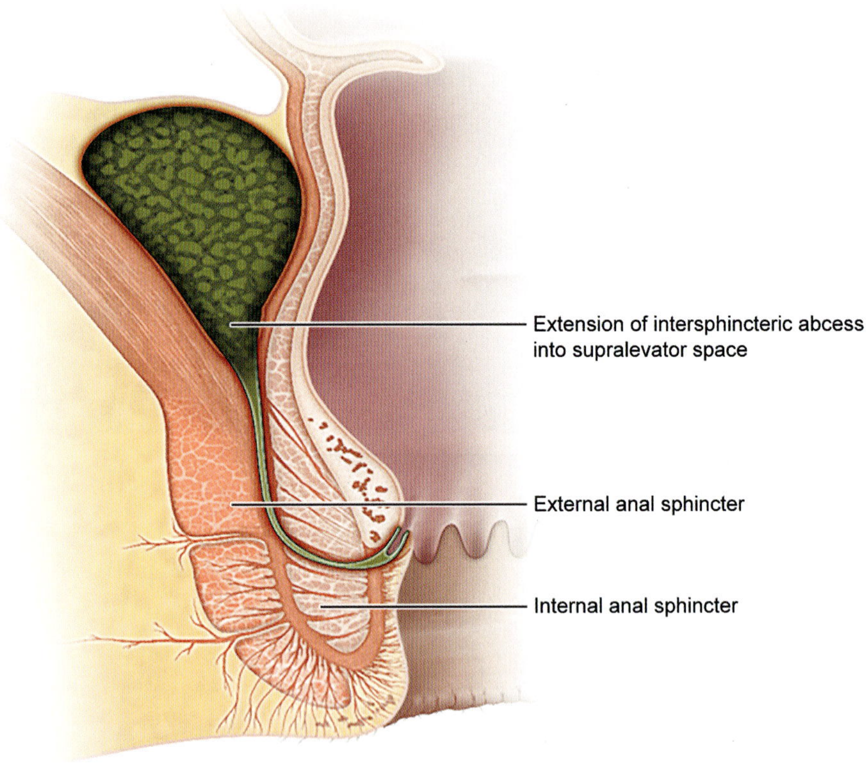

Fig. 5.10A: Diagrammatic representation of a supralevator abscess. A) Upward extension of an intersphincteric abscess to supralevator space

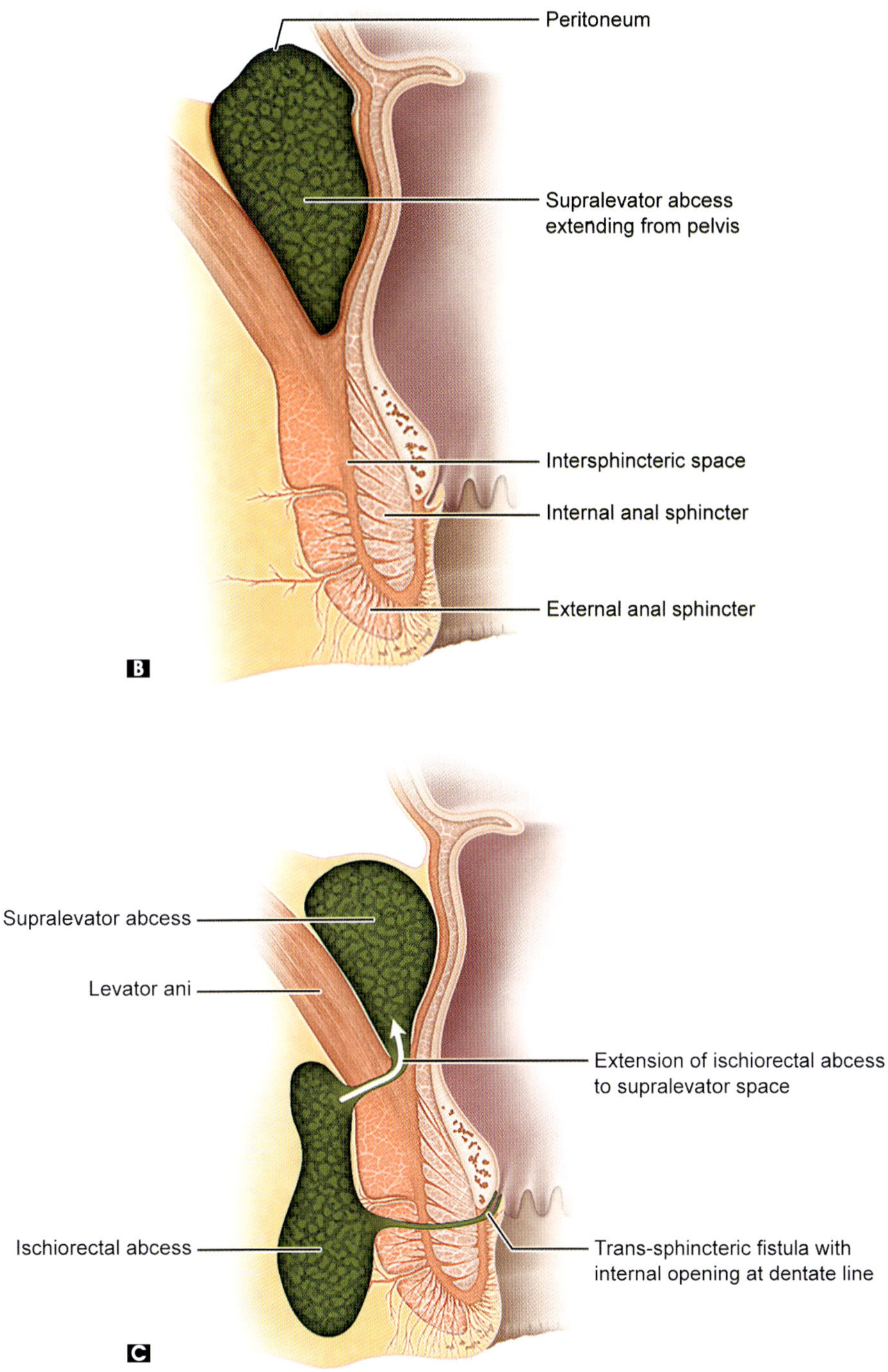

Fig. 5.10(B-C): Diagrammatic representation of a supralevator abscess. B) Downward extension of pelvic infection leading to supralevator abscess formation. C) Extension of an ischiorectal abscess to supralevator space with a communicating trans-sphincteric fistula

MANAGING SUPRALEVATOR ABSCESS

Instrumentation: Figure 5.2A-D

Type of anaesthesia: Spinal/General

Position of the patient: Lithotomy

Ischiorectal Abscess Extending Upwards to the Supralevator Space

Proper evaluation of the tract is essential before draining the abscess. It is a good practice to get the MRI done. Ask the radiologist to mark the abscess cavity on the most medial aspect, for easy access for abscess drainage (Fig. 5.11A-C).

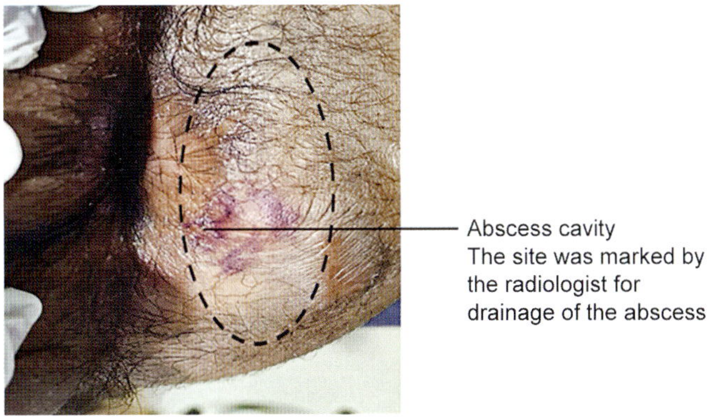

Fig. 5.11A: An abscess cavity with a marked site for incision and drainage

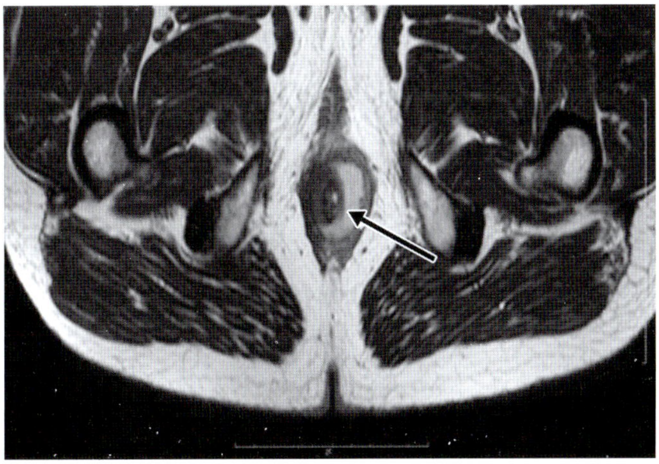

Fig. 5.11B: Axial T2W image of MRI image showing left intersphincteric abscess extending from 1 o'clock to 7o' clock position. (Image courtsey: Dr Dhawal Kaushal Radiologist)

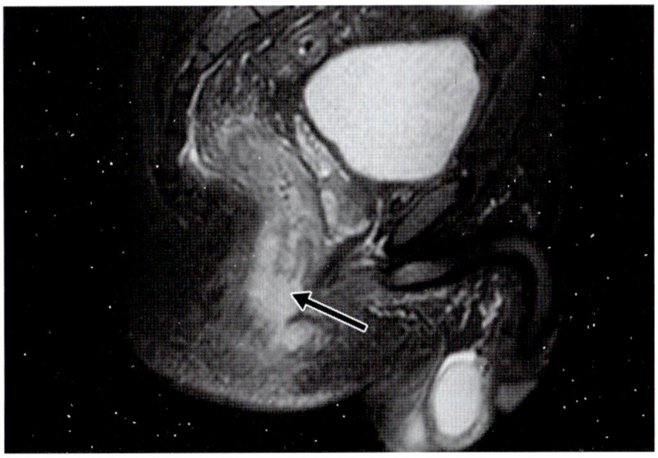

Fig. 5.11C: STIR Sagittal MRI image showing ischioanal abscess extending across the levator to reach upto the ischiorectal fossa (Image courtesy: Dr Dhawal Kaushal, Radiologist)

Steps of the Procedure

Step 1: A needle is inserted, and pus is aspirated from the most medial part of the abscess cavity at the site of the marking (Fig. 5.12A). Hydrogen peroxide and methylene blue are injected into the abscess cavity. In an abscess of cryptoglandular origin, bubbles can be seen emerging from the internal opening at the dentate line.

Step 2: A half-cut proctoscope is inserted in the anal canal to locate the internal opening (Fig. 5.12B). In some cases, bubbles may emerge from the distal part of the rectum above the anorectal ring, indicating an upward extension of the tract opening into the distal rectum (Fig. 5.12C, D).

Step 3: A small incision of approximately 3mm is given at the site of needle aspiration, which can be widened later (Fig. 5.12E). A blunt artery or a sinus forceps is inserted, and the blades are separated for complete drainage of pus (modified Hilton's technique as shown in Fig. 5.12F). The pus can be seen oozing out of the drainage site (Fig. 5.12G).

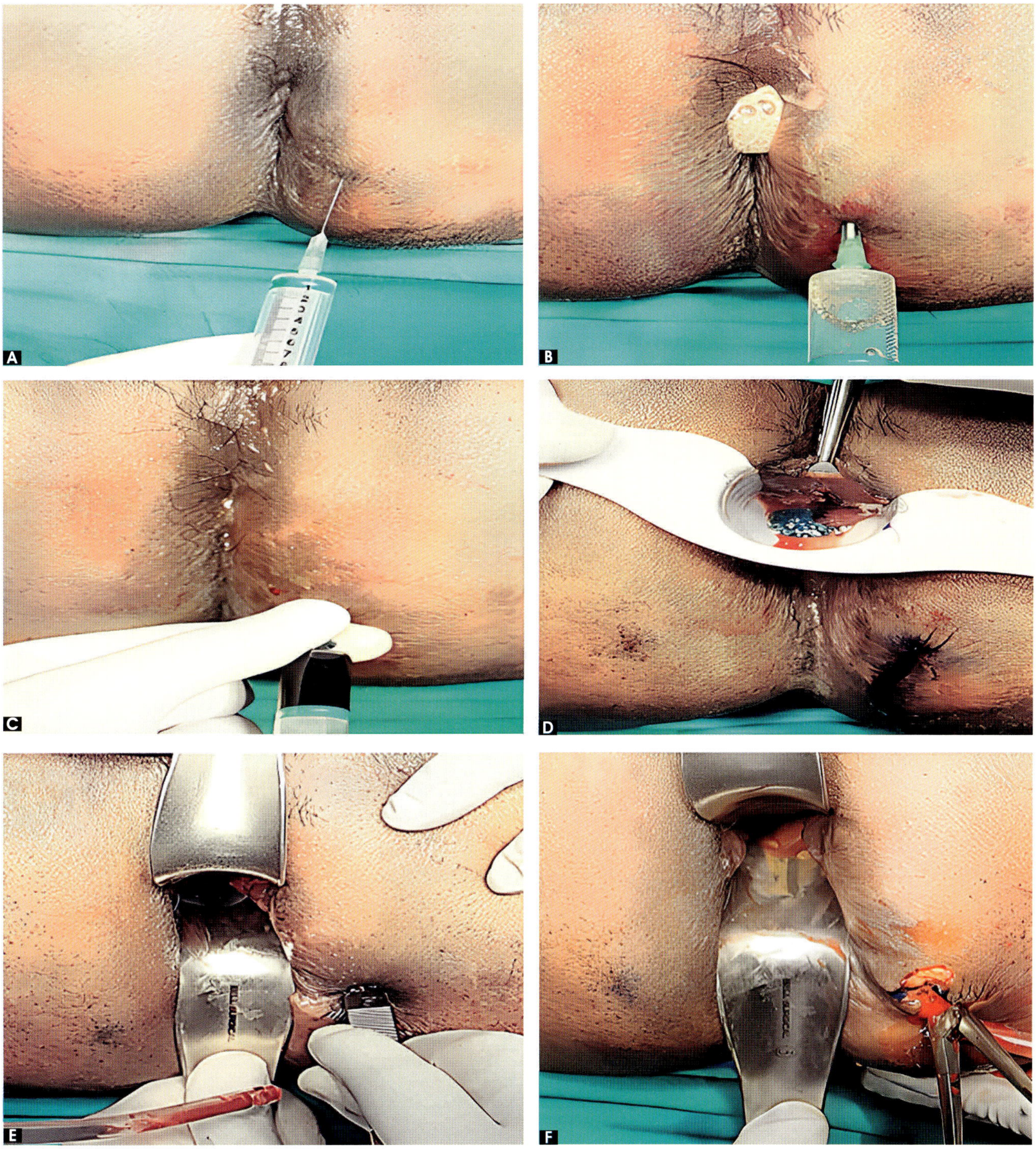

Fig. 5.12(A-F): Management of ischiorectal abscess extending upwards to the supralevator space. A) Needle aspiration of the pus from the most medial part. B). Injecting hydrogen peroxide in the abscess cavity. C) Injecting methylene blue in the abscess cavity. D) Bubbles emerge from the internal opening and distal part of the rectum, indicating an upward extension of the tract. E) A stab incision at the site of the marked abscess. F) Opening of abscess cavity by modified Hilton's method to drain the pus and the necrotic material

Step 4: After the drainage, the necrotic material is removed, and the depth of the abscess cavity is assessed by inserting a large blunt forceps (Fig. 5.12H). The internal opening is excised in a communicating fistula tract.

Step 5: A primary fistulotomy is done after assessing the extent of the external anal sphincter involved (Fig. 5.12I). The extension of cryptogenic origin, opening in the distal rectum, is curetted and irrigated. The internal opening in the distal rectum is closed using Vicryl 2-0.

Step 5: Finally, the abscess cavity is curetted and irrigated, and a Foley's catheter is placed for 72 hours for drainage and irrigation (Fig. 5.12J, K).

Tips and Tricks

- As mentioned in the drainage of an ischiorectal abscess, one should not insert a finger in the abscess cavity to break the loculi.
- Drainage of the abscess, followed by primary fistulotomy in the trans-sphincteric fistula tract, is the best approach. If the extent of the involvement of EAS cannot be assessed due to edema, placement of seton is a good option.
- Unnecessary probing should always be avoided. If the hydrogen peroxide and methylene blue are not seen coming out of the internal opening, and no internal opening can be made out on DRE, it is better to drain only the abscess. If the fistula tract appears later, it can be managed in a second surgical procedure.
- While removing the drain, some surgeons prefer to withdraw the drain gradually over the next few weeks. This is a good approach as the abscess cavity heals slowly. The abscess cavity collapses over time.

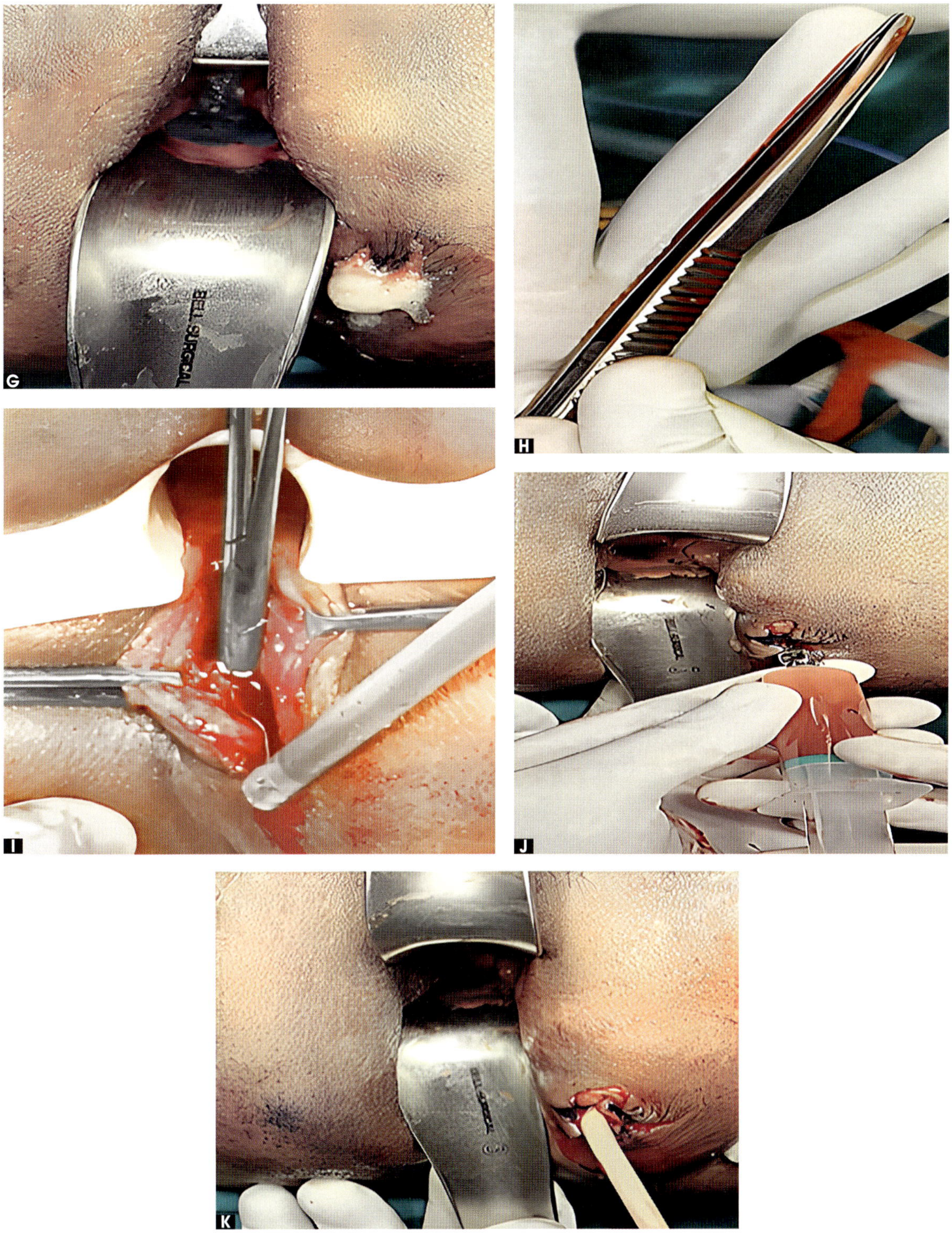

Fig. 5.12(G-K): Management of ischiorectal abscess extending upwards to the supralevator space. G) Pus coming out of the abscess cavity. H) Assessing the depth of the abscess cavity. I) Primary fistulotomy after drainage of an abscess. J) Irrigation of the abscess cavity. K) Placement of drain in the abscess cavity

Supralevator Abscess Extending from Intersphincteric Abscess

These abscesses are of cryptoglandular origin, with the internal opening at 6 o'clock. Excision of the internal opening and drainage of the abscess through a transanal approach is most appropriate in these cases.

The procedural steps are the same as described for managing an intersphincteric abscess.

Supralevator Abscess Secondary to Abdominopelvic Disease

In this type of supralevator abscess, the collection is secondary to abdominopelvic disease. The abscess can be drained by a CT-guided transrectal or transabdominal approach (Fig. 5.13).

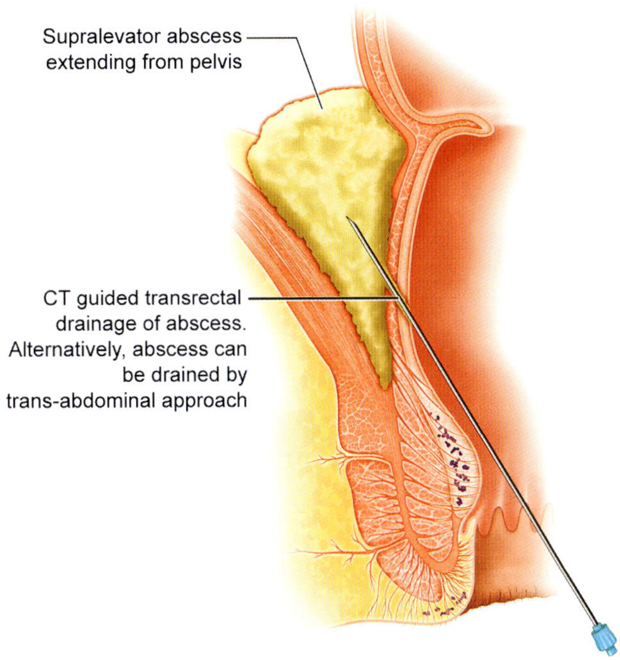

Fig. 5.13: Drainage of supralevator abscess by CT-guided transanal approach, formed due to downward extension of pelvic infection

Tips and tricks of drainage of Supralevator Abscess—A Paradigm shift

- If the supralevator abscess has developed from the upward extension of an intersphincteric abscess, always drain the abscess through the anal canal after widening the internal opening (Fig. 5.14A, B).
- For drainage of subsequent collection, a low-end fistulotomy should be done at 6 o'clock, up to the anal verge.

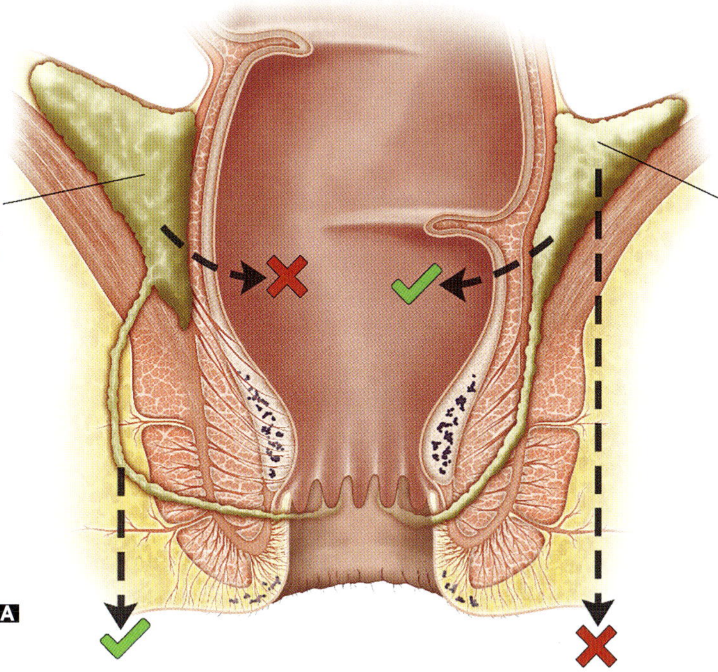

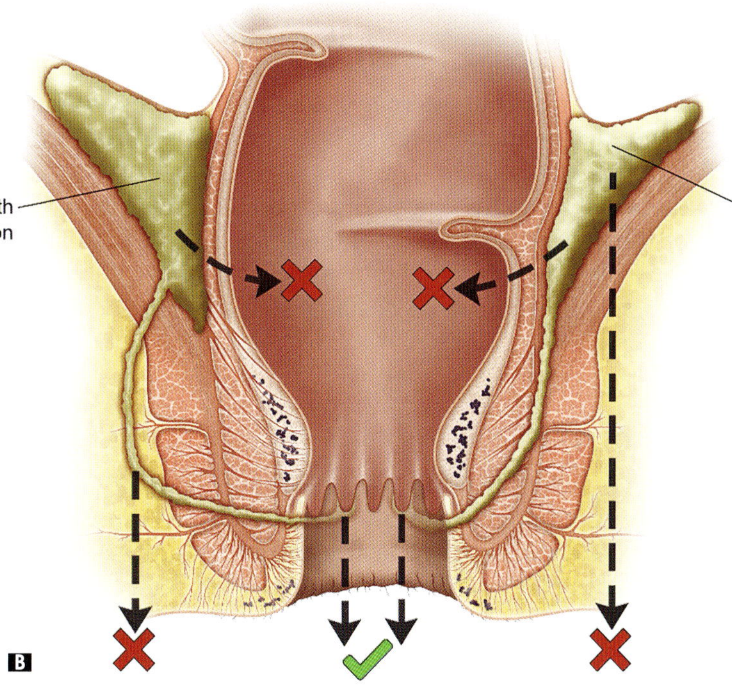

Fig. 5.14A, B: Diagrammatic representation of drainage of a supralevator abscess. A) Drainage of supralevator abscess into the rectum or perineum, as previously suggested. B) Drainage of supralevator abscess by the trans-anal opening of intersphincteric space with fistulotomy from dentate line to the anal verge, irrespective of inter-sphincteric or trans-sphincteric extension as presently suggested

DEEP POSTANAL ABSCESS

The deep postanal space infection often communicates through the ischiorectal fossa on both sides and may present as a horseshoe abscess (Fig. 5.15). Most of the time, recurrences after fistula surgery occur because the deep postanal abscess is missed or inadequately drained during surgery.

MANAGING DEEP POSTANAL ABSCESS

There are two techniques to open the deep postanal space.

Hanley's Technique

The original Hanley's technique advocates the extension of posterior fistulotomy upto the deep postanal space. A longitudinal incision is continued downwards between the subcutaneous part of EAS and the coccyx to reach the deep postanal space. The space is loosely packed for 24 hours for drainage of the collection (Fig. 5.16).

The disadvantage of this technique is postoperative anal incontinence which may be transient but associated with significant discomfort to the patient. This technique may also result in a keyhole deformity.

Modified Hanley's Technique

In the modified Hanley's technique, the anococcygeal ligament is incised halfway between the coccyx tip and the subcutaneous part of the external anal sphincter to access the deep postanal area. The anococcygeal ligament is incised vertically, and the superficial external anal sphincter fibres are split open using a blunt artery forceps. A draining seton is inserted through the internal opening and retrieved from the drainage incision of the postanal space.

If the deep postanal abscess extends into the connecting ischiorectal region forming a horseshoe abscess, a bilateral incision is made over the abscess. The cavity of the abscess is curetted and irrigated. A seton can be placed, which is tightened at regular intervals to aid in complete healing.

The stepwise surgical approach to open the deep postanal space is mentioned under the management of a horseshoe abscess.

DEEP ANTERIOR ANAL SPACE ABSCESS

The deep anterior abscess is formed when the intersphincteric abscess ruptures through the superficial and deep part of the external anal sphincter into the deep anterior anal space. Rupture of the abscess into the lower part of the vagina can lead to a rectovaginal fistula. The abscess may extend superior to the triangular ligament between the bulbospongiosus and the ischiocavernosus muscles (Fig. 5.17).

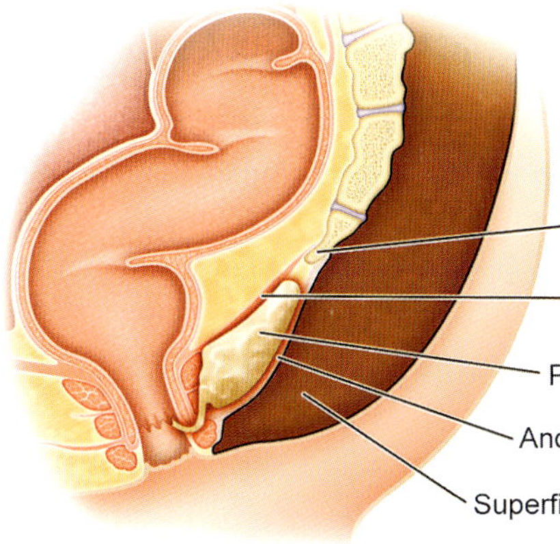

Fig. 5.15: The postanal abscess is inferior to the levator, posterior to the deep part of the external sphincter, and superior to the superficial part of the external sphincter muscle

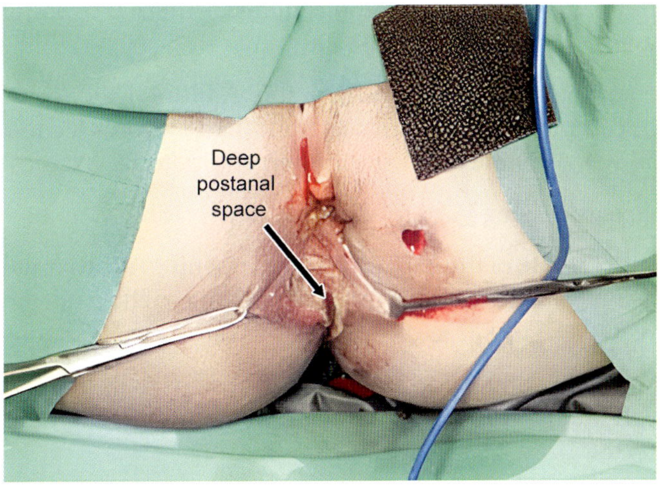

Fig. 5.16: Drainage of the deep post-anal abscess. Extension of posterior fistulotomy to the deep postanal space

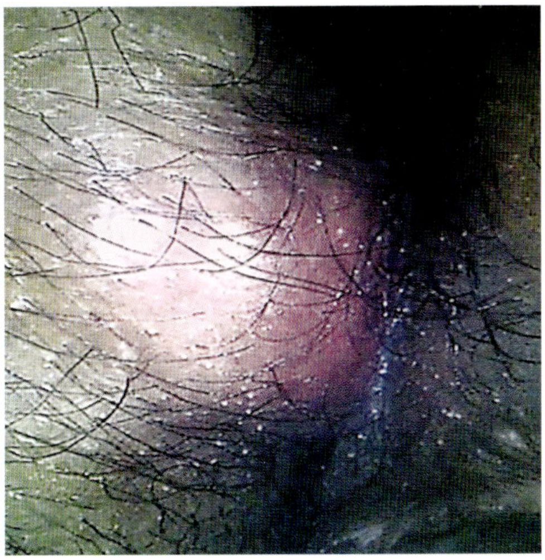

Fig. 5.17: Anterior abscess

MANAGING ANTERIOR ABSCESS WITH A COMMUNICATING FISTULA IN MALES

In males, the deep anterior space abscess is managed by anterior fistulotomy.

Instrumentation: As mentioned in Fig. 5.2A–D.

Type of anaesthesia: Spinal/General

Position of the patient: Lithotomy

Steps of the Procedure

Step 1: In an anterior abscess, the patient is always catheterized to prevent injury to the urethra which lies in close proximity.

Step 2: The abscess is palpated, and the pus is aspirated (Fig. 5.18A). Hydrogen peroxide is injected into the cavity. In an abscess of cryptoglandular origin, bubbles emerge from the internal opening at the dentate line. If no bubbles appear, hydrogen peroxide may be injected through the internal opening (Fig. 5.18B). An increase in the size of the abscess indicates a communicating fistula.

Step 3: A small incision is given at the site of needle aspiration. A blunt artery or a sinus forceps is inserted, and the blades are separated for complete drainage of pus (modified Hilton's technique). The pus can be seen oozing out of the incision (Fig. 5.18C). After the drainage, the necrotic material is removed by thorough curetting.

Step 4: The internal opening is excised using Park's technique (Fig. 5.18D).

Step 5: A probe is inserted through the site of the excised internal opening. A proximal fistulotomy is done over the probe by extending the incision from the excised internal opening to the anal verge (Fig. 5.18E). The distal fistula tract is curetted and irrigated (Fig. 5.18F,G).

Step 6: A counter incision is given on the other side of the scrotal abscess to drain any residual pus (Fig. 5.18H). An eye probe is inserted through the fistulotomy wound and taken out through the scrotum, and a draining seton using silk is placed (Fig. 5.18I, J).

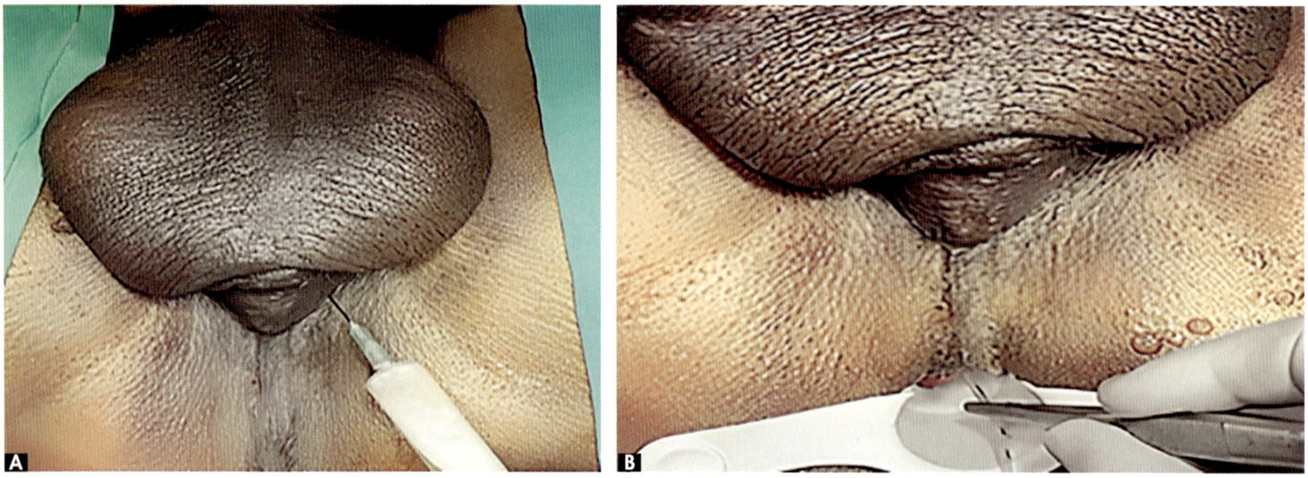

Fig. 5.18(A-B): Management of anterior abscess with communicating fistula in males. A) Pus is aspirated, and hydrogen peroxide is injected into the abscess cavity. B) Hydrogen peroxide injected through the internal opening

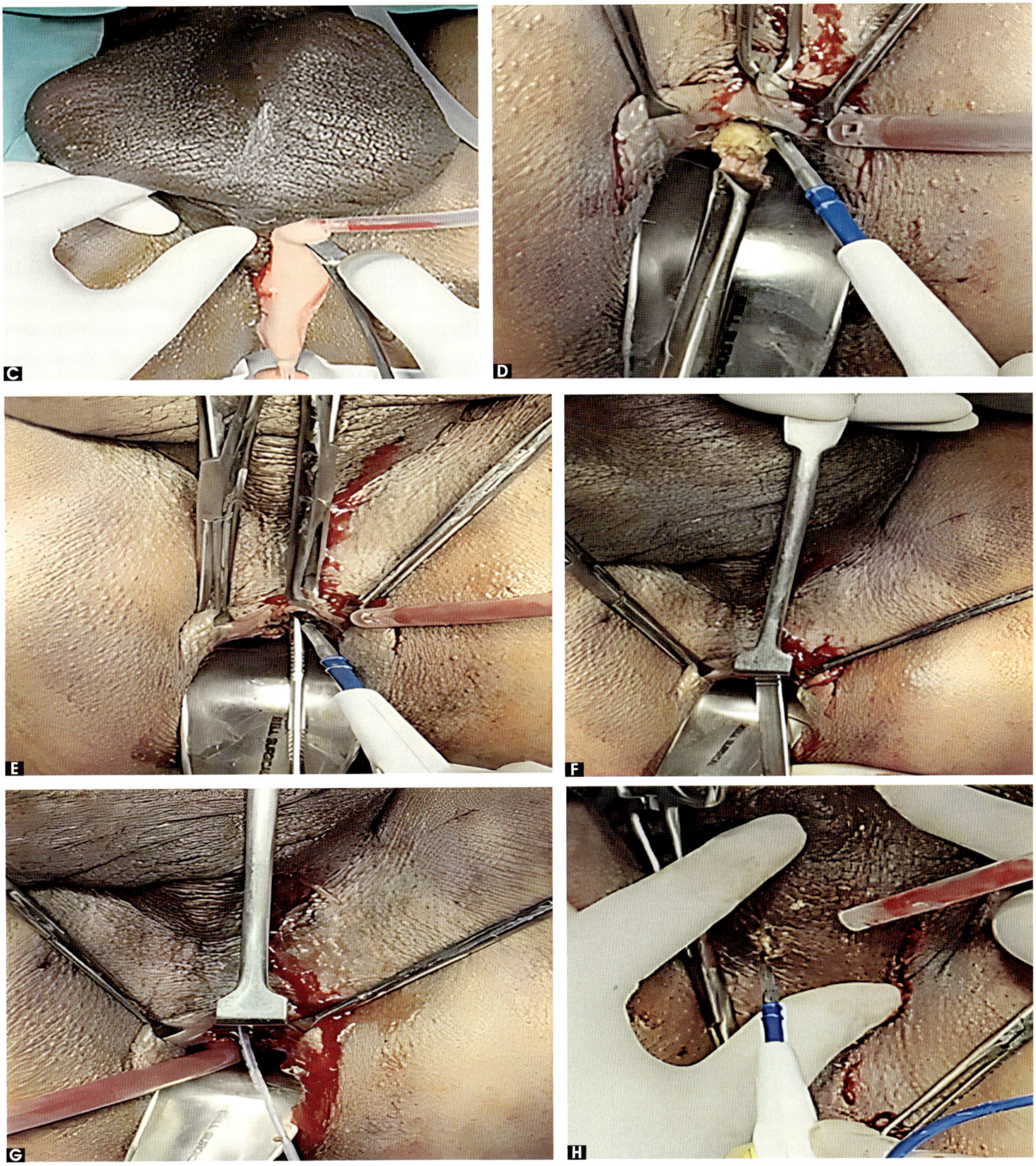

Fig. 5.18(C-H): Management of anterior abscess with communicating fistula in males. C) Incision given over the abscess cavity and pus drained. D) Excision of the internal opening. E) Proximal fistulotomy is done over the probe. F) Curetting of the communicating fistula tract. G) Irrigation of the tract. H) Counter incision made on the other side of the abscess cavity

Step 7: A corrugated drain is placed in the abscess cavity for drainage, which is removed after 72 hours (Fig. 5.18K). The margins of the proximal fistulotomy wound are marsupialized (Fig. 5.18L).

Step 8: Local infiltration of 0.5% bupivacaine and pudendal nerve block is given to reduce postoperative pain (Fig. 5.18M, N, O).

The final wound at the end of the procedure is shown in Fig. 5.18P.

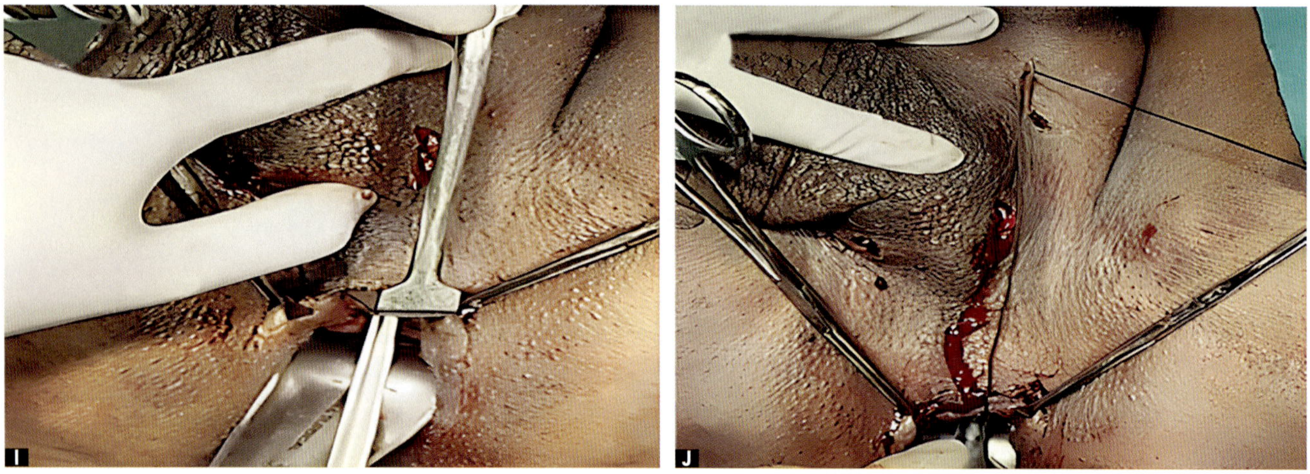

Fig. 5.18(I-J): Management of anterior abscess with communicating fistula in males. I) Probe inserted from the internal opening into the fistula tract. J) Placement of seton

Scan QR Code for Video on
Management of Anterior Abscess in Males
VIDEO 21

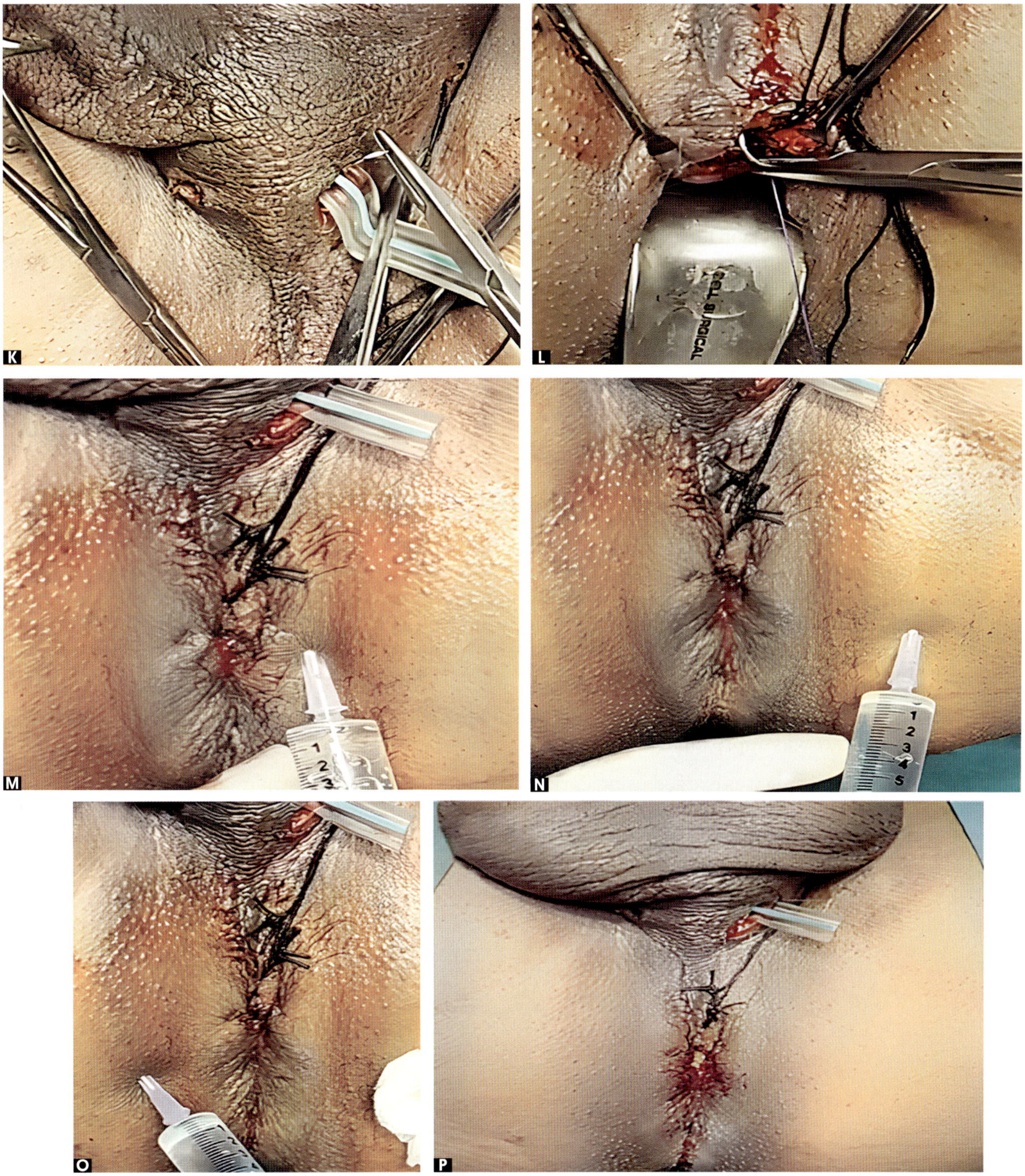

Fig. 5.18(K-P): Management of anterior abscess with communicating fistula in males.K) Placement of corrugated drain. L) Marsupialization. M) Local infiltration. N) Pudendal nerve block at 3 o'clock. O) Pudendal nerve block at 9 o'clock. P) Final postoperative image

Anterior Abscess in Females

While operating for an anterior abscess in females, the crucial step is to prevent injury to the perineal body. Drainage of an abscess with seton placement in the intersphincteric space is recommended. The seton can be tightened every three to four weeks. However, after an anterior abscess is drained and the fistula tract matures, a fistulotomy can be carried out with primary sphincter repair.

Alternatively, drainage of the abscess with proximal fistulotomy can also be done.

Case Discussion—Managing Anterior Abscess with A Communicating Fistula in Females

A female patient was operated on for anterior abscess drainage by a colleague. The patient had a communicating anterior curvilinear fistula tract which was not dealt with. Subsequently, the drained abscess cavity did not heal, becoming a chronic non-healing wound (Fig. 5.19).

An MRI imaging is a must before taking such cases for surgery.

Instrumentation: As mentioned in Fig. 5.2A, B

Type of anaesthesia: Spinal anaesthesia/General

Position of the patient: Lithotomy

Steps of the Procedure

Below is a generalized protocol that should be followed in all such cases.

Step 1: The first and crucial step is establishing communication between the non-healing wound and the anal canal. Hydrogen peroxide is injected through the open wound to visualize the bubbles in the anal canal. If no bubbles are seen, inject the hydrogen peroxide through the internal opening with a 6F infant feeding tube. In this case, the internal opening was present anteriorly at 12 o'clock. Once hydrogen peroxide was injected through the internal opening, the bubbles could be seen in the open wound, indicating a communicating anterior fistula (Fig. 5.19A).

Step 2: Methylene blue was injected through the internal opening, and the tract was demarcated (Fig. 5.19B). The length of the tract was approximately 3 cm.

Step 3: The internal opening was excised using Park's technique (Fig. 5.19C). The margins of the chronic wound were refreshed, and the base was thoroughly curetted to convert a chronic wound into an acute one (Fig. 5.19D). A probe was inserted through the open wound up to the excised internal opening, and fistulotomy was done over the probe (Fig. 5.19E, F).

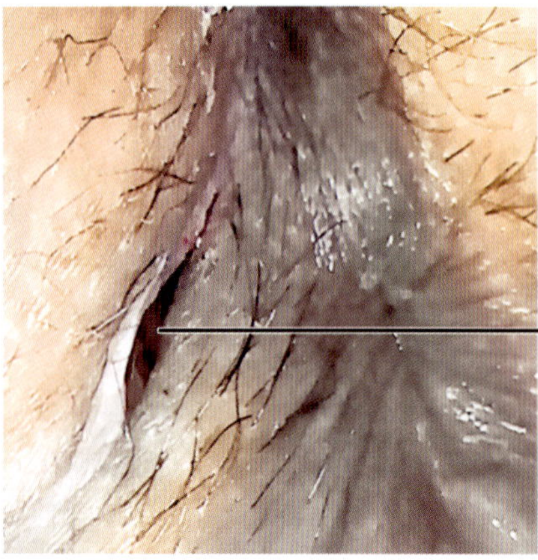

Fig. 5.19: Chronic wound formation after drainage of an anterior abscess in a female

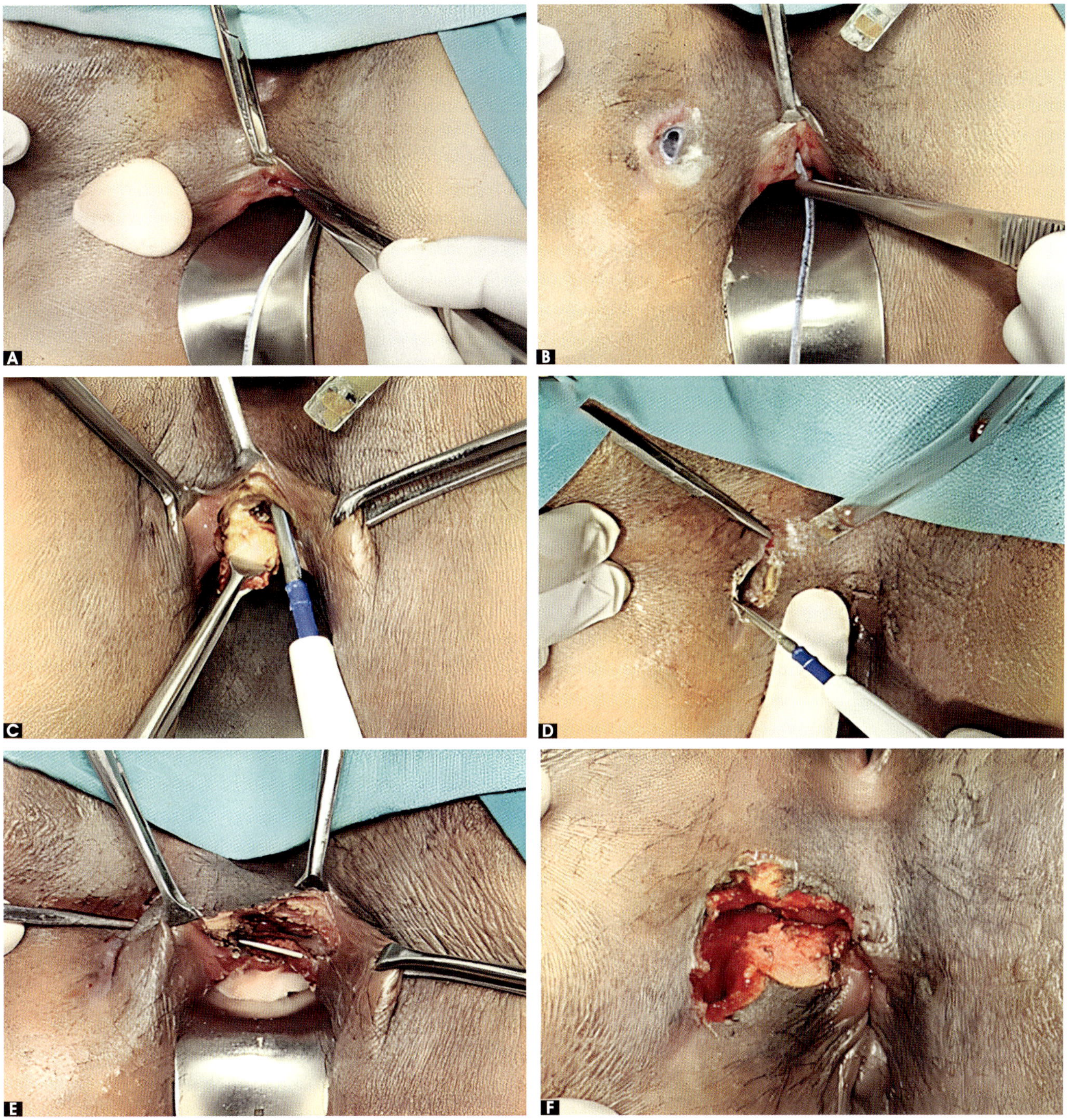

Fig. 5.19(A-F): Managing anterior abscess with a communicating fistula in females. A) Injecting hydrogen peroxide through the internal opening. Bubbles are seen at the open wound, indicating a communicating fistula. B) Methylene blue injected through the internal opening to demarcate the fistula tract. C) Excision of internal opening by Park's technique. D) Refresing the margins of the chronic wound. E) Insertion of the curved probe from the open wound to the excised internal opening. F) Fistulotomy is done over the probe

Methylene blue stained unhealthy granulation tissue could be seen in the open tract. Thorough curetting and wound irrigation was done to remove the unhealthy granulation tissue (Fig. 5.19G).

Step 4: To prevent anal incontinence, a primary sphincter repair was performed using a 2-0 PDS suture (Fig. 5.19H, I).

Step 5: The wound was irrigated (Fig. 5.19J). Local infiltration of bupivacaine was done, followed by a pudendal nerve block (Fig. 5.19K, L, M).

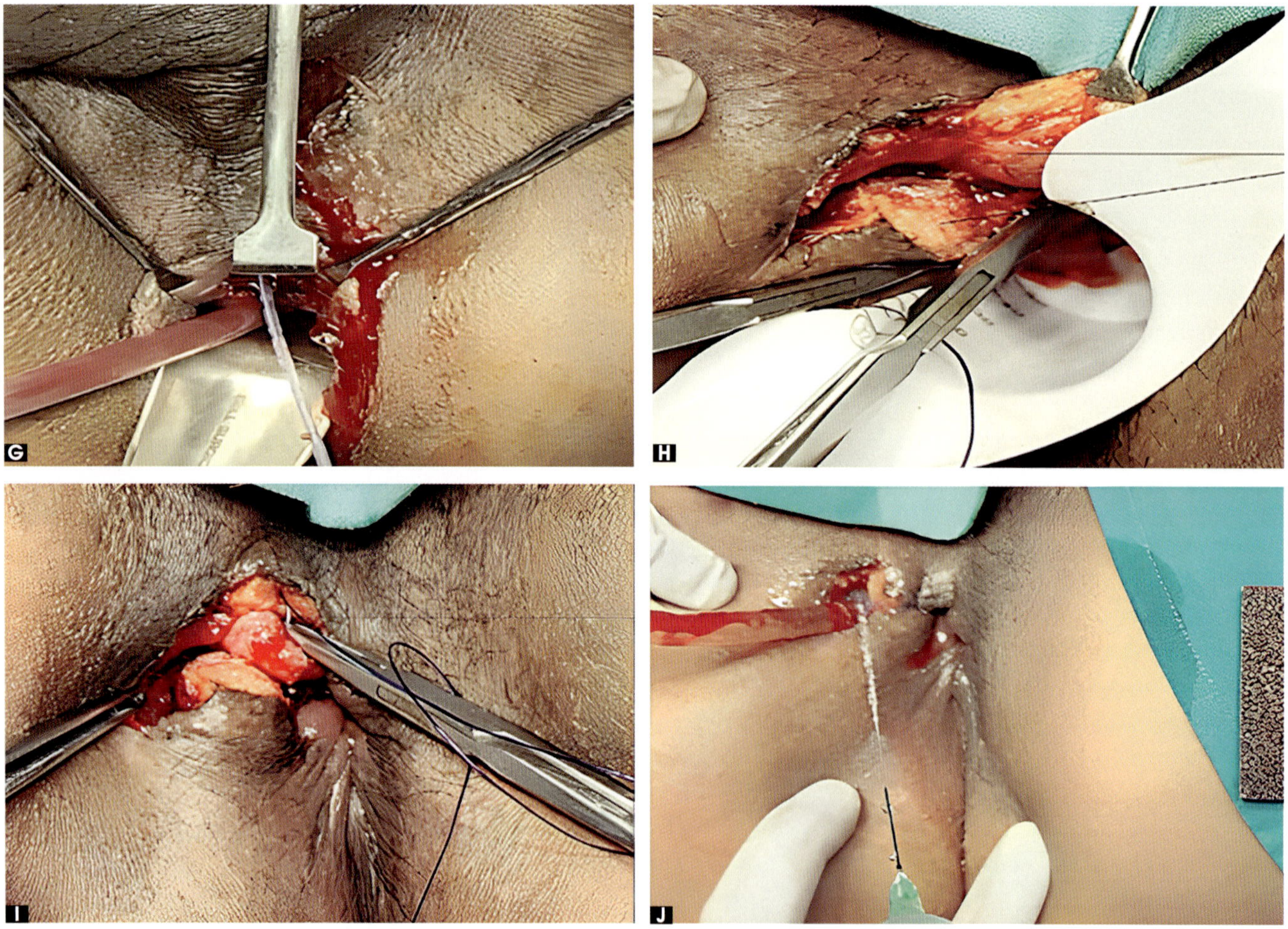

Fig. 5.19(G-H): Managing anterior abscess with a communicating fistula in females. G) Curetting of the fistula tract and the open wound. H) Per-operative image showing the margins of the incised external anal sphincter. I) Primary sphincter repair is done using 2-0 PDS. J) Irrigation of the wound. K) Local infiltration of bupivacaine

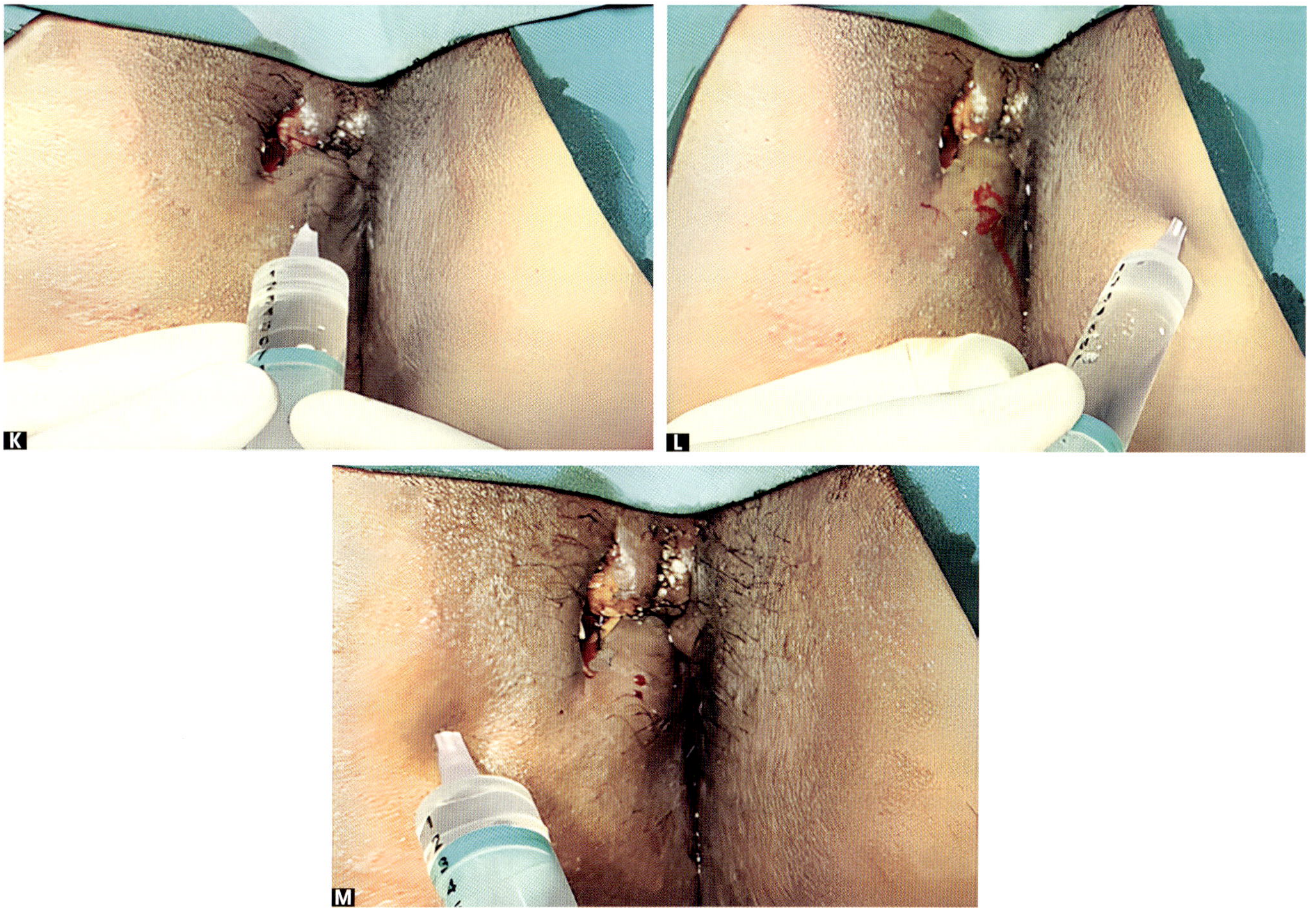

Fig. 5.19(I-M): Managing anterior abscess with a communicating fistula in females. L) Pudendal nerve block at 3 O'clock. M) Pudendal nerve block at 9 o'clock

Tips and Tricks

- Inadequate drainage may lead to fistula formation.
- An anterior abscess in females should be drained with care because of the presence of the perineal body.

Learning Points

Contraindications for primary fistulotomy in an abscess associated with a communicating fistula

- A primary fistulotomy is not recommended for those with Crohn's disease or in immunocompromised patients.
- Primary fistulotomy should be avoided in a trans-sphincteric fistula where the anatomy of the sphincters is ill defined due to sepsis.
- If more than 50% of the external sphincter is involved laterally or posteriorly, or 30% of the external sphincter is involved anteriorly, fistulotomy is not advisable. In such situations, a draining seton is the best option.
- One should avoid anterior fistulotomy in females as the perineal body is weak. The length of the external sphincter anteriorly in females is half compared to males.

SUPERFICIAL POSTANAL SPACE ABSCESS

The abscess is managed in the same way as a perianal abscess.

HORSESHOE ABSCESS

When one branch of a horseshoe abscess spontaneously bursts into the skin, an incomplete or a semi-horseshoe fistula develops. In contrast, the bursting of both the branches leads to a complete horseshoe fistula.

A horseshoe abscess can be anterior or posterior and extends below the anorectal ring.

The posterior horseshoe "abscess originates in the postanal space in the midline crypt" (Fig. 5.20). Since both ischiorectal spaces communicate with the postanal space," the pus extends through both the ischiorectal spaces. The pus may extend anteriorly to encircle the lower anorectal area. It may form a fistula tract with secondary openings in the labia, scrotum, and thigh (Fig. 5.21). Posteriorly, the abscess can extend towards the sacrotuberous ligament and gluteus maximus.

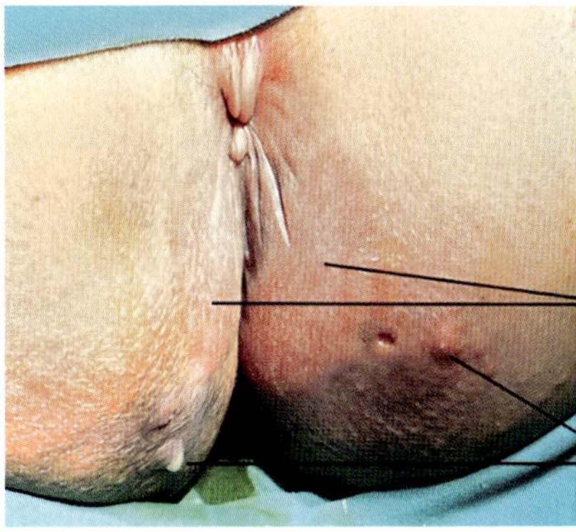

Fig. 5.20: Horseshoe abscess

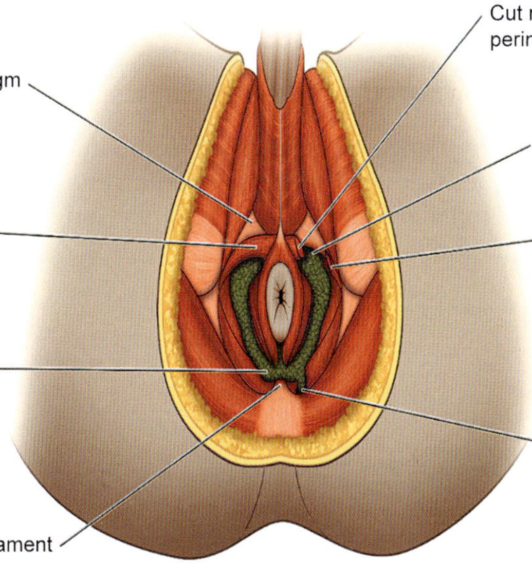

Fig. 5.21: Extension of horseshoe abscess anteriorly and posteriorly

MANAGING HORSESHOE ABSCESS AND THE OPENING OF THE DEEP POSTANAL SPACE

Instrumentation: As mentioned in Fig. 5.2A, B

Position of the patient: Lithotomy position/Jack-knife

Type of anaesthesia: Spinal anaesthesia/General

Steps of the Procedure

Step 1: A needle is inserted into the abscess cavity, and pus is aspirated. To assess whether the abscess cavity is associated with a communicating fistula tract, hydrogen peroxide is injected through both sides of the horseshoe abscess to visualize the bubbles in the anal canal and the communicating horseshoe tract. Methylene blue is injected to demarcate the tracts and the internal opening (Fig. 5.22A–D). In the presence of multiple abscesses or associated tracts, hydrogen peroxide and methylene blue should be injected through all the tracts for demarcation.

Step 2: The horseshoe abscess is drained on both the sides by giving a stab incision (Fig. 5.22E).

Step 3: The internal opening is excised by Park's technique. Once the internal opening is excised, the deep intersphincteric space is opened, which lies below the internal opening and is the central nidus of infection. A low-end posterior fistulotomy is carried out at 6 o'clock (Fig. 5.22F). Thorough curetting and wound irrigation is done to remove the unhealthy granulation tissue.

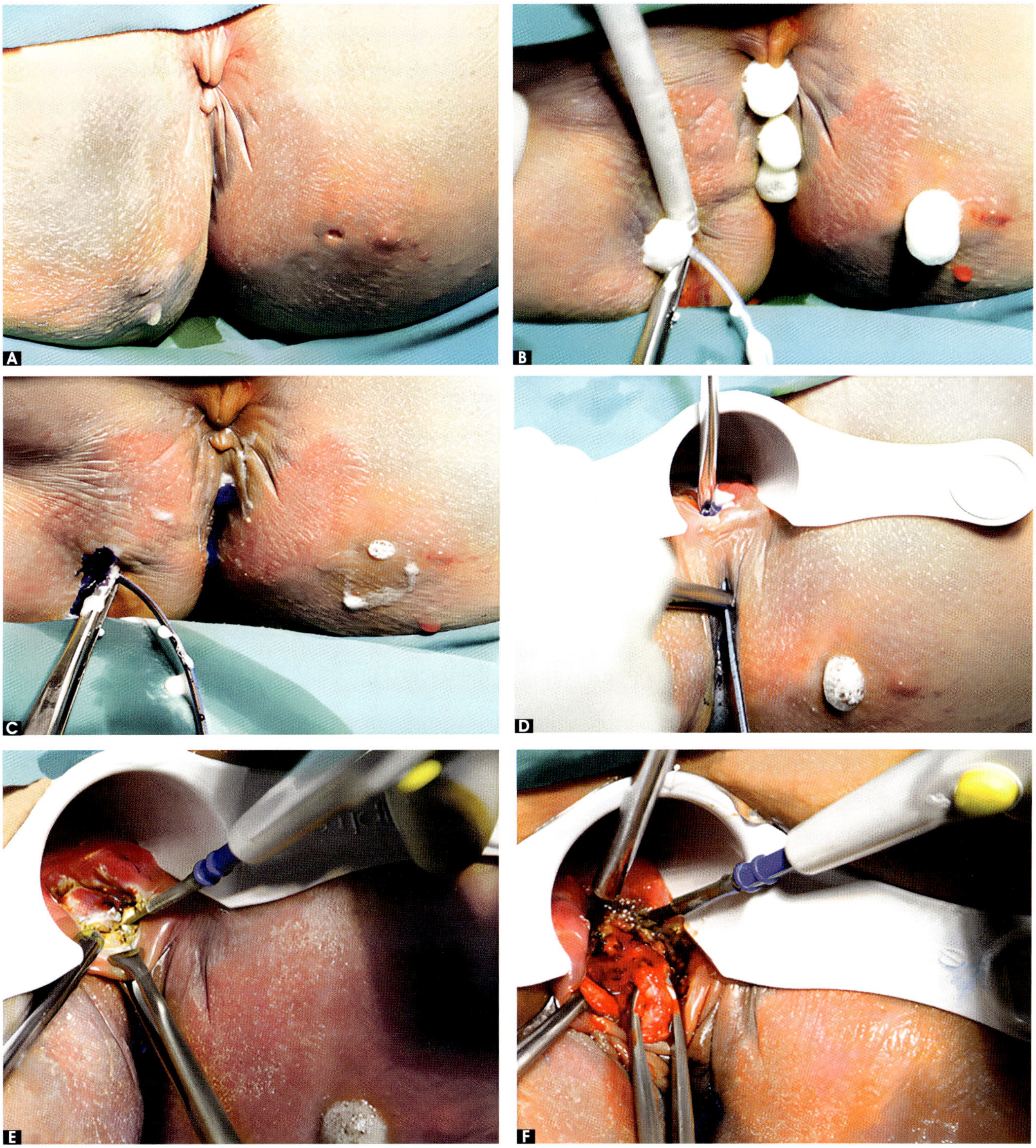

Fig. 5.22A–F: Drainage of Horseshoe abscess with communicating fistula tracts. A) Presence of horseshoe abscess at 5 and 7 o'clock. B, C, D) After aspirating pus, injecting hydrogen peroxide and methylene blue through the abscesses and the external opening at 6 o'clock. The bubbles of hydrogen peroxide and methylene blue are seen coming out through all the intercommunicating tracts and the internal opening. E) Demarcation of the internal opening to be excised. F) Excision of the internal opening using Park's technique

Step 4: The posterior fistulotomy wound is extended midway between the anal verge and the coccyx, and the deep postanal space is opened to separate the horseshoe tract (Hanley's procedure). The space is curetted and irrigated (Fig. 5.22G, H, I).

Step 5: One can place draining setons or opt for coring of the tracts (Fig. 5. 22 J, K, L, M).

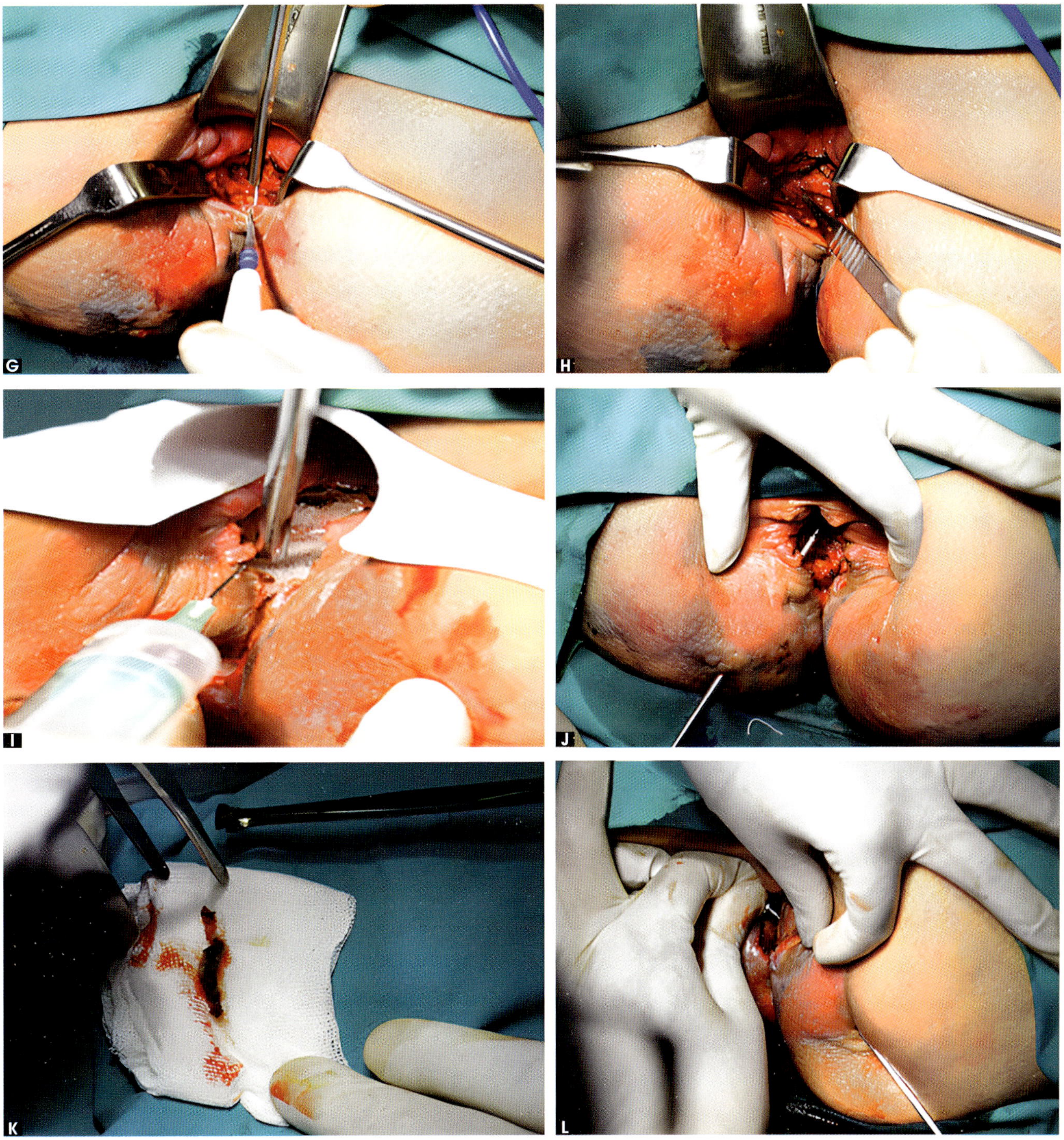

Fig. 5.22G–L: Drainage of Horseshoe abscess with communicating fistula tracts. G) Extending the posterior fistulotomy wound posteriorly to open the deep postanal space (Hanley's procedure). H, I). Curetting and irrigation of the postanal space. J, K, L) Coring of both the limbs of fistula tracts using FiXcision

A fixcision instrument is inserted through one of the tracts and brought out of the deep postanal space. The tract is cored out, and the inside tunnel created after coring is closed using 2-0 vicryl (5.22 N). The same procedure is repeated on the other side.

Step 6: Fistulotomy wound is marsupiliazed (Fig. 5.22O).

Step 7: To reduce postoperative pain, local infiltration and pudendal nerve block using bupivacaine 0.5% are given at the end of the procedure. The final wound picture is shown in Fig. 5.22 P.

The completely healed wound is shown in Fig. 5.22Q.

Learning Point

- A chronic horseshoe abscess can often resurface as an acute abscess with the development of a new tract. Hence the deep postanal space must be explored.

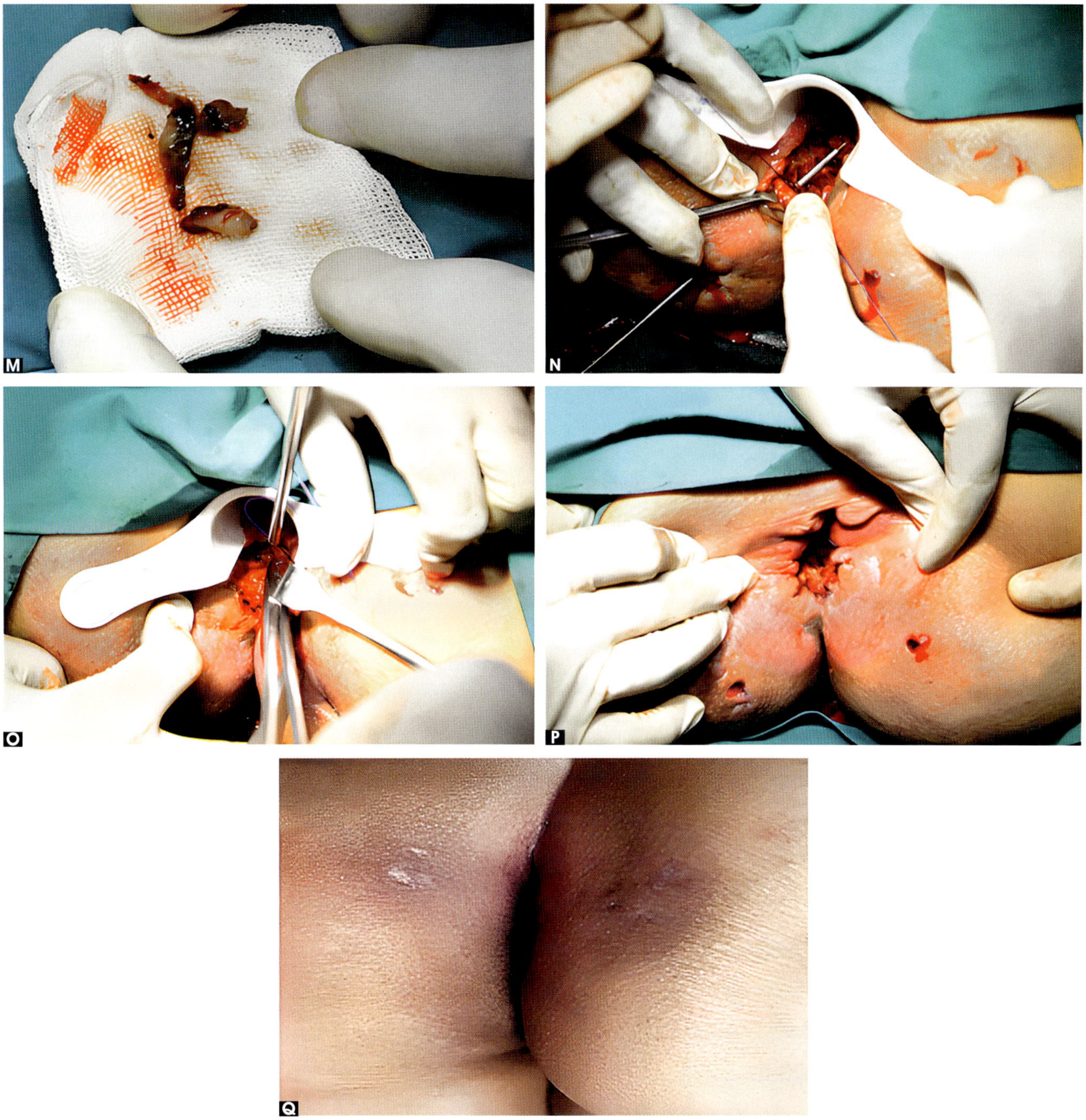

Fig. 5.22M–Q: Drainage of Horseshoe abscess with communicating fistula tracts. M) Coring of both the limbs of fistula tracts using Fixcision. N). Closure of the tunnel after FiXcision. O) Marsupialization of the fistulotomy margins. P) Final picture after surgery. Q) Complete healing of wound in three months

MANAGING HORSESHOE INTERSPHINCTERIC ABSCESS WITH SUPRALEVATOR EXTENSION

The horseshoe abscess is named after its characteristic U-shaped collection that extends semi-circumferentially around the internal anal sphincter in the intersphincteric space. MRI remains one of the confirmatory diagnostic tool in such cases (Fig. 5.23).

Instrumentation: As mentioned in Fig. 5.2A, B

Position of the patient: Lithotomy/Jack-knife

Type of anaesthesia: Spinal/General

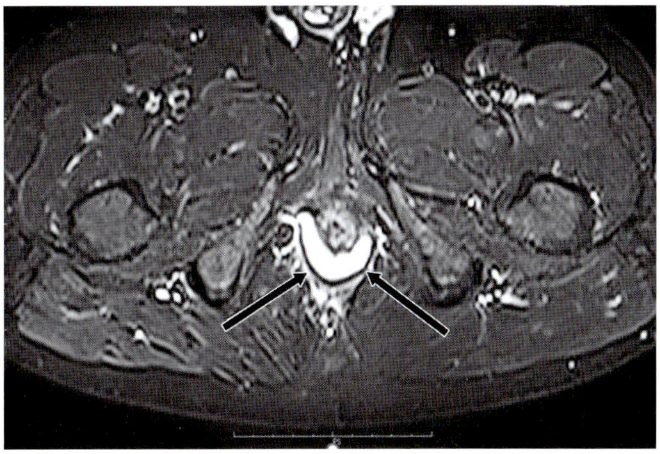

Fig. 5.23: STIR Axial image of Horseshoe shaped intersphincteric abscess marked with arrows (Image *Courtesy:* Dr Dhawal Kaushal, Radiologist)

Steps of the Procedure

Step 1: A half-cut proctoscope is inserted in the anal canal, and a bulge is seen in the intersphincteric space above the dentate line (Fig. 5.24A). The internal opening is identified, which is felt as an induration at the dentate line (Fig. 5.24B).

Step 2: The internal opening is excised by Park's technique, and the intersphincteric and deep intersphincteric space is opened (Fig. 5.24C). Pus can be seen oozing out of the intersphincteric abscess (Fig. 5.24D).

Step 3: The intersphincteric space towards 4 o'clock is opened, followed by the opening of intersphincteric space towards 8 o'clock (Fig. 5.24 E). The intersphincteric space is opened upto the anorectal ring on both sides. While operating, one should always palpate the anorectal ring (Fig. 5.24F). The opened intersphincteric space is curetted and irrigated (Fig. 5.24G).

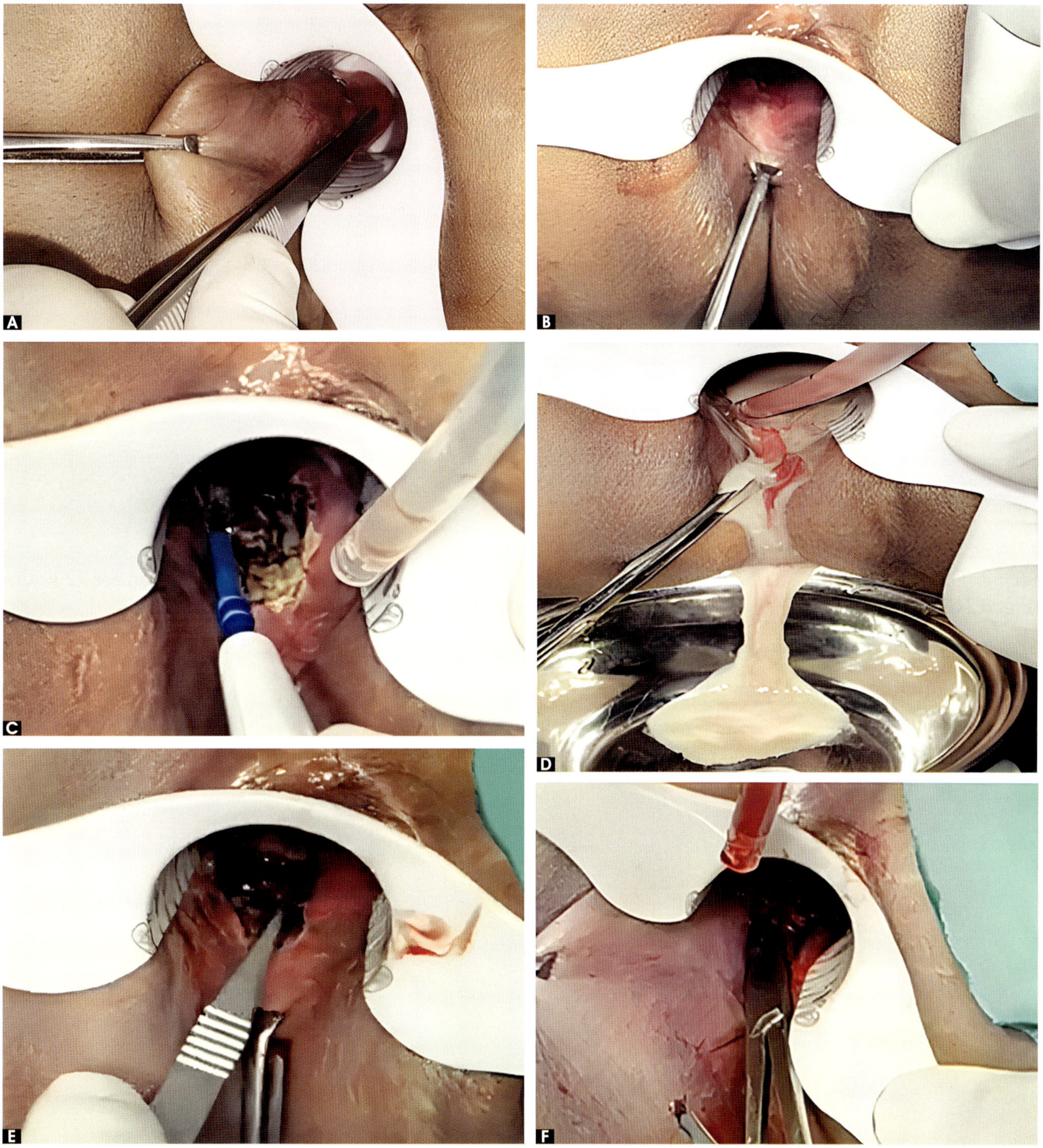

Fig. 5.24(A-F): Managing horseshoe intersphincteric abscess with supralevator extension. A) Insertion of half-cut proctoscope in the anal canal, and a bulge is seen in the intersphincteric space above the dentate line. B) Identification of the internal opening which is felt as induration at the dentate line. C) Excision of the internal opening by Park's technique. D) Opening of the intersphincteric and deep intersphincteric space and pus oozing out of the intersphincteric abscess. E) Opening of the intersphincteric space towards 4 o'clock, followed by the opening of intersphincteric space towards 8 o'clock. F) Palpation of the anorectal ring

Step 4: The supralevator extension is curetted and irrigated, and a drain is placed for irrigation for 72 hours (Fig. 5.24H, I).

Step 5: Posterior fistulotomy is done at 6 o'clock to drain the collection, if any (Fig. 5. 24J).

Step 6: Fistulotomy wound is marsupiliazed (Fig. 5.24K).

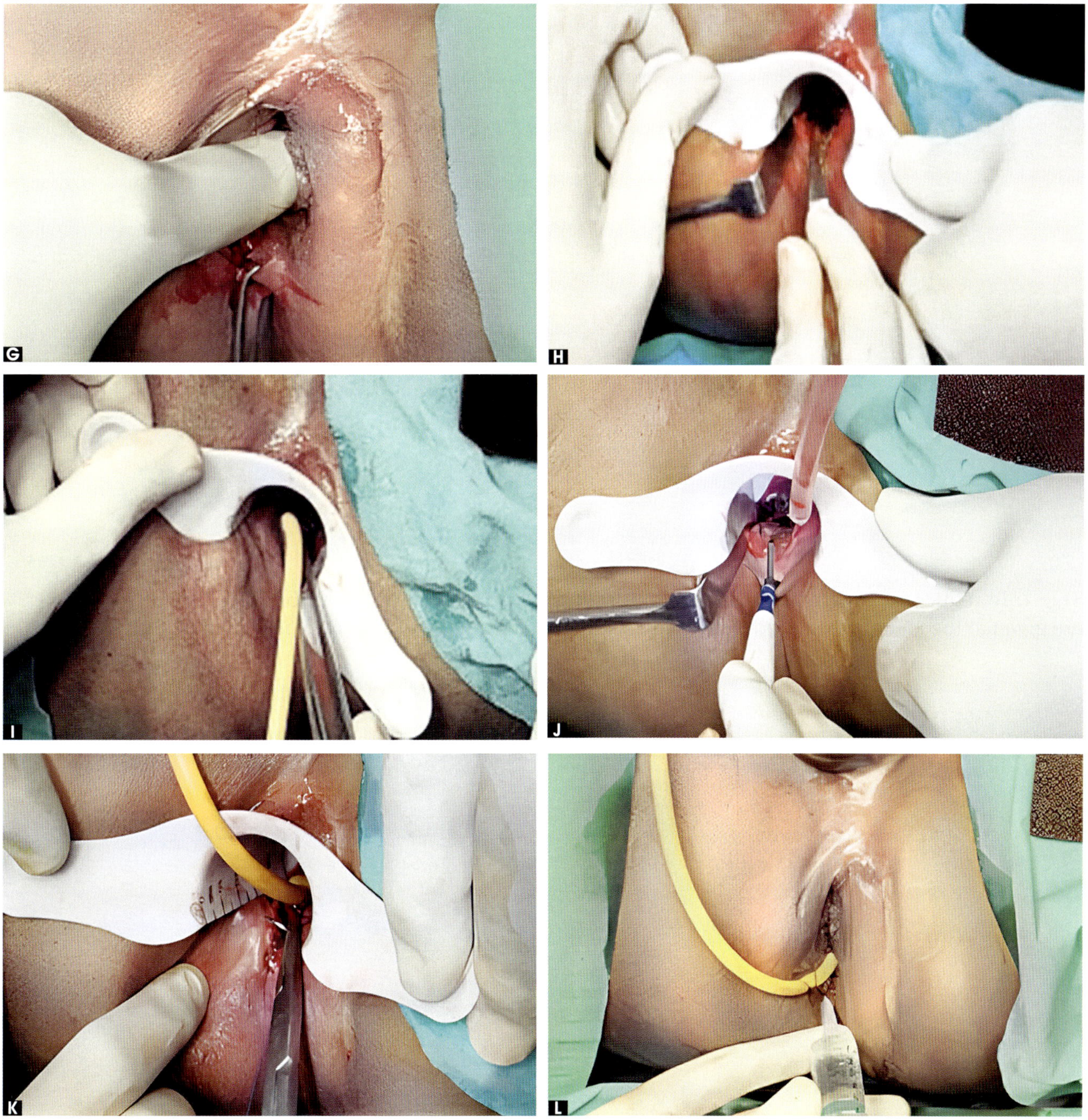

Fig. 5.24(G-L): Managing horseshoe intersphincteric abscess with supralevator extension. G) Curretting and irrigation of the intersphincteric space. H, I) Curretting and irrigating the supralevator extension and placement of the drain for irrigation for 72 hours. J) Posterior fistulotomy is done at 6 o'clock to drain the collection. K) Marsupiliazation of fistulotomy wound. L) Local infiltration and pudendal nerve block

Step 7: To reduce postoperative pain, the local infiltration and pudendal nerve block using bupivacaine 0.5% are given at the end of the procedure (Fig. 5.24L, M, N). The final wound image is shown in Fig. 5.24O.

Scan QR Code for Video on

Intersphincteric Horseshoe Abscess with Supralevator Extension

VIDEO 22

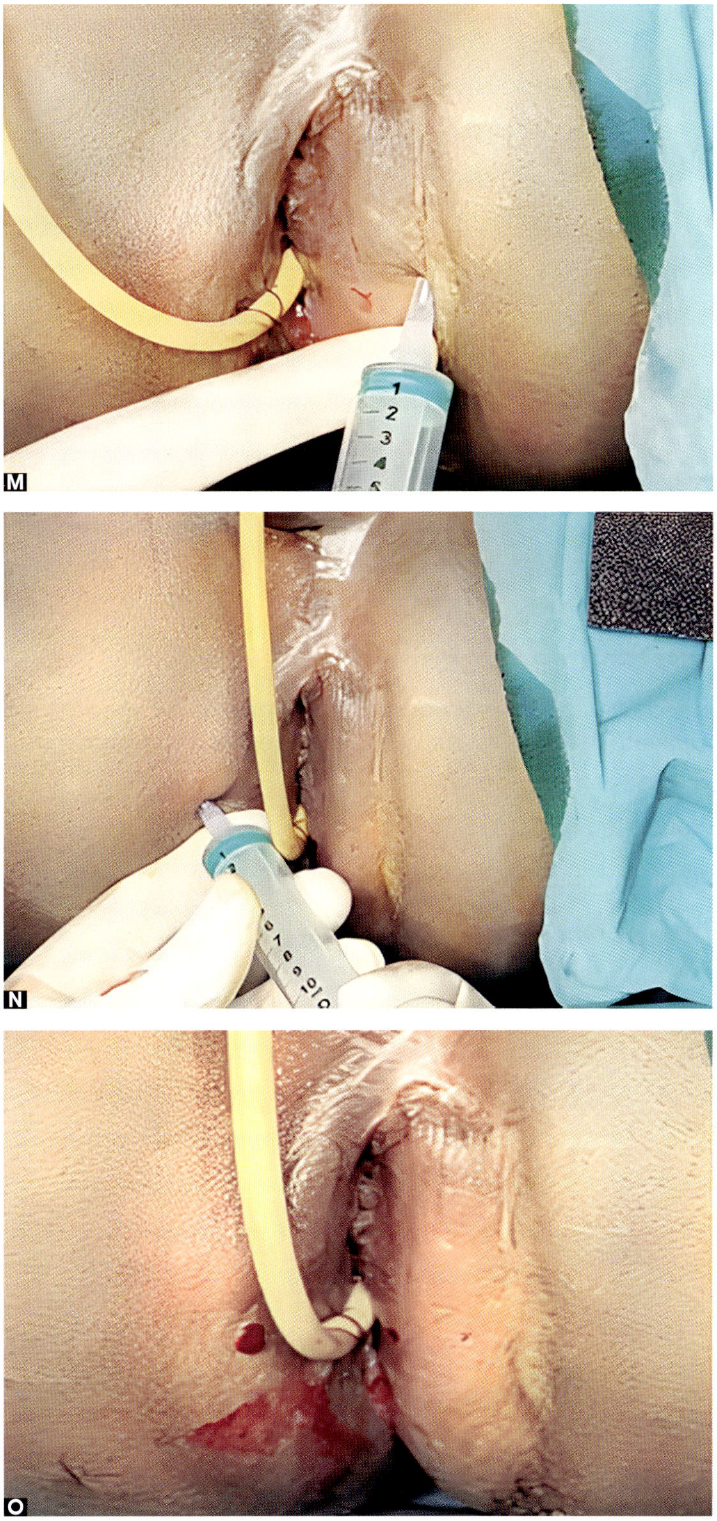

Fig. 5.24(M-O): Managing horseshoe intersphincteric abscess with supralevator extension. M) Local infiltration and pudendal nerve block. O) Final wound picture

MANAGING HORSESHOE SUPRALEVATOR ABSCESS

The abscess from the ischiorectal space can extend upto the supralevator space. A posterior spread can lead to a posterior horseshoe supralevator abscess. Usually, there is present a communicating trans-sphincteric fistula (Fig. 5.25A, B).

Instrumentation: As mentioned in Fig. 5.2A, B

Position of the patient: Lithotomy/Jack-knife

Type of anaesthesia: Spinal/General

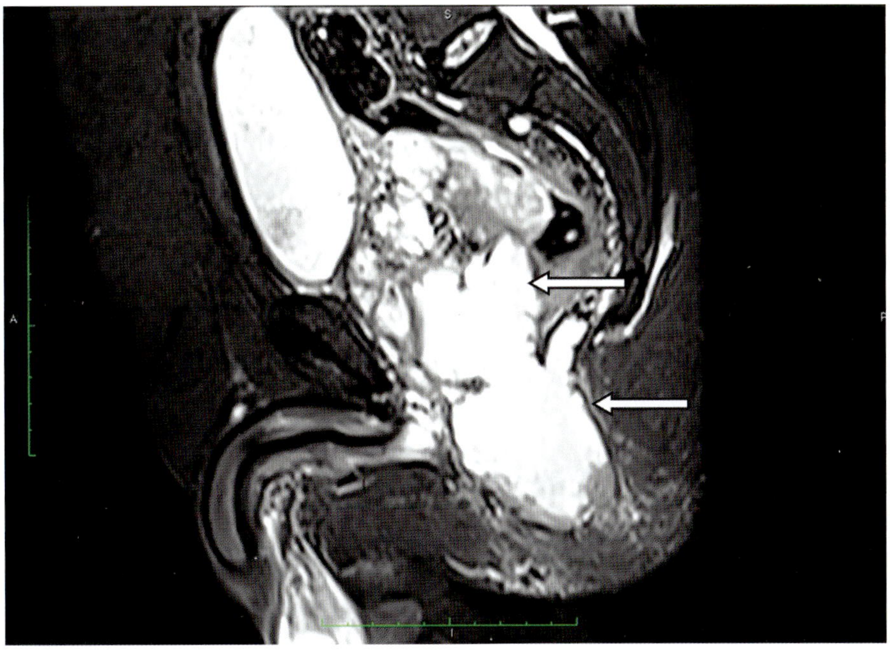

Fig. 5.25A: MRI images of horseshoe suprasphincteric abscess. A) Sagittal MRI image showing ischioanal abscess extending across the levator ani muscle to reach supralevator space

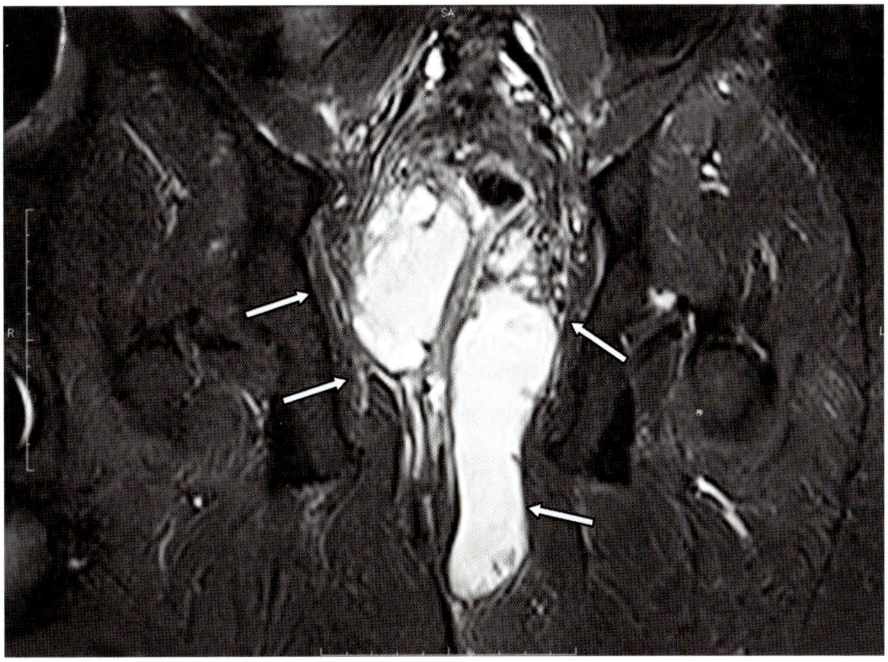

Fig. 5.25B: Coronal MRI image showing left ischioanal abscess extending across the levator ani muscle to reach the right supralevator space to cross the midline. (*Images courtesy:* Dr Dhawal Kaushal, Radiologist)

Case Presentation

A 51-year-old gentleman presented with the complaints of painful swelling in the gluteal region and fever for the last 10 days. He was treated on antibiotics by a local physician, but the pain increased. On examination an abscess could be palpated in the left ischiorectal region. The MRI revealed a large ischiorectal collection with horseshoe supralevator extension, with internal opening at 6 o'clock and a communicating trans-sphincteric fistula (Fig. 25A, B).

The extent of external anal sphincter involved and the extension of horseshoe abscess in the supralevator space were two major concerns at the time of surgery. The procedure planned was drainage of ischiorectal and supralevator abscesses with placement of drain in the supralevator space with primary fistulotomy for trans-sphincteric fistula.

Steps of the Procedure

Step 1: A 21G needle on a syringe was inserted into the ischiorectal abscess through the most medial part of the abscess cavity, as close to the anal verge as possible (Fig. 5.26A). The pus was aspirated, and the hydrogen peroxide was injected into the abscess cavity (Fig. 5.26B). In this case, the internal opening was palpated on DRE, and bubbles could not be seen emerging (Fig. 5.26C). An attempt to inject hydrogen peroxide through the internal opening failed.

Step 2: A small nick was given on the most medial aspect of the abscess using 11 number blade at the pus aspiration site (Fig. 5.26D). A blunt artery forceps was inserted into the abscess cavity, and the pus was drained by modified Hilton's method (Fig. 5.26E). A finger was inserted and seen going upwards towards the levators (Fig. 5.26F).

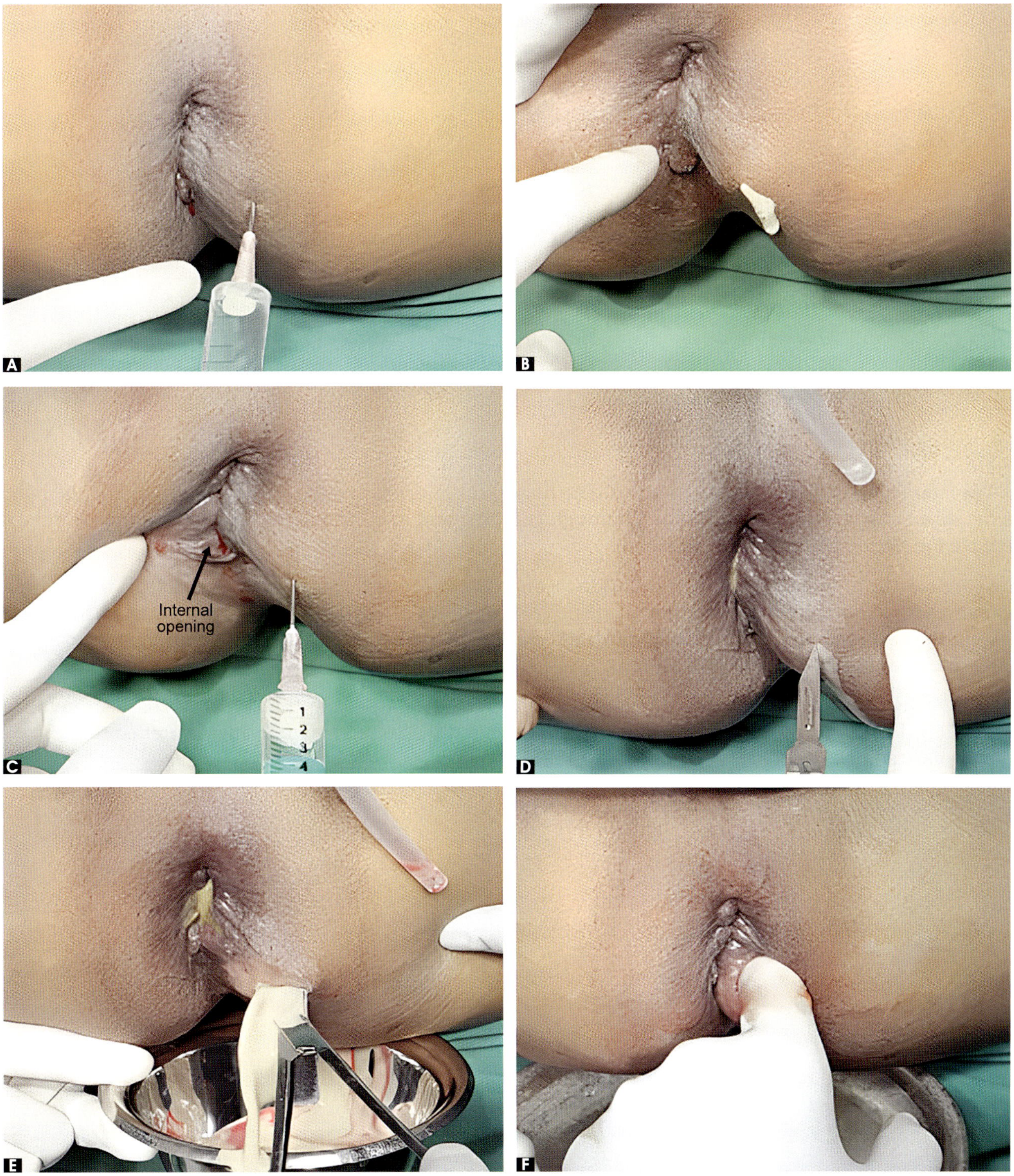

Fig. 5.26A-F: Managing horseshoe supralevator abscess with trans-sphincteric fistula. A) Aspiration of pus from the medial part of the abscess cavity. B) Injecting hydrogen peroxide into the abscess cavity. C) Bubbles could not be seen emerging. D) Drainage of the ischiorectal abscess. E) Insertion of a blunt artery into the abscess cavity. F) A finger is inserted upwards towards the levators

The lateral part of EAS could be palpated. The finger was inserted into the anal canal to look for any bulge in the supralevator space on both sides. Thorough curetting and irrigation of the abscess cavity were done to remove the necrotic material (Fig. 5.26G).

Step 3: An attempt to inject hydrogen peroxide through the internal opening failed (Fig. 5.26H). The internal opening was excised by Park's technique (Fig. 5.26I). A blunt artery forceps was passed from the site of ischiorectal abscess drainage medially towards the excised internal opening. The forceps tip could be palpated at the site of excision of the internal opening.

Step 4: A primary fistulotomy was done over the forceps after assessing the extent of the EAS involved (Fig. 5.26J). The unhealthy granulation tissue at the base of the fistulotomy wound was curetted (Fig. 5.26K). The primary sphincteric repair was done using PDS 2-0 (Fig. 5.26L).

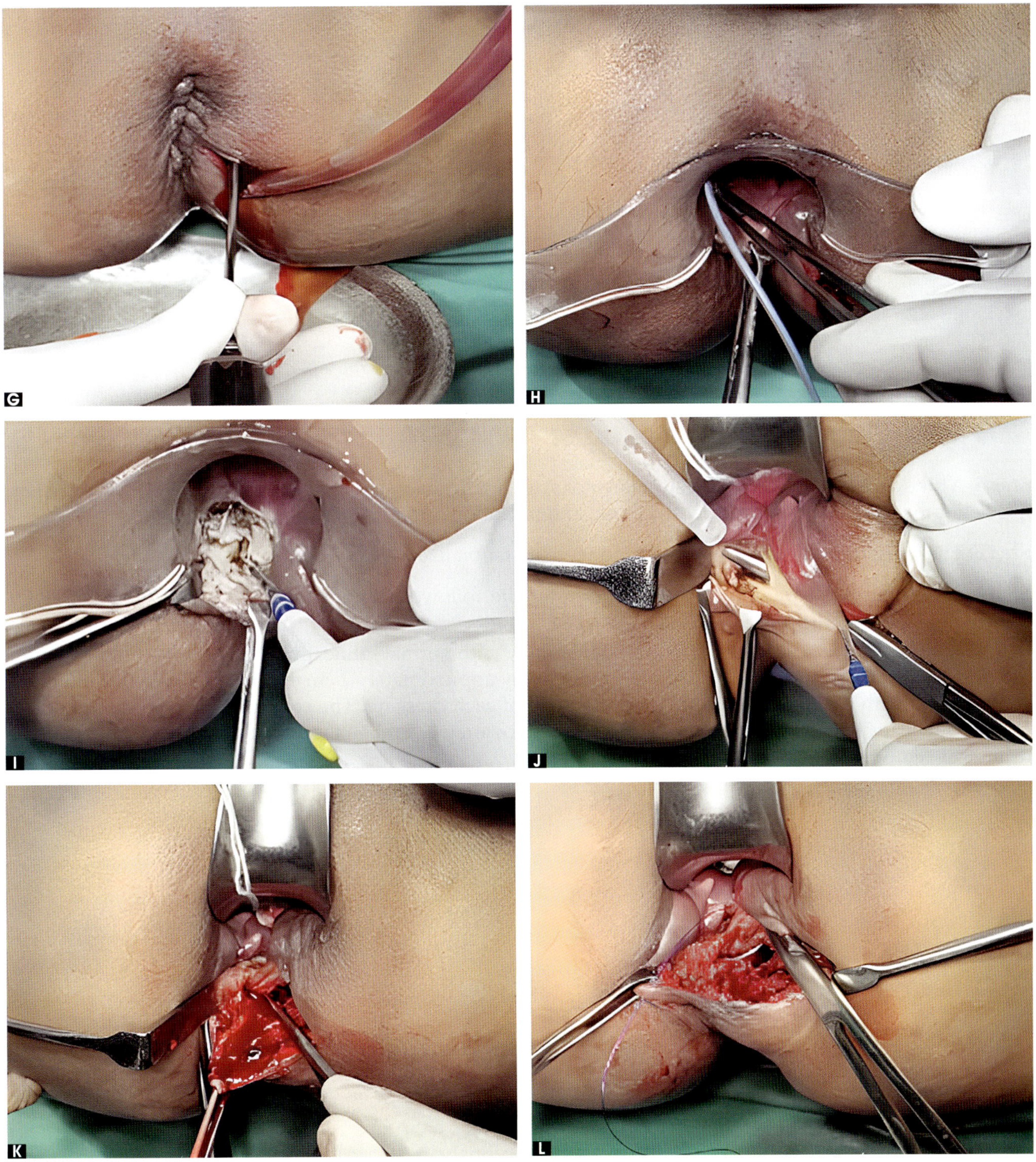

Fig. 5.26G-L: Managing horseshoe supralevator abscess with trans-sphincteric fistula. G) Curetting and irrigation of the abscess cavity. H) Injecting hydrogen peroxide through the internal opening. I) Excision of the internal opening. J) Primary fistulotomy done. K) Curetting of unhealthy granulation tissue. L) The primary sphincteric repair is done using PDS 2-0

Step 5: A tube drain was placed in the supralevator space for drainage and irrigation (Fig. 5.26M). In such cases, it is better to leave the drain for at least a week, and irrigation can be done daily.

Step 6: The margins of the fistulotomy wound were marsupialized (Fig. 5.26N).

Step 7: Bupivacaine 0.5% was infiltrated at the operated site, followed by pudendal nerve block (Fig. 5.26O, P, Q). The final image after the procedure is shown in Fig. 5.26R.

Postoperatively, the abscess cavity was irrigated daily with normal saline, through the tube drain. From the 3rd day onwards, the drain was pulled out gradually by approximately 2 cm every day. The collection in the bag attached with the drain was recorded at the time of each dressing. The collection dropped substantially from about 40 to 50 ml on 1st postoperative day to approximately 5 ml on the 7th postoperative day, when the drain was removed.

Scan QR Code for Video on
Managing Horseshoe Supralevator Abscess with Trans-Sphincteric Fistula
VIDEO 23

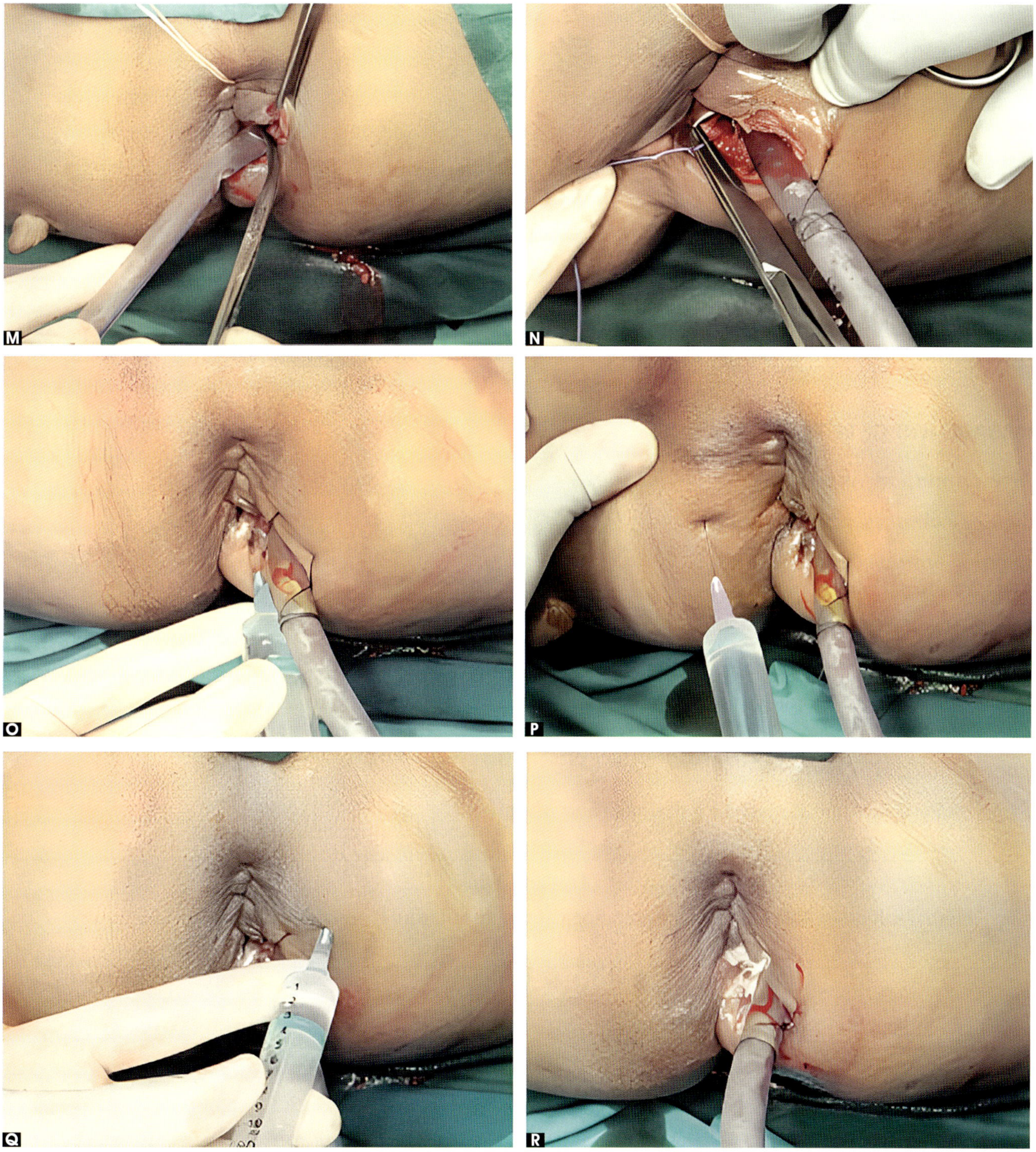

Fig. 5.26M-R: Managing horseshoe supralevator abscess with trans-sphincteric fistula. M) Placement of tube drain in the supralevator space. N) Marsupialization of the fistulotomy margins. O, P, Q) Local infiltration of bupivacaine and pudendal nerve block. R) Final image after the procedure

RETRORECTAL ABSCESS

If a high intramuscular abscess is left unattended, it may rupture the longitudinal muscle above the level of puborectalis and form a retrorectal abscess.

MANAGEMENT OF RETRORECTAL ABSCESS

Instrumentation: As mentioned in Fig. 5.2A-D.

Type of anaesthesia: Spinal/General

Position of the patient: Lithotomy

Steps of the Procedure

Step 1: A probe is passed from the internal opening into the retrorectal abscess (Fig. 5.27A, B).

Step 2: Internal sphincterotomy is done over the probe to prevent fistula formation.

Step 3: The abscess cavity is drained, and a blunt artery forceps is inserted to widen the opening and to drain pus (Modified Hilton's technique).

Step 4: A Penrose drain is placed for drainage and irrigation.

> **Tips and Tricks**
>
> The internal sphincterotomy inhibits the pathological process of fistula formation and resolves the supralevator infection.

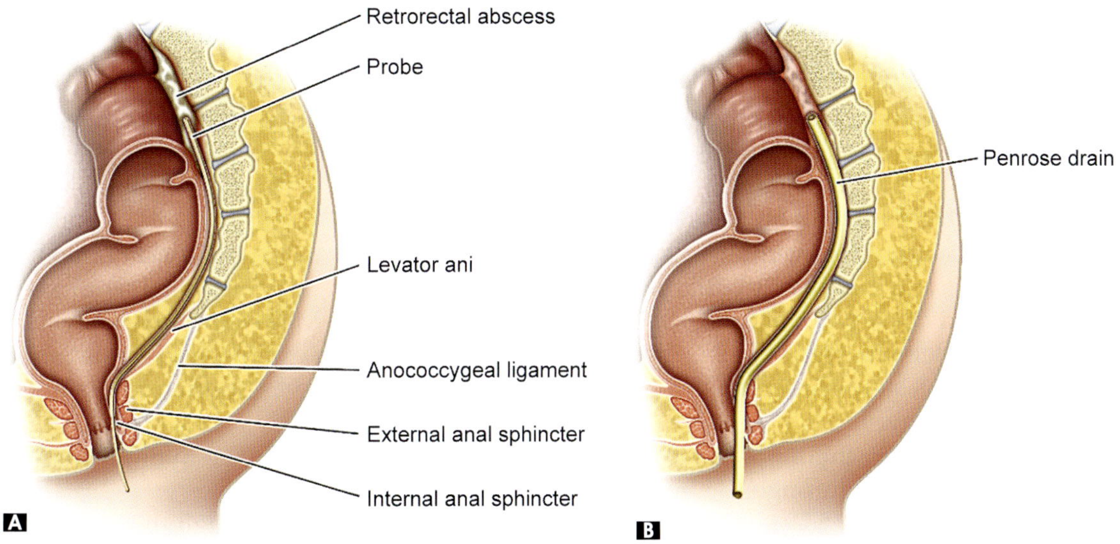

Fig. 5.27(A, B): Management of retrorectal abscess. A) Insertion of a probe in the retrorectal space followed by internal sphincterotomy for drainage of the abscess. B) Placement of Penrose drain for drainage and irrigation

BURST PERIANAL ABSCESS—A CASE PRESENTATION

A male patient, aged 34, came to the hospital in the emergency at night. He had severe pain in the perianal region for the last three days and difficulty sitting. On examination, there was a tender swelling in the perianal region at 7 o'clock near the anal verge. The patient was febrile, and the leucocyte counts were raised. Since the patient was in pain, DRE could not be done.

The importance of surgical intervention was conveyed, but he wanted to be treated conservatively. At night, the abscess burst open, and the severity of the pain decreased. The following day on digital rectal examination, internal opening could be palpated at 6 o'clock. The patient underwent an MRI examination which showed a communicating low intersphincteric fistula. The need for surgery was again explained to the patient, to which he agreed. Since it was a simple intersphincteric fistula with an abscess, it was decided to drain the abscess with a primary fistulotomy.

The patient was placed in the lithotomy position under spinal anaesthesia. The hydrogen peroxide and methylene blue were injected through the burst perianal abscess cavity, and bubbles were seen coming out from the internal opening (Fig. 5.28A, B). A blunt artery forceps was inserted through the burst abscess site, brought out of the internal opening, and a primary fistulotomy was done (Fig. 5.28C, D). The internal opening was excised by Park's technique (Fig. 5.28E).

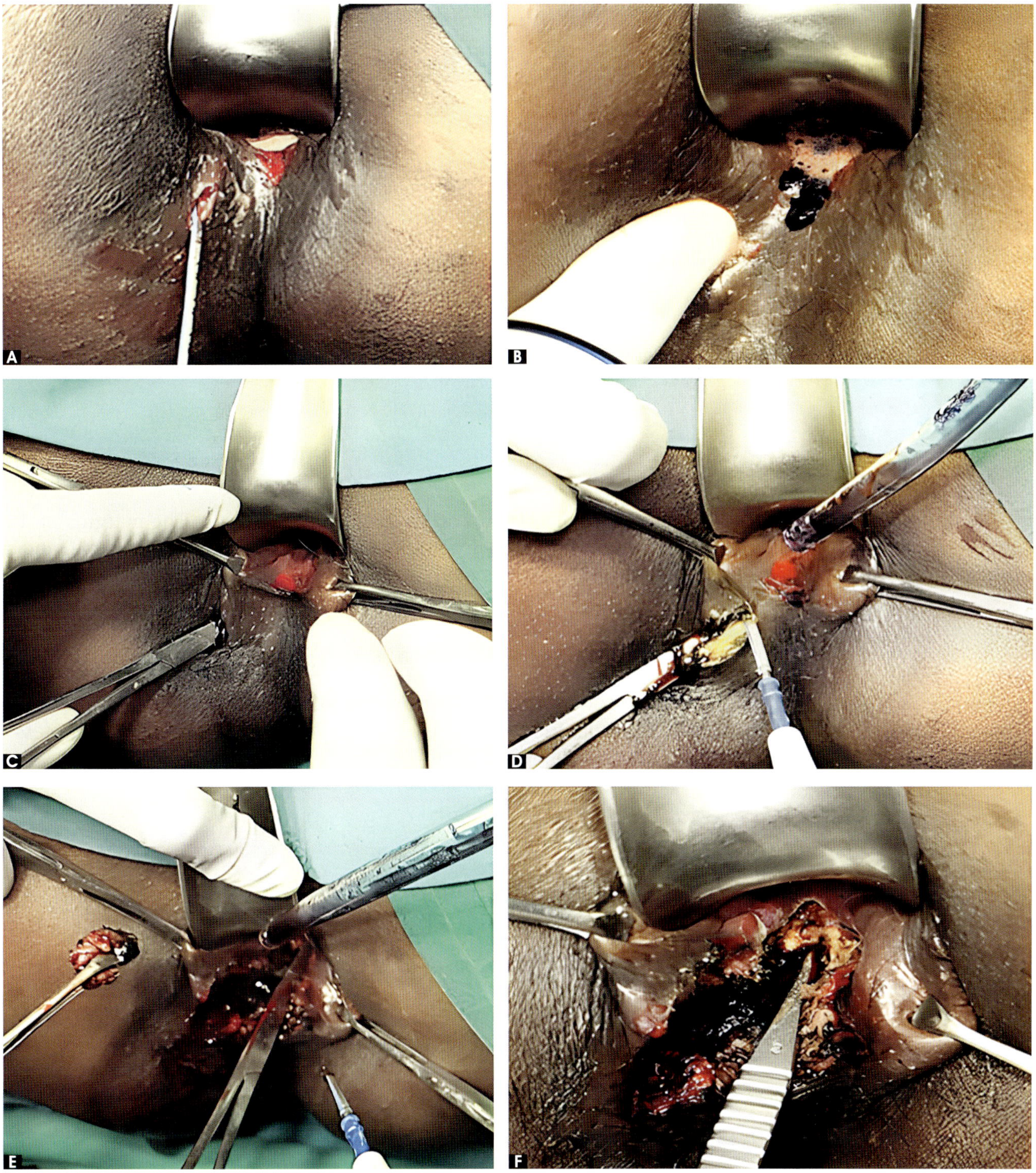

Fig. 5.28(A–F): Management of burst perianal abscess with a communicating intersphincteric fistula. A) Injecting hydrogen peroxide through the burst perianal abscess and bubbles seen at the internal opening at 6 o'clock. B) Demarcation of tract with methylene blue. C) Insertion of blunt artery forceps through burst abscess wound. D) Primary fistulotomy carried out over the forceps. E) Excision of internal opening. F) Curetting and irrigation of the laid open tract and the abscess cavity

The abscess cavity and the opened tract were curetted and irrigated (Fig. 5.28F, G). The margins of the fistulotomy tract were marsupialized (Fig. 5.28H). Local infiltration of 0.5% bupivacaine was done, and a pudendal nerve block was given to reduce postoperative pain (Fig. 5.28I, J, K).

Conclusion

An abscess is always managed by incision and drainage. The incision should be given as close to the anal verge as possible so that the subsequent fistula formed, if any, is small. Primary fistulotomy and abscess drainage should be carried out after assessing the extent of the external anal sphincter involved.

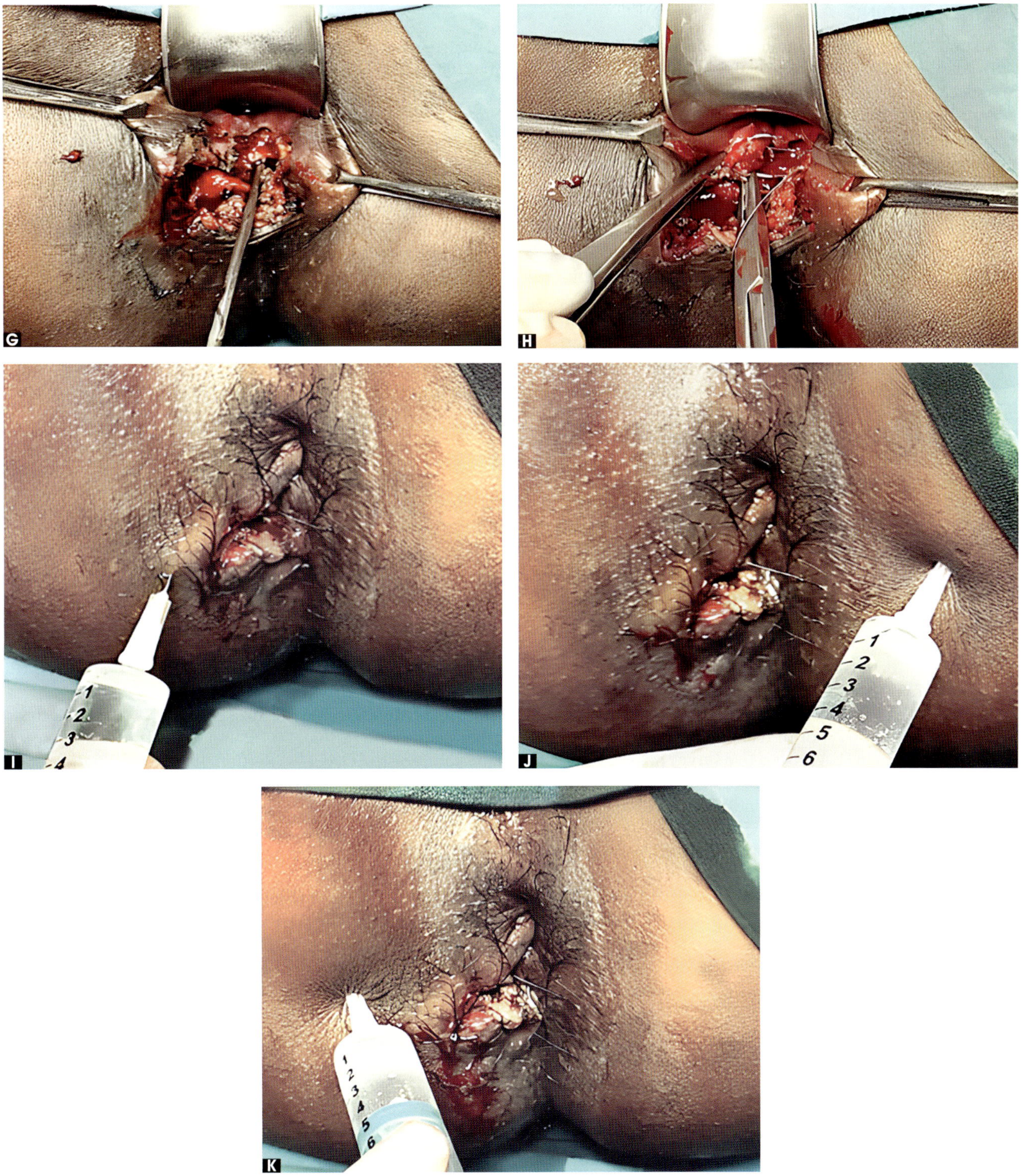

Fig. 5.28(G–K): Management of burst perianal abscess with a communicating intersphincteric fistula. G) Curetting and irrigation of the laid open tract and the abscess cavity. H) Marsupialization of the fistulotomy wound margins. I, J, K) Local infiltration of bupivacaine and pudendal nerve block at 3 and 9 o'clock

FURTHER READING

- Adamo K, Sandblom G, Brännström F, Strigård K. Prevalence and recurrence rate of perianal abscess--a population-based study, Sweden 1997-2009. Int J Colorectal Dis. 2016 Mar;31(3):669–73. doi 10.1007/s00354-015-2500-7. Epub 2016 Jan 14. PMID: 26765004.
- Aspects_of_fistula-in-ano PDF by PJ Lunnis.
- Brett E.Ruffo, Anorectal abscess, Chapter 13,pg372, Colorectal Surgery 2015 Corman
- Eisenhammer, S. (1966). The anorectal fistulous abscess and fistula. Diseases of the Colon and Rectum, 9(2), 91–106.
- EISENHAMMER S. The internal anal sphincter; its surgical importance. S Afr Med J. 1953 Mar 25;27(13):266-70. PMID: 13076663.
- EISENHAMMER S. The internal anal sphincter and the anorectal abscess. Surg Gynecol Obstet. 1956 Oct;103(4):501–6. PMID: 13360660.
- Goligher JC, Ellis M, Pissidis AG. A critique of anal glandular infection in the etiology and treatment of idiopathic anorectal abscesses and fistulas. Br J Surg. 1967 Dec;54(12):977–53. doi: 10.1002/bjs.1500541202. PMID: 6066322.
- Hamilton CH. Anorectal problems: the deep postanal space--surgical significance in horseshoe fistula and abscess. Dis Colon Rectum. 1975 Nov-Dec;15(5):642–5. Doi: 10.1007/BF02604265. PMID: 1192906.
- Hanley PH. (1975). Anorectal abscess fistula. Surgical Clinics of North America, 55(3): 457–503.
- Hanley PH. Reflections on anorectal abscess fistula: 1954. Dis Colon Rectum. 1955 Jul;25(7):525–33. doi 10.1007/BF02554105. PMID: 3593945.[PubMed]
- Herand Abcarian Relationship of Abscess and Fistula. Anal Fistula: Principles and Management, DOI 10. 1007/975-1-4614-9014-2-3
- Lockhart-Mummery JP. Fistula in ano. Lancet 1936; 227, 5573: 657–660.
- ML Prasad, DR Read, and H Abcarian, "Supralevator abscess: diagnosis and treatment," Diseases of the Colon and Rectum, vol. 24, no. 6, pp. 456–461, 1951. View at:[Google Scholar]
- Millan M, García-Granero E, Esclápez P, Flor-Lorente B, Espí A, Lledó S. Management of intersphincteric abscesses. Colorectal Dis. 2006 Nov;8(9):777–80. doi: 10.1111/j.1463-1318.2006.01035.x. PMID: 17032324.
- MORGAN CN. The surgical anatomy of the ischiorectal space. Proc R Soc Med. 1949 Mar;42(3):159–200. PMID: 15126956; PMCID: PMC2051231.
- Parks AG. (1961). Pathogenesis and treatment of fistula-in-ano. British medical journal, 1(5224), 463.
- Parks AG, Gordon PH, Hardcastle JD. A classification of fistula-in-ano. Br J Surg. 1976 Jan;63(1):1–12. doi: 10.1002/bjs.1500630102. PMID: 1267567.
- PARKS AG. Pathogenesis and treatment of fistula-in-ano. Br Med J. 1961 Feb 15;1(5224):463–9. Doi: 10.1136/bmj.1.5224.463. PMID: 13732550; PMCID: PMC1953161.
- Ramanujam PS, Prasad ML, Abcarian H, Tan AB. Perianal abscesses and fistulas. A study of 1023 patients. Dis Colon Rectum. 1954 Sep;27(9):593–7. doi 10.1007/BF02553545. PMID: 6465199.[PubMed]
- Read DR Abcarian H. A prospective survey of 474 patients with anorectal abscesses. Dis Colon Rectum. 1979 Nov-Dec;22(5):566–5. doi 10.1007/BF02557005. PMID: 527452.
- Rezmovitz J, MacPhee I, Schwindt G. Horseshoe abscesses in primary care. Can Fam Physician. 2019 Jul;65(7):476–478. PMID: 31300429; PMCID: PMC6738465.
- Robinson AM Jr, DeNobile JW. Anorectal abscess and fistula-in-ano. J Natl Med Assoc. 1955 Nov;50(11):1209-13. PMID: 3074175; PMCID: PMC2571535.
- Sanyal S, Khan F, Ramachandra P. Successful management of a recurrent supralevator abscess: a case report. Case Rep Surg. 2012;2012:571639. Doi: 10.1155/2012/571639. Epub 2012 May 7. PMID: 22649747; PMCID: PMC3357932.
- Sigmon DF, Emmanuel B, Tuma F. Perianal Abscess. 2021 Jun 29. In: StatPearls [Internet]. Treasure Island (FL): StatPearls Publishing; 2022 Jan. PMID: 29053652.
- Tarasconi A, Perrone, G., Davies, J. et al. Anorectal emergencies: WSES-AAST guidelines. World J Emerg Surg 16, 45 (2021). https://doi.org/10.1156/s13017-021-00354-x
- Turner SV, Singh J. Perirectal Abscess. 2021 Aug 11. In: StatPearls [Internet]. Treasure Island (FL): StatPearls Publishing; 2022 Jan–. PMID: 29939672.[PubMed]
- Téoule P, Seyfried S, Joos A, Bussen D, Herold A. Management of retrorectal supralevator abscess-results of a large cohort. Int J Colorectal Dis. 2018 Nov;33(11):1589–1594. doi: 10.1007/s00384-018-3094-7. Epub 2018 May 29. PMID: 29845388.
- Ustynoski K, Rosen L, Stasik J, Riether R, Sheets J, Khubchandani IT. Horseshoe abscess fistula. Seton treatment. Dis Colon Rectum. 1990 Jul;33(7):602–5. doi: 10.1007/BF02052216. PMID: 2361430.
- Vasilevsky CA, Gordon PH.Benign anorectal: Abscess and fistula. InWolffBG, Fleshman JW, Beck De, et al., editors: The ASCRS Textbook Of colon and rectal surgery. New York 2007, Springer Science, business media, LLC,p192
- Whiteford MH. Perianal abscess/fistula disease. Clin Colon Rectal Surg. 2007 May;20(2):102–9. doi 10.1055/s-2007-977455. PMID: 20011354; PMCID: PMC2750152.[PubMed]

Chapter

6

Management of Fistula in ANO

The fistula in ano is an abnormal passage that develops between the inner lining of the anal canal or rectum and the perianal skin. An anorectal fistula may be simple or complex. The management depends upon the type of fistula and the surgeon's expertise.

A thorough evaluation and assessment of the fistulas in relation to the anal sphincters is necessary for the management. Surgical procedures such as fistulotomy or fistulectomy remain the gold standard. However, sphincter-saving techniques are becoming popular as the sphincter integrity is preserved.

The fistulas can be evaluated and classified based on their location and relation with the sphincters. One should remember that irrespective of the external opening, the internal opening is usually present posteriorly at 6 o'clock at the dentate line.

Goodsall's Rule

Goodsall's rule describes the typical path followed by the fistula, which helps to locate the internal opening. An imaginary transverse line in the middle of the anal orifice divides the anal canal into anterior and posterior halves, describing the fistula as anterior and posterior (Fig. 6.1).

According to the rule, if an external opening is present anterior to the transverse line, it will have a straight radial tract. If an external opening is posterior to the transverse line, it will have a curved tract.

An exception to the rule is an external opening 3 cm from the anal verge anteriorly.

Types of Fistulas based on their Relation with the Sphincters (Park's Classification)

The fistula in ano is classified into four primary types based on the anatomy and its relationship to the sphincter muscles (Fig. 6.2).

TYPES OF FISTULAS

- **Intersphincteric:** The fistula is present in the intersphincteric plane. It may present in six different ways.
- **Trans-sphincteric:** The fistula extends beyond the external sphincter into the ischiorectal space. Depending on the extent of the external anal sphincter involved, it can be subclassified into:
  - Low trans-sphincteric
  - High trans-sphincteric
- **Suprasphincteric:** The fistula tract crosses the inter-sphincteric plane above the puborectalis and then moves downwards to the ischiorectal fossa into the skin via the levator plate.
- **Extrasphincteric:** The fistula tract enters the perianal skin from the rectum outside the sphincter complex, travelling through the levator and ischiorectal fat.

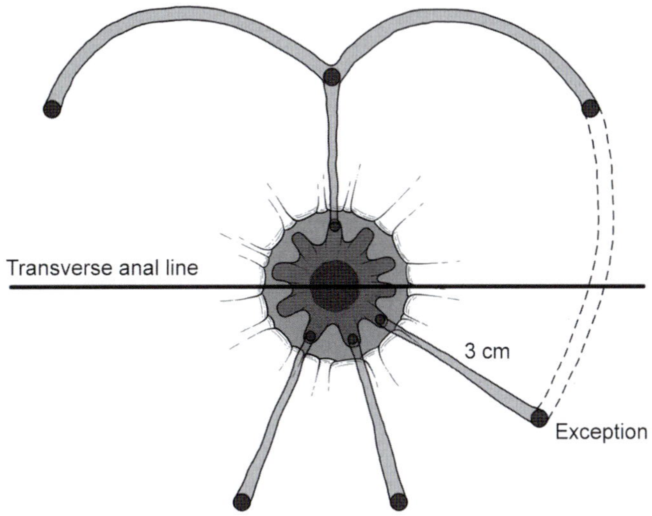

Fig. 6.1: Goodsall's rule

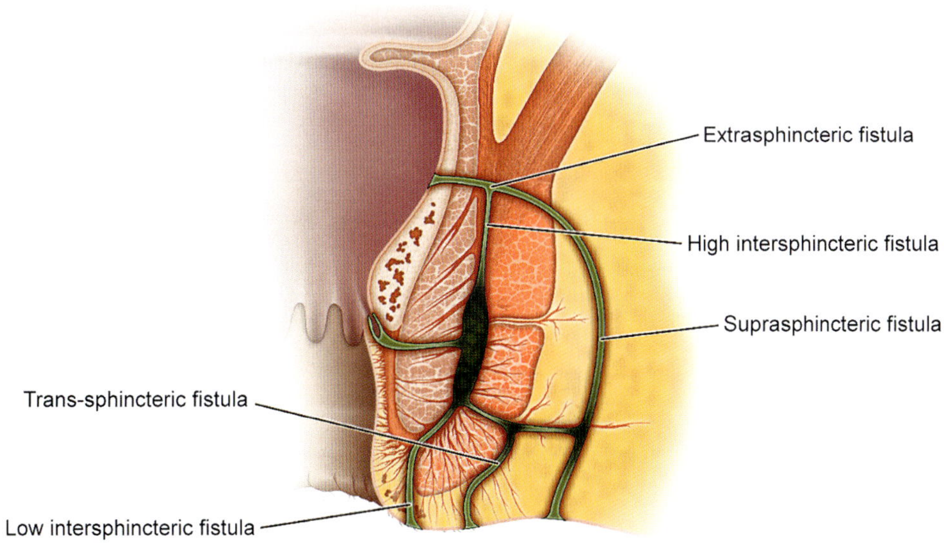

Fig. 6.2: Park's classification

1. Inter-sphincteric Fistula

It begins on the dentate line and travels across the intersphincteric space before opening into the perianal area. It may be low or high. The incidence reported is 70%.

This fistula can be further categorized into six types based on its path.

A-1 Type: Simple Intersphincteric Fistula

The tract travels down to the anal verge from the intersphincteric plane (Fig. 6.3A). It is also referred to as a simple low fistula.

A-2 Type: Intersphincteric Fistula having a High Blind Tract

The intersphincteric fistula has an upward extension and ends blindly Fig. 6.3B. It is also referred to as a high intersphincteric fistula.

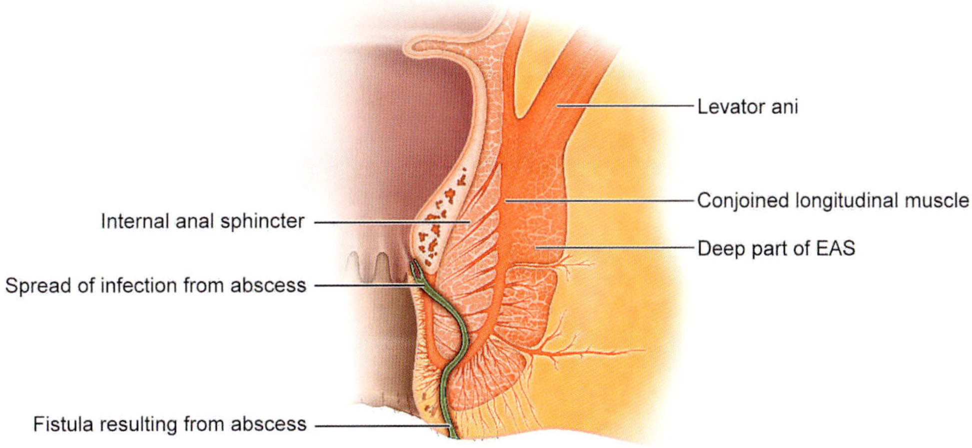

Fig. 6.3A: A-1 type of intersphincteric fistula

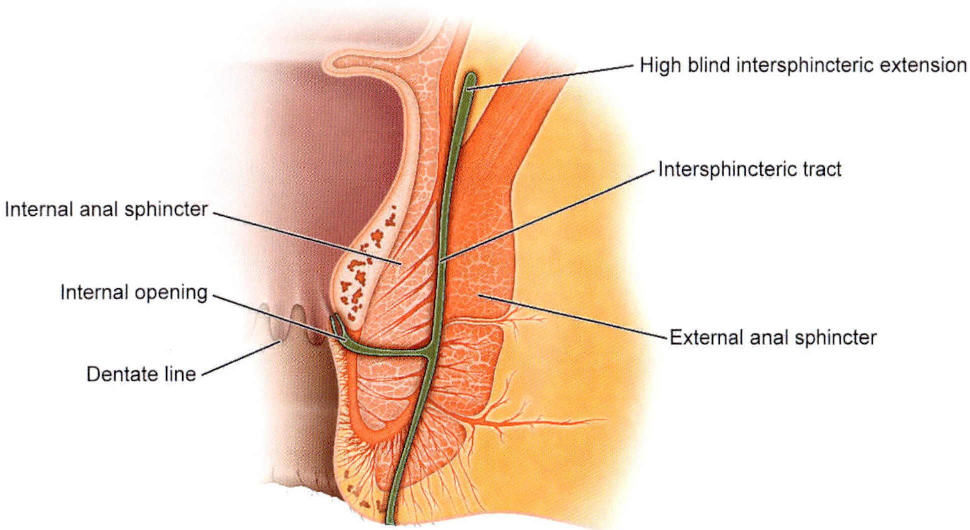

Fig. 6.3B: A-2 type of intersphincteric fistula with a high blind tract

A-3 Type: Intersphincteric Fistula with a Rectal Opening

The intersphincteric fistula has an upward extension that opens into the rectum (Fig. 6.3C).

A-4 Type: Intersphincteric Fistula with No Perianal Opening

The intersphincteric tract extends upwards into the intersphincteric plane without an external opening. The upward extension may end blindly or open into the rectum (Fig. 6.3D).

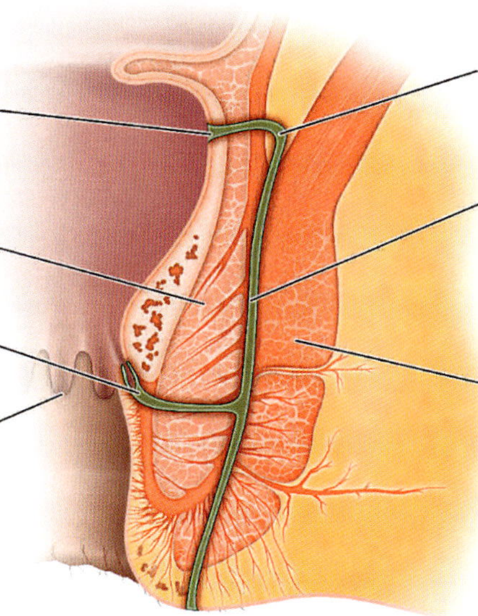

Fig. 6.3C: A-3 type of intersphincteric fistula with rectal opening

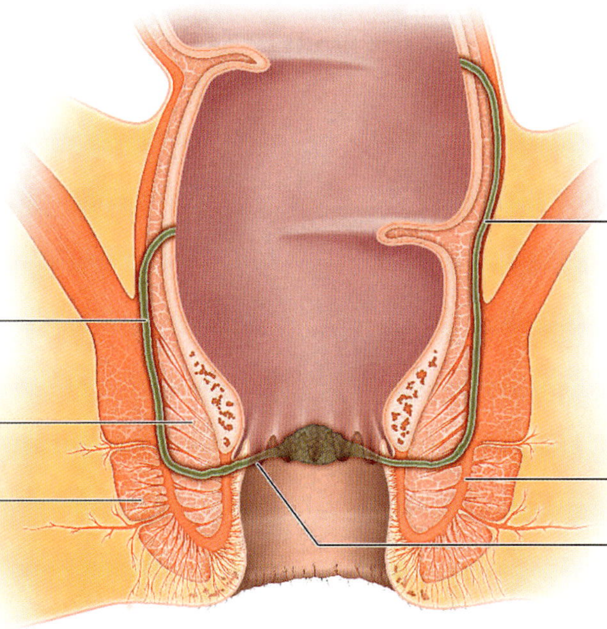

Fig. 6.3D: A-4 type of intersphincteric fistula without perineal opening

A-5 Type: Intersphincteric Fistula with Pelvic Extension

The tract extends upwards through the intersphincteric space above the levators to enter the pelvis (Fig. 6.3E). There is no caudal extension towards the anal verge.

A-6 Type: Intersphincteric Fistula Secondary to Pelvic Infection

The infection from the pelvic disease travels downwards to reach the intersphincteric plane. As there is no communication with the anal canal, it is not an anal fistula in the true sense (Fig. 6.3F).

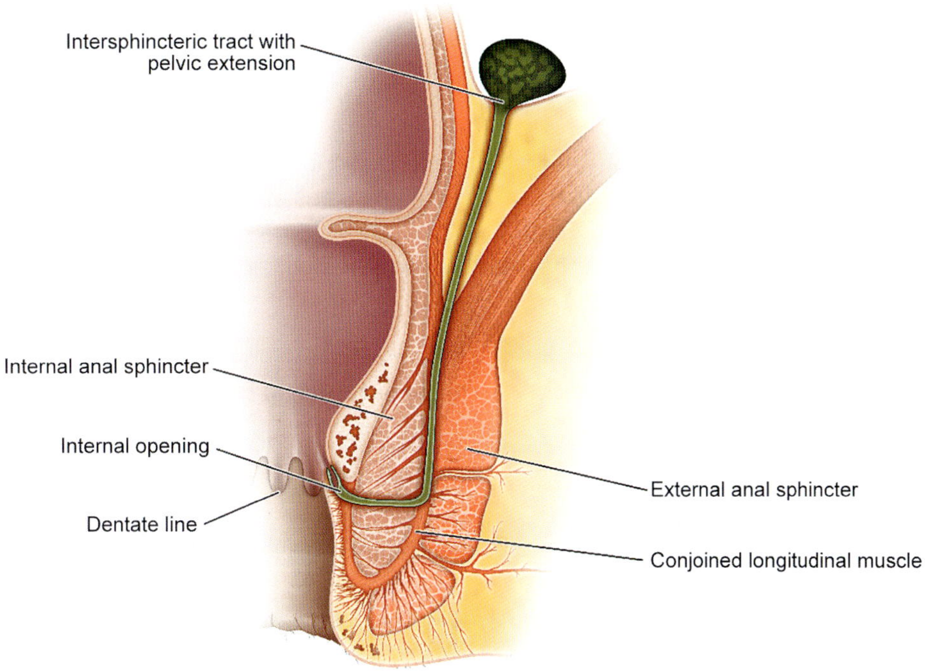

Fig. 6.3E: A-5 type of intersphincteric fistula with pelvic extension

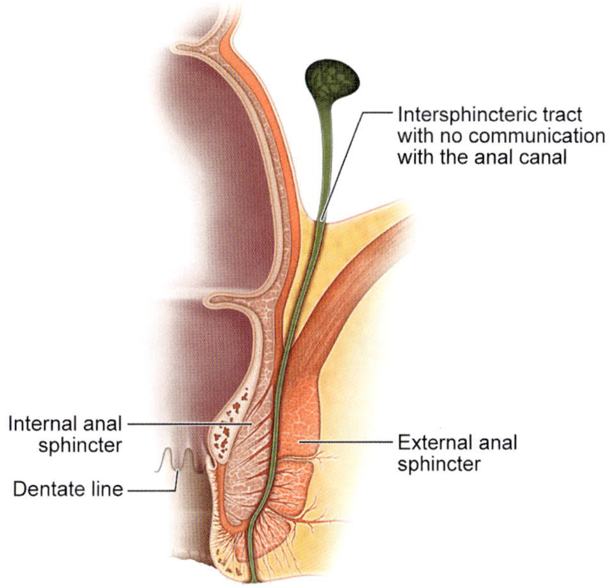

Fig. 6.3F: A-6 type of intersphincteric fistula secondary to pelvic infection

2. Trans-sphincteric Fistula

Trans-sphincteric fistula extends beyond the internal and external sphincters. The incidence reported is 20–25%. When the external sphincter involved is less than 30%, it is a low trans-sphincteric fistula, and when more than 30% is involved, it is a high trans-sphincteric fistula.

The trans-sphincteric fistula may be uncomplicated or complicated.

B-1 Type: Uncomplicated

The tract traverses through the external sphincter, enters the ischiorectal fossa from the intersphincteric plane, and then opens into the skin (Fig. 6.4).

B-2 Type: Complicated Trans-sphincteric Fistula

The tract gives an upward extension that may cross the levator ani muscle or travel to the apex of the ischiorectal fossa (Fig. 6.5).

Another type of trans-sphincteric fistula may present with an upward intersphincteric extension (Fig. 6.6). This type of fistula was not mentioned in the original Park's classification.

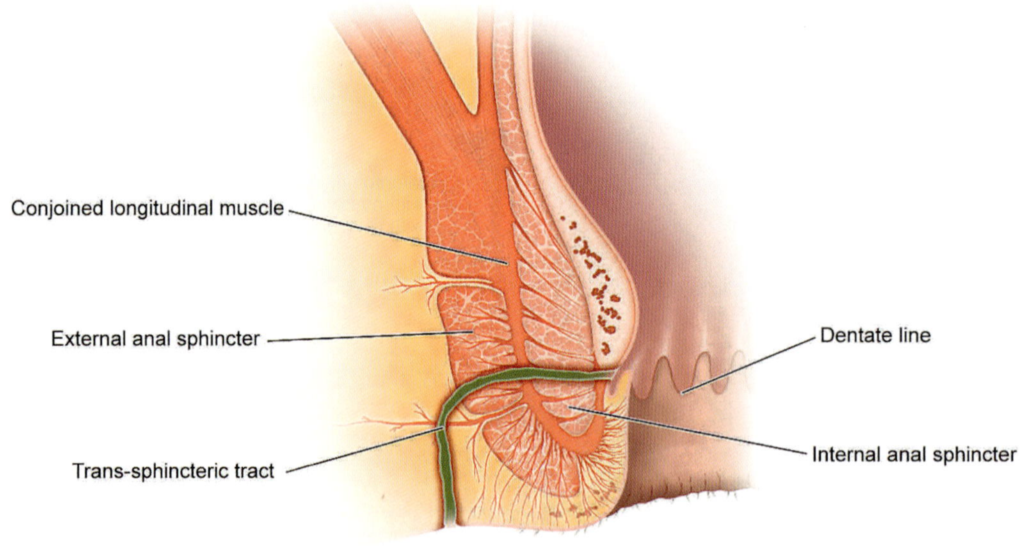

Fig. 6.4: B-1—Uncomplicated trans-sphincteric fistula

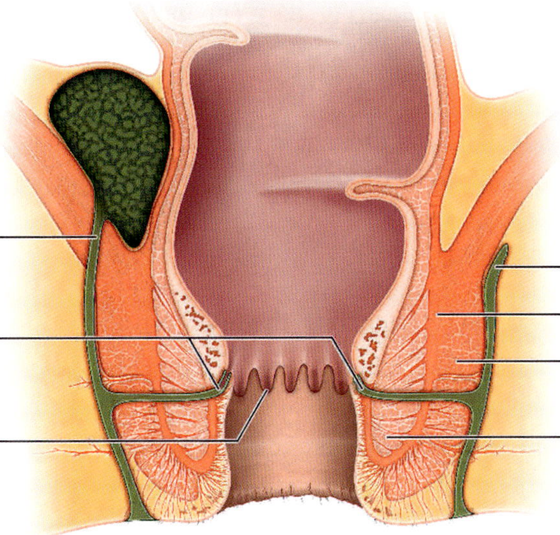

Fig. 6.5: B-2—High blind tract or tract with upward extension

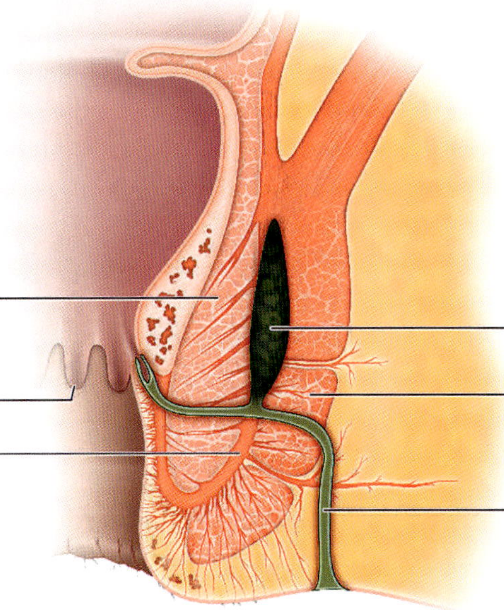

Fig. 6.6: Trans-sphincteric tract with upwards intersphincteric extension

3. Suprasphincteric Fistula

The tract extends beyond the anal sphincter complex (Fig. 6.7). The incidence reported is 2 to 5%.

4. Extrasphincteric Fistula

The external opening in an extrasphincteric tract is present in the perianal skin, while the internal opening is above and outside the sphincter complex (Fig. 6.8).

SIMPLE AND COMPLEX FISTULA

As per the American Society of Colon and Rectal Surgeons, the fistulas may be simple and complex.

Simple Fistula

- Low intersphincteric or low trans-sphincteric fistula

Complex Fistula

- Recurrent fistula
- Fistula involving more than 30% to 50 % of the sphincter
- Anterior fistula in females
- Fistula with multiple openings
- Fistula with pre-existing incontinence
- Fistula associated with inflammatory bowel disease
- Fistula secondary to radiation
- Fistula associated with an abscess

St. James Classification (Based on radiological findings)

- Grade I: Simple intersphincteric linear tract
- Grade II: Abscess with an intersphincteric tract
- Grade III: Trans-sphincteric tract
- Grade IV: Abscess associated with trans-sphincteric tract
- Grade V: Supralevator extensions

MANAGEMENT OF FISTULA IN ANO

Once evaluated, fistulas are managed surgically, and the technique depends on the presentation of the disease. While treating a fistula, one has to deal with three features of the fistula:

- First, the internal opening
- Second, the fistula tract
- Third, the external opening

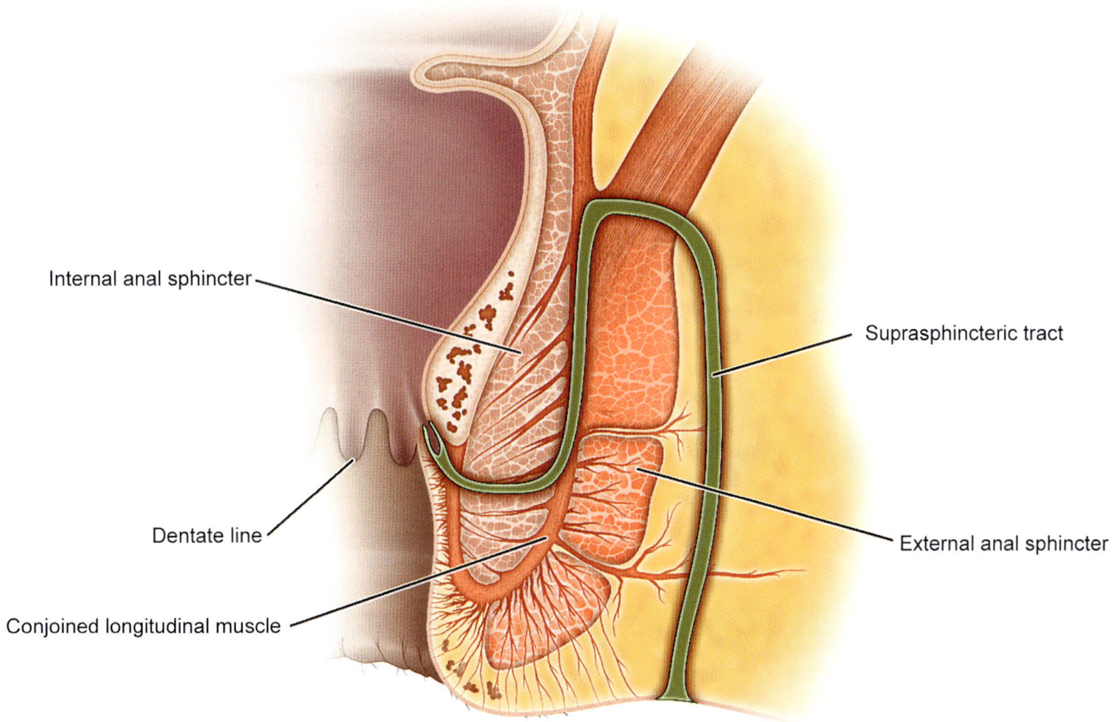

Fig. 6.7: Suprasphincteric tract

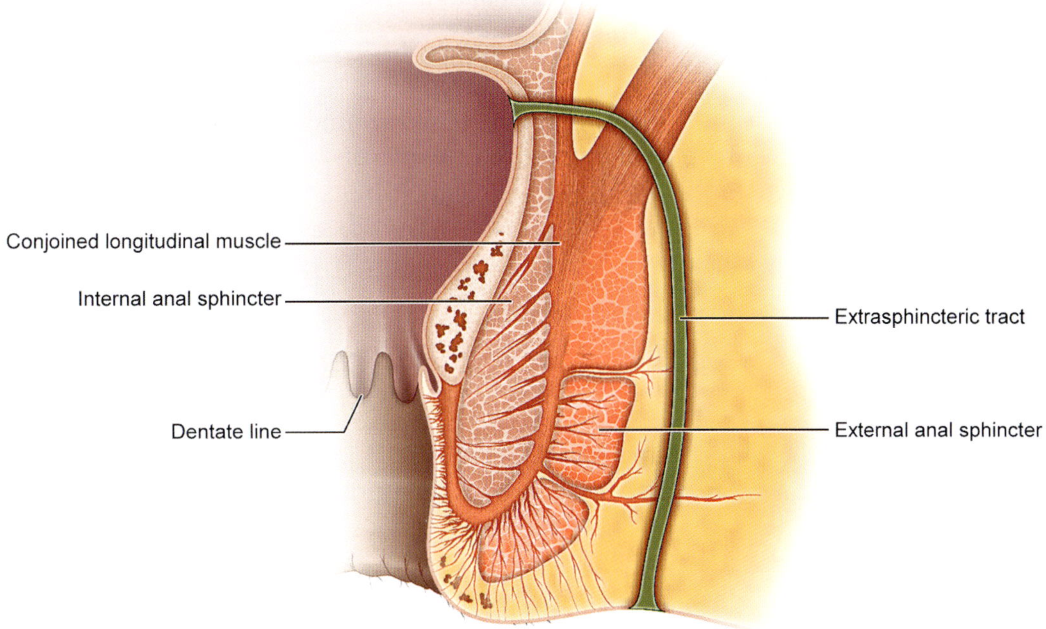

Fig. 6.8: Extrasphincteric tract

The internal opening is the nidus of infection and should be excised. As discussed in the chapter on abscesses, the techniques are:

- Park's technique
- Eissenhammer technique

The procedures for the management of fistula in ano are:

- **Sphincter cutting**
  - Fistulotomy
  - Fistulectomy
- **Sphincter saving procedures**
  - Seton placement (draining)
  - Fistula plug
  - Advancement flap
  - Fistula laser closure (FilaC)
  - Ligation of Intersphincteric Fistula Tract (LIFT)
  - Video-assisted ablation of Fistula Tract (VAAFT)
- **Hybrid procedures**
  - Distal laser and proximal SLOFT (DLPS)
  - Distal laser and proximal SLOFT with distal tract coring (DCPS)
  - Distal laser with proximal LIFT
  - VAAFT with LIFT with laser ablation of the distal tract (VA-LIFT)
  - Distal coring with proximal fistulotomy with laser ablation (DCPF)

Principle Behind Marsupialization

Marsupialization is a technique where the margins of the incised wound are stitched from the interior to the exterior surface. This technique is not a part of any procedure but can be performed as an add-on in routine practice (Fig. 6.9).

Advantages

- Prevents the bridging of the margins of the fistula tract.
- Prevents early skin closure. Since the skin heals faster than mucosa, the underlying raw area can give rise to recurrence.
- Decreases the size of the wound.
- Maintains hemostasis from the edges of the wound.
- Avoids trapping of the fecal matter underneath the wound margins.

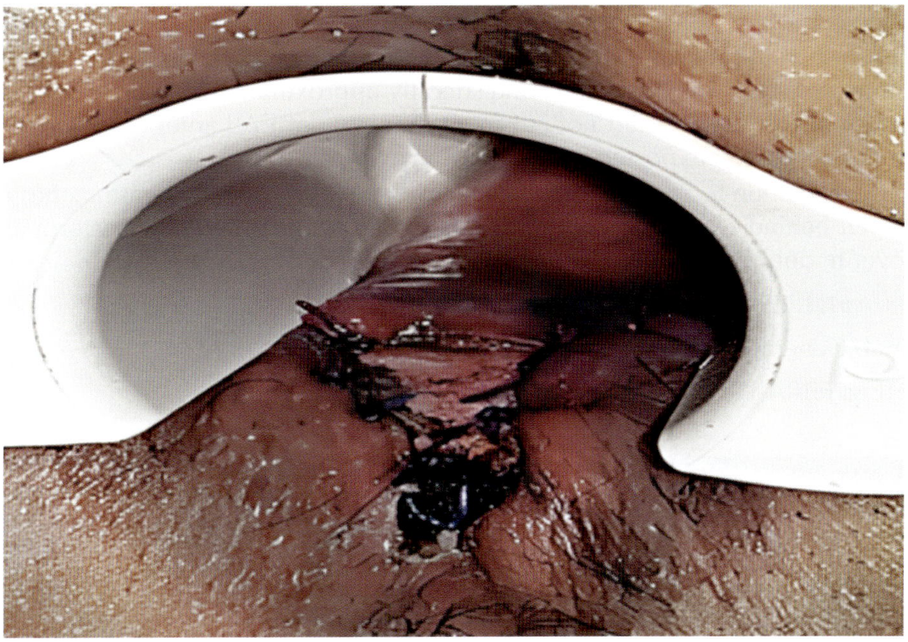

Fig. 6.9: Marsupialization of the wound margins

SPHINCTER CUTTING PROCEDURES

Fistulotomy

Depending on the level of the sphincter cut, the fistulotomy can be referred to as low or high. A low fistulotomy is when less than 30% of the EAS is cut, and a high fistulotomy is when 50% sphincter is cut.

One should be aware that under no circumstance should the deep part of EAS be cut, as it will lead to fecal incontinence.

When 50% of the EAS is cut, primary sphincter repair can be done to avoid anal incontinence.

Assessment of Extent of involvement of EAS

While operating, it is very difficult to know how much EAS has been cut. A surgeon should keep two important landmarks in mind:

- The dentate line is approximately 2 cm from the anal verge. It roughly corresponds to the junction of EAS's superficial and deep parts.
- While operating for fistulotomy, one should always follow the anorectal ring. This acts as a guide to how much EAS sphincter has been cut. Posteriorly and laterally, approximately 50% of the EAS can be cut without fear of fecal incontinence. One should not cut more than 30% of EAS anteriorly since the length of EAS anteriorly is half as compared to posterior part of the anal canal.

MRI is the best investigation to assess EAS involvement. Moreover, while operating, the crucial part is how much sphincter is left behind rather than how much has been cut. It is better to perform a sphincter-saving procedure whenever in doubt or opt for a seton placement.

Position of the patient: Lithotomy

Anaesthesia: Spinal/General/Pudendal nerve block

Instrumentation (Fig. 6.10A-D)

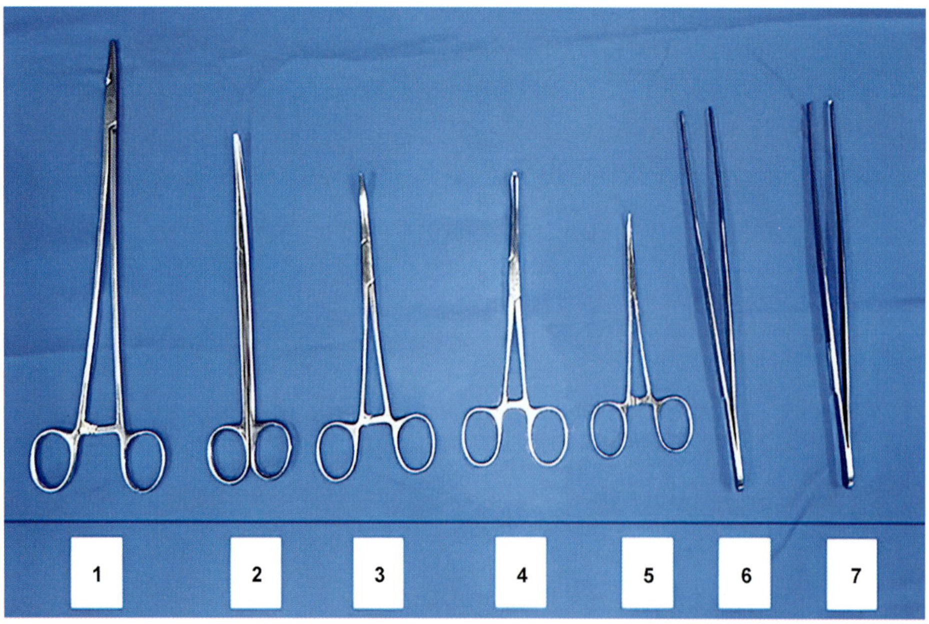

Fig. 6.10A: Instrumentation. 1) Needle holder. 2) Scissors. 3) Blunt artery forceps. 4) Allis forceps. 5) Mosquito forceps. 6) Plain forceps. 7) Tooth forceps

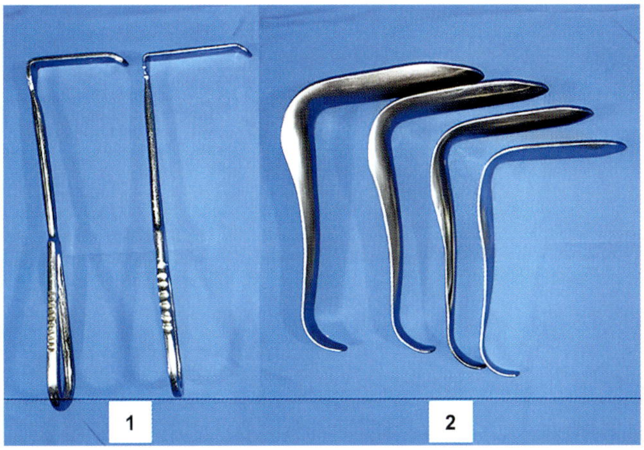

Fig. 6.10B: Instrumentation. 1) A pair of right-angle retractors. 2) Sim's speculum

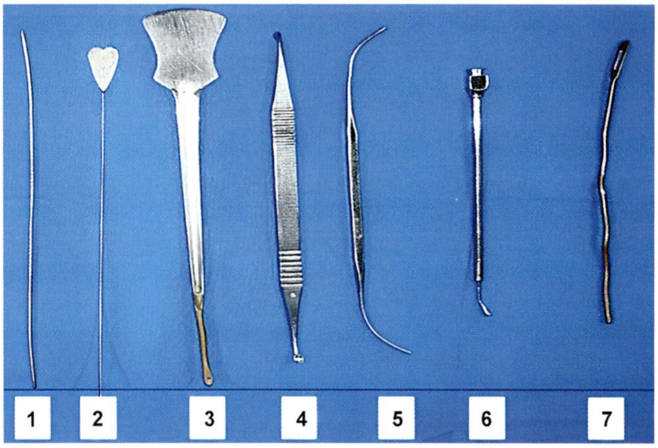

Fig. 6.10C: Instrumentation. 1) Hager's dilator 3mm. 2) Lockhart mummery probe. 3) Eye probe for seton placement. 4) Curette. 5) Curved probe. 6) Irrigation cannula. 7) Malleable metal probe

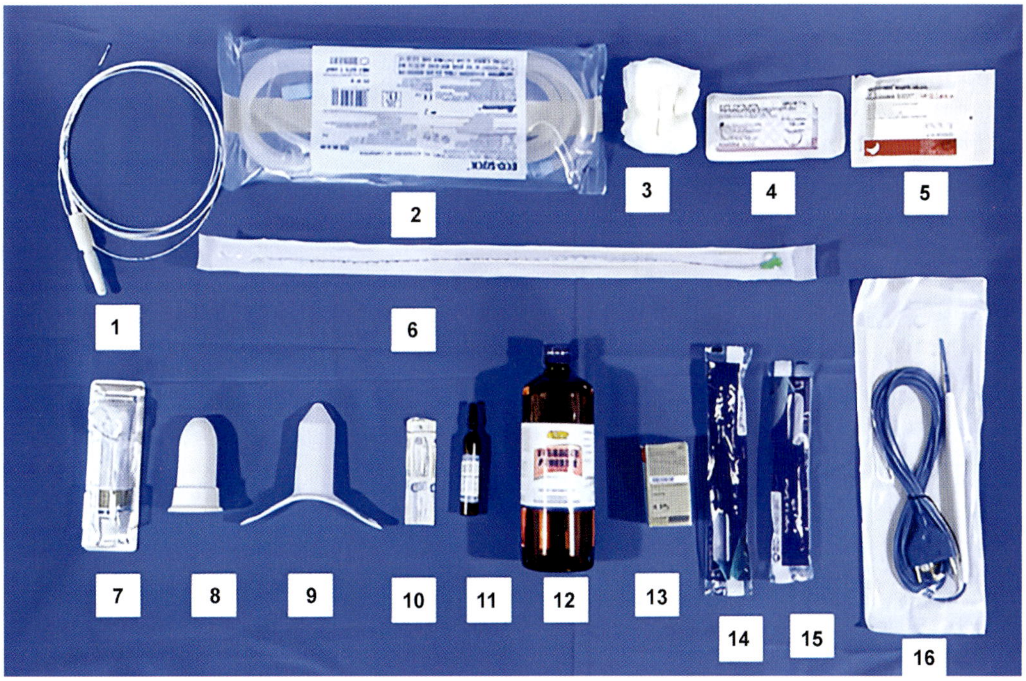

Fig. 6.10D: Instrumentation. 1) Laser fibre 36 degrees radial. 2) Suction tip. 3) Gauze pieces. 4) Vicryl 2-0. 5) Cautery tip cleaner. 6) Infant feeding tube. 7) Xylocaine jelly. 5) Circular anal dilator. 9) Half-cut proctoscope. 10) Surgical blade 11 number. 11) Methylene blue ampule. 12) Hydrogen peroxide. 13) Injection bupivacaine 0.5%. 14) Disposable syringe 10 ml. 15) Disposable syringe 5 ml. 16) Cautery pencil

Steps of the Procedure (Low Fistulotomy)

Step 1: The tract is identified and demarcated by injecting hydrogen peroxide and methylene blue through the external opening. The bubbles emerge from the internal opening (Fig. 6.11A, B).

Step 2: A probe is inserted gently into the tract through the external opening and brought out through the internal opening (Fig. 6.11C). The overlying tract is divided over the probe Fig. 6.11D). The unhealthy granulation tissue at the base of the opened tract is curetted and irrigated. Other branches, if any, demarcated by methylene blue are identified and excised.

Step 3: The deep intersphincteric space is identified by the white color fibres of the IAS anteriorly and the superficial part of the EAS posteriorly (Fig. 6.11E). The space is scooped out to remove the underlying infected tissue, followed by irrigation.

Step 4: The wound base is then curetted and left open to heal by secondary intention. Marsupialization of the fistulotomy wound edges is done (Fig. 6.11F). A pudendal nerve block can be given to reduce postoperative pain.

Scan QR Code for Video on
Fistulotomy

VIDEO 24

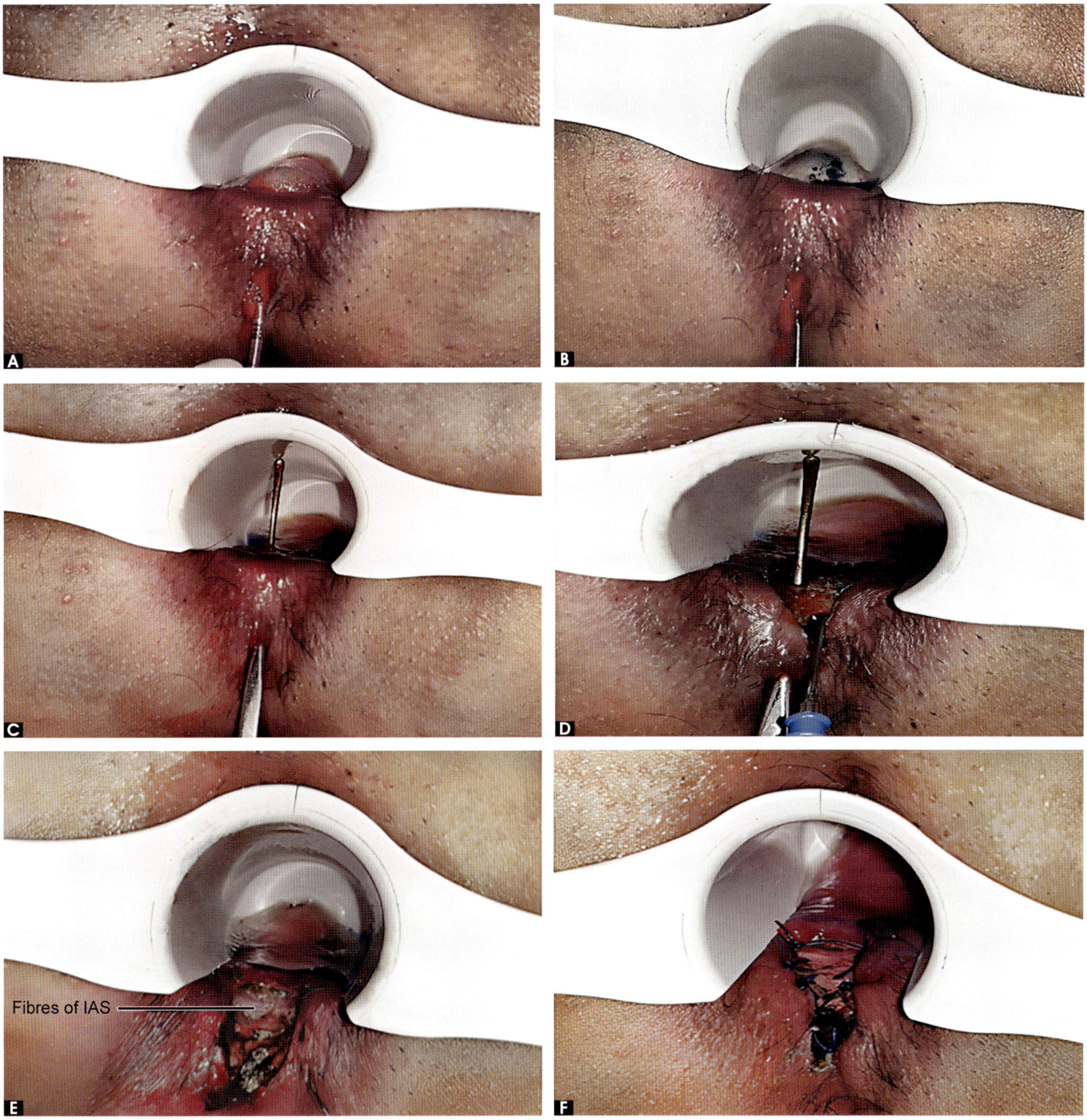

Fig. 6.11(A-F): The technique of low fistulotomy. A) Injecting hydrogen peroxide through an external opening. Bubbles are seen coming out of the internal opening at the dentate line. B) Demarcation of the fistula tract by injecting methylene blue. C) The probe is entered via the external opening and brought out through the internal opening. D) Laying open of fistula tract over the probe using monopolar electrocautery. E) Fistulotomy wound showing fibres of EAS. F) Marsupialization of the fistulotomy wound edges

Steps of the Procedure (High Fistulotomy)

Steps 1 to 3 remain the same

Step 4: Once the superficial part of the EAS is incised, primary sphincter repair is carried out using PDS 2-0. The mucosa can be approximated with Vicryl 3-0 (Fig. 6.12A-D). The stitches over the incised sphincter are always taken in a figure of 8 or horizontal mattress technique, for approximation.

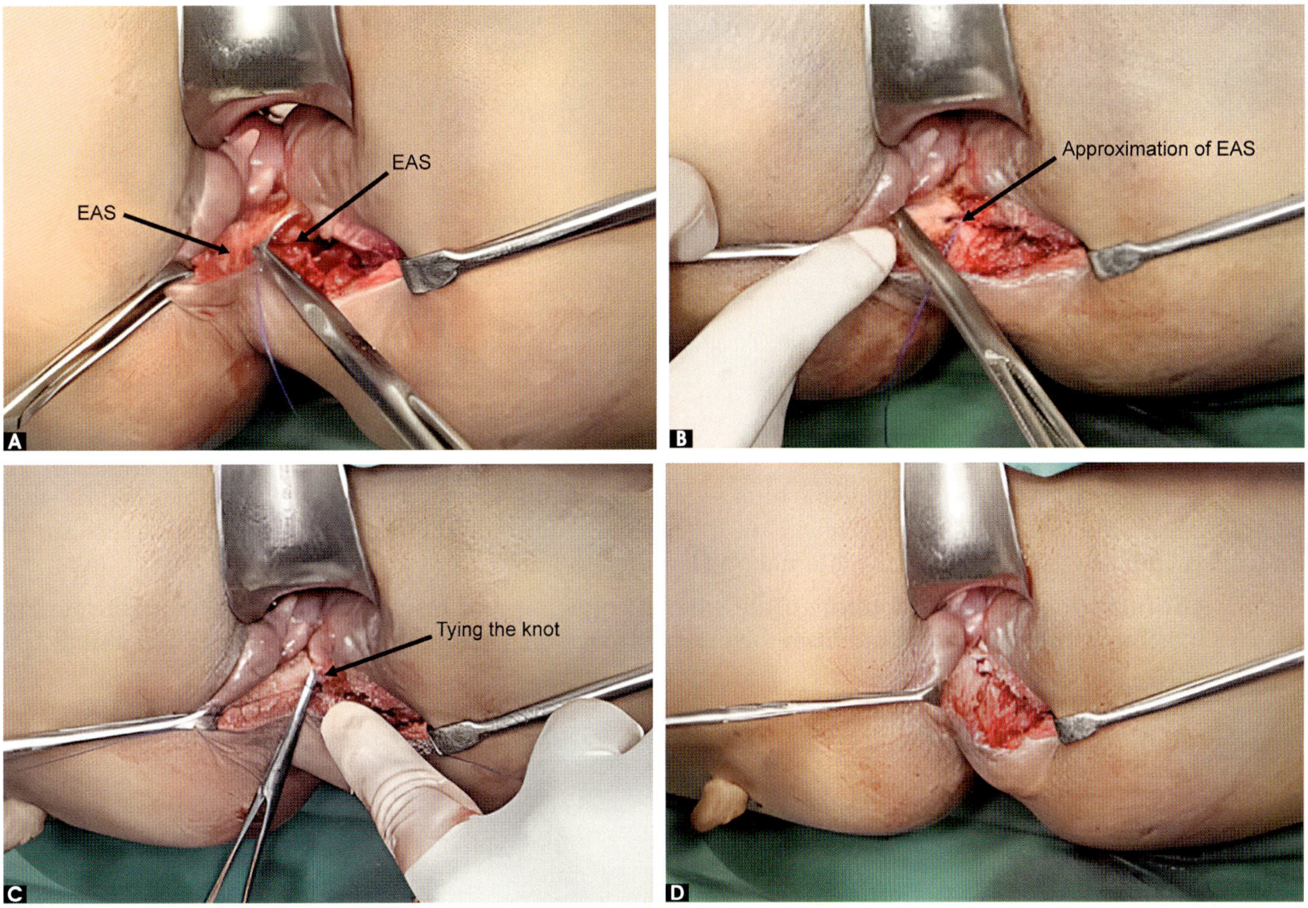

Fig. 6.12(A-D): Primary sphincter repair. A) Insertion of PDS 2-0 through the margins of EAS. B, C) Approximation of the cut margins of the superficial part of the EAS. D) Final wound after primary sphincter repair

Fistulectomy

Fistulectomy refers to the excision of the tract.

Steps of the Surgical Procedure

Step 1: Hydrogen peroxide and methylene blue are injected from the external opening. Bubbles can be seen emerging from the internal opening (Fig. 6.13A, B). The half-cut proctoscope or one-sided Sim's speculum is inserted to identify the location of the internal opening (Fig. 6.13C).

Step 2: A fistula probe is inserted through the external opening and brought out of the internal opening (Fig. 6.13D). The fistula tract is excised from the external to internal opening over the probe (Fig. 6.13E, F, G).

Scan QR Code for Video on
Fistulectomy

VIDEO 25

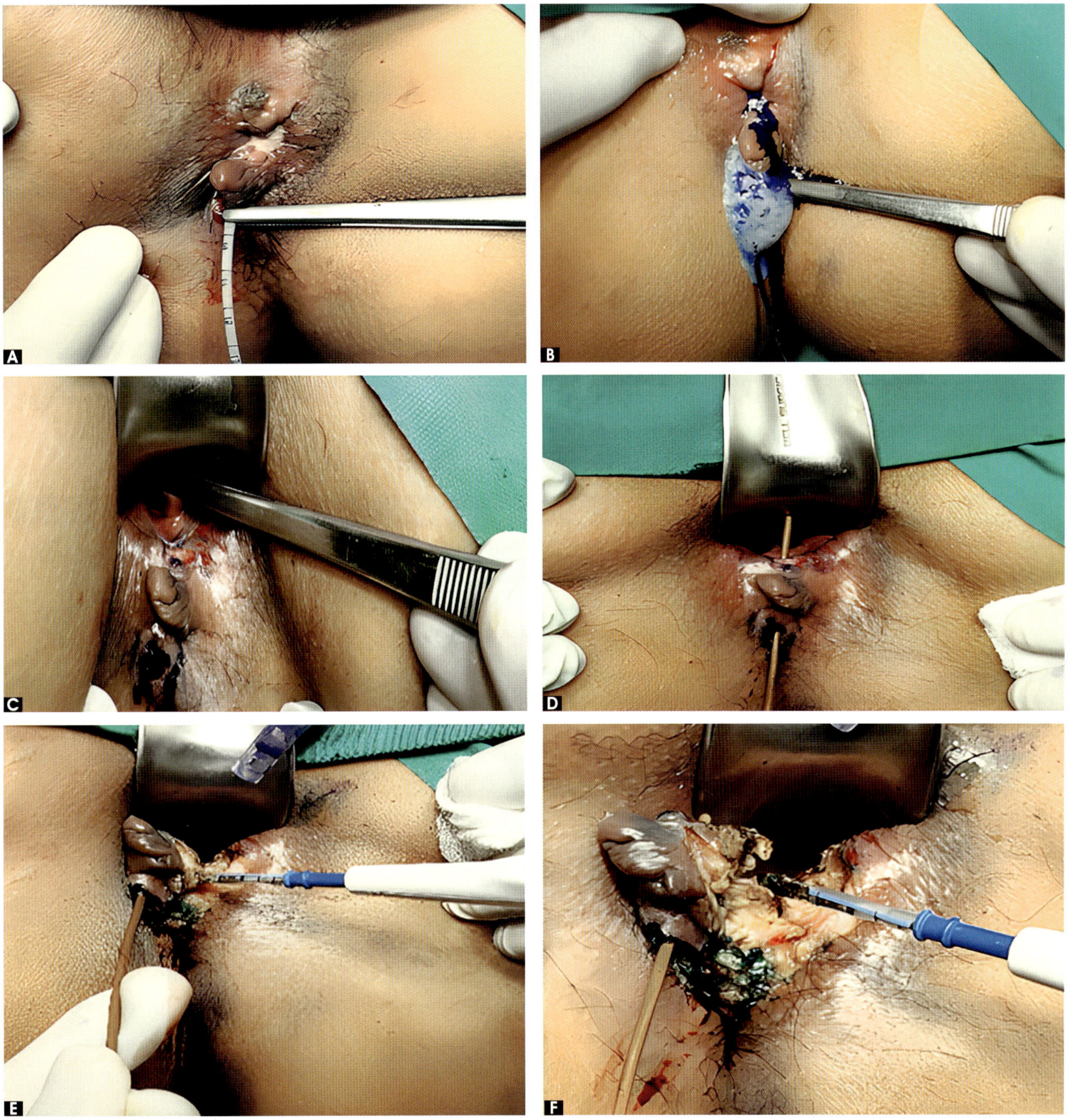

Fig. 6.13(A-F): Technique of fistulectomy. A) Injecting hydrogen peroxide and methylene blue through the external opening. B) Bubbles can be seen emerging from the internal opening. C) Insertion of Sim's speculum to identify the location of the internal opening. D) Insertion of a fistula probe through the external opening and tip of the probe brought out of the internal opening. E) The fistula tract excised over the probe. F) The excised fistula tract

Step 3: After complete excision of the tract, the wound is thoroughly curetted, irrigated, and marsupialization of the margins is done (Fig. 6.13H, I, J).

Step 4: Bupivacaine 0.5% is infiltrated locally, followed by a pudendal nerve block to reduce postoperative pain (Fig. 6.13K, L, M).

The vent created in the EAS should be closed during fistulectomy for the trans-sphincteric fistula.

A glance at fistula management is mentioned in Table 6.1 to Table 6.3

TABLE 6.1: MANAGEMENT OF INTERSPHINCTERIC FISTULA—AT A GLANCE

Type of intersphincteric fistula	*Amount of sphincter to be cut*
A-1 Simple intersphincteric fistula	Lower half of the IAS
A-2 Intersphincteric fistula with high blind tract	Low fistulotomy with the division of IAS upto the anorectal ring
A-3 Intersphincteric fistula with an opening in the lower rectum	Low fistulotomy with the division of IAS up to the anorectal ring
A-4 High intersphincteric fistula without perineal opening	Laying open of intersphincteric tract upto the anorectal ring with fistulotomy at 6 o'clock.
A-5 High intersphincteric fistula with pelvic extension	Low-end fistulotomy with the opening of intersphincteric space and curetting of pelvic extension
A-6 Intersphincteric fistula extending from pelvic disease	Manage pelvic disease

TABLE 6.2: MANAGEMENT OF TRANS-SPHINCTERIC FISTULA—AT A GLANCE

Type of Trans-sphincteric fistula	*Amount of sphincter to be cut*
B-1 Uncomplicated	The superficial and subcutaneous parts of the EAS and the lower part of the IAS.
B-2 Trans-sphincteric fistula with a high blind tract	Fistulotomy up to the superficial part of the EAS with primary sphincter repair. The upper extension is curetted

TABLE 6.3: MANAGEMENT OF SUPRASPHINCTERIC AND EXTRASPHINCTERIC FISTULA—AT A GLANCE

Type of fistula	*Amount of sphincter to be cut*
Suprasphincteric fistula	Avoid sphincter cutting. Intersphincteric space can be opened up to the anorectal ring, and a seton can be placed.
Extrasphincteric fistula	Avoid sphincter cutting. Treat the primary cause. Seton can be placed.

Tips and tricks

- There may be a transient postoperative anal incontinence due to division of the lowermost part of the external anal sphincter.
- In a high fistulotomy, primary sphincter repair should be performed to prevent anal incontinence.
- Before fistulotomy, it is advisable to assess the anal tone and the extent of the external sphincter involved.
- It is important to preserve the external sphincter between the internal opening and the levator ani. The aim is to preserve at least 2–2.5 cm of the external sphincter.
- The internal opening and the surrounding tissue can be excised through the anal approach. This helps eliminate the primary source of infection in the deep intersphincteric space with a decreased chance of recurrence.
- Explore the deep intersphincteric space thoroughly, as the infection can extend due to the ramifications of the anal glands.
- When opening the intersphincteric space, the entire internal sphincter can be cut open upto the anorectal ring, without the risk of incontinence.

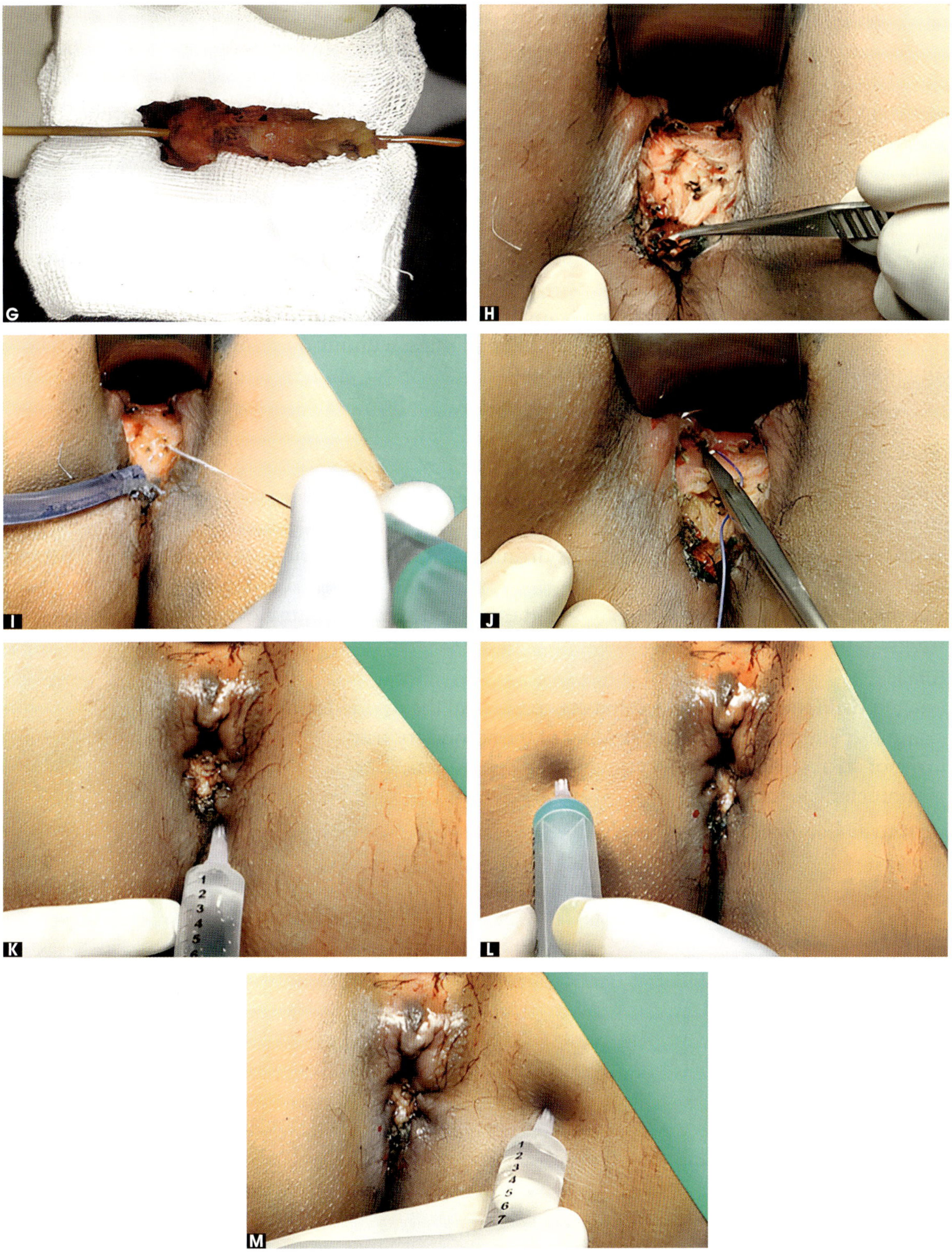

Fig. 6.13(G-M): Technique of fistulectomy. G, H, I,J) Curetting, irrigation and marsupialization of the margins. K, L, M) Infiltration of Bupivacaine 0.5% locally, followed by a pudendal nerve block to reduce postoperative pain

Sphincter-saving Procedures

The sphincter-saving techniques are minimally invasive procedures for treating a fistula. They aim to obliterate the epithelialized tracts and the internal fistulous openings without dividing the sphincters. The various minimally invasive techniques are described below.

SETON PLACEMENT

Seton is a thin, flexible material that keeps the fistula open and allows it to heal over time.

Principle

- Draining the pus and sepsis control before starting definitive treatment
- Stimulating fibrosis
- The cutting seton leads to slow transection of the external sphincter muscle by pressure necrosis. A cutting seton should not be considered a sphincter-saving procedure.

Indications

- Two staged fistulotomy where the seton is used to heal the divided sphincter
- In a complex fistula to promote the healing of the secondary tracts
- Drainage of an abscess, thus preventing further sepsis
- Trans-sphincteric fistula

Instrumentation: Figure 6.10A-D

Types of Setons (Fig. 6.14)

- Kshar-sutra
- Rubberband
- Silk
- Vessel loop

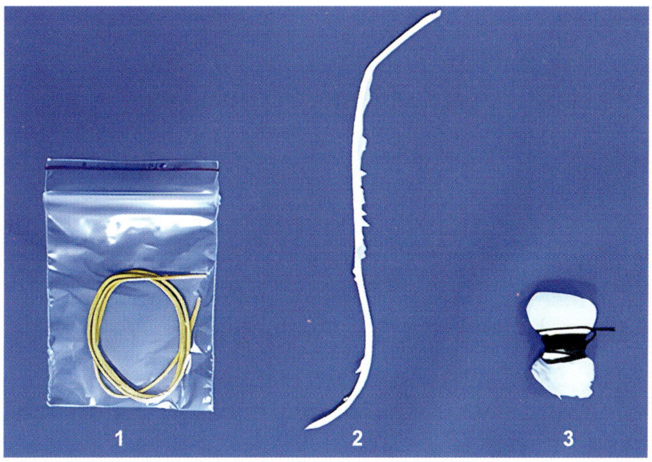

Fig. 6.14: Types of setons: 1) Kshar-sutra. 2) Rubberband. 3) Silk

Position of the patient: Lithotomy

Anaesthesia: Spinal/General/Pudendal nerve block.

Inserting or changing a seton without anaesthesia can be painful.

Steps of the Procedure

Step 1: The tract is identified and demarcated by injecting hydrogen peroxide and methylene blue through the external opening, and bubbles are observed coming out of the internal opening.

Step 2: A probe with an eye is inserted from the internal opening, brought out through the external opening, and a seton is passed into the tract (Fig. 6.15A, B). Alternatively, the probe may be inserted from the external to the internal opening.

Step 3: The seton is secured using a knot on the external end. When a draining seton is used, it is left loose, whereas it is tightened for cutting seton (Fig. 6.15C, D).

The draining seton may be changed after 4 weeks, whereas the cutting seton is tightened at regular intervals.

Scan QR Code for Video on
Placement of Draining Seton
VIDEO 26

Scan QR Code for Video on
Changing of the Seton
VIDEO 27

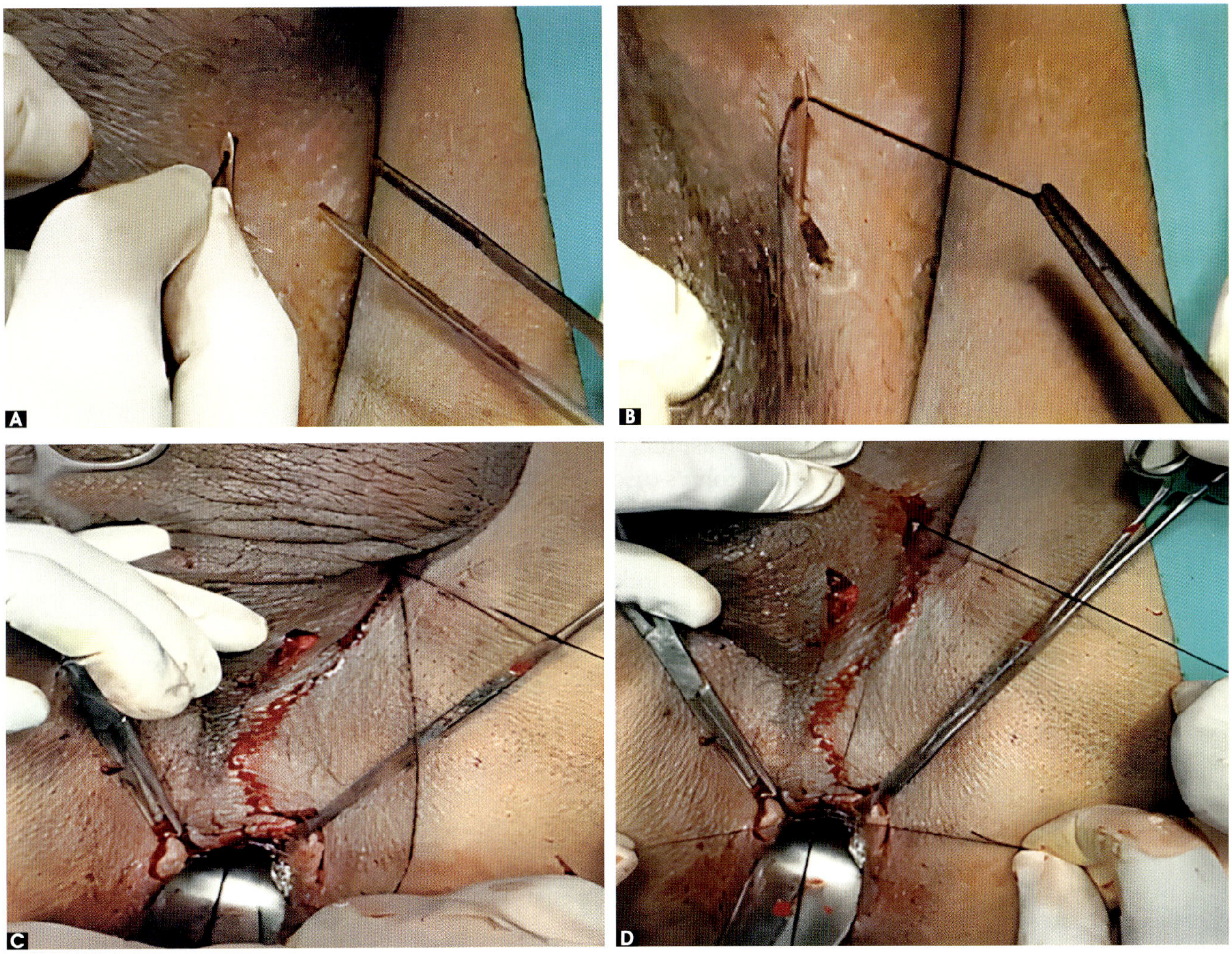

Fig. 6.15(A-D): Placement of draining seton. A) The probe is brought out of the external opening. B) Silk thread taken inside through the eye of the probe. C) Both ends brought together at the internal opening. D) Loose seton left inside for drainage

FISTULA LASER CLOSURE (FILAC)

Principle

The epithelized fistula tract is ablated with a diode laser, and the internal opening is closed.

Indications

- Fistula with a long tract
- Intersphincteric, trans-sphincteric and suprasphincteric fistula
- Extrasphincteric fistula associated with Crohn's disease
- Anterior fistula in females
- Complex or high fistula
- In patients with weak sphincters, to prevent incontinence

Contraindications

- Fistula associated with an abscess
- Fistula with a small tract (less than 3 cm in length)

Instrumentation: Figures 6.10A-D

Equipment: Figure 6.16

- Laser equipment
- 360-degree corona radial fibre

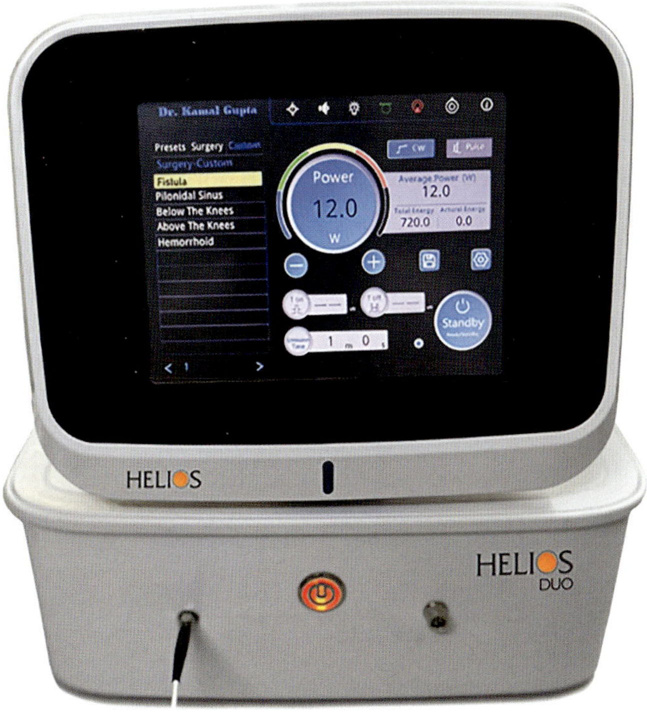

Fig. 6.16: Diode laser 1470

Energy/Dosage/Fibre

- Continuous mode with the dosage of 12 W per mm per sec
- 360-degree corona radial fibre

Steps of the Procedure

Step 1: Hydrogen peroxide and methylene blue are injected from the external opening to identify the internal opening. Bubbles can be seen coming out of the internal opening (Fig. 6.17A).

Step 2: The tract is curetted, and the necrotic material is removed (Fig. 6.17B).

Step 3: A 360-degree corona radial laser fibre is inserted from the external to the internal opening (Fig. 6.17C).

Step 4: The fibre is activated, and the energy is delivered radially. The unhealthy granulation tissue and the epithelized tract are laser ablated (Fig. 6.17D).

Step 5: The tract is again curetted, followed by irrigation with normal saline to remove the debris.

Step 6: The internal opening is closed using Polyglactin 2-0. A circumambulation stitch taken with the probe inside the tract is a good way of closing, as it ensures complete closure of the internal opening (Fig. 6.17E). Before tying the knot, the probe is pulled out. A jerk indicates proper closure of the internal opening. Few fibres of the IAS are included for proper anchoring of the suture.

Step 7: The external opening is widened for drainage (Fig. 6.17F).

The final image at the end of the procedure is shown in Fig. 6.17G.

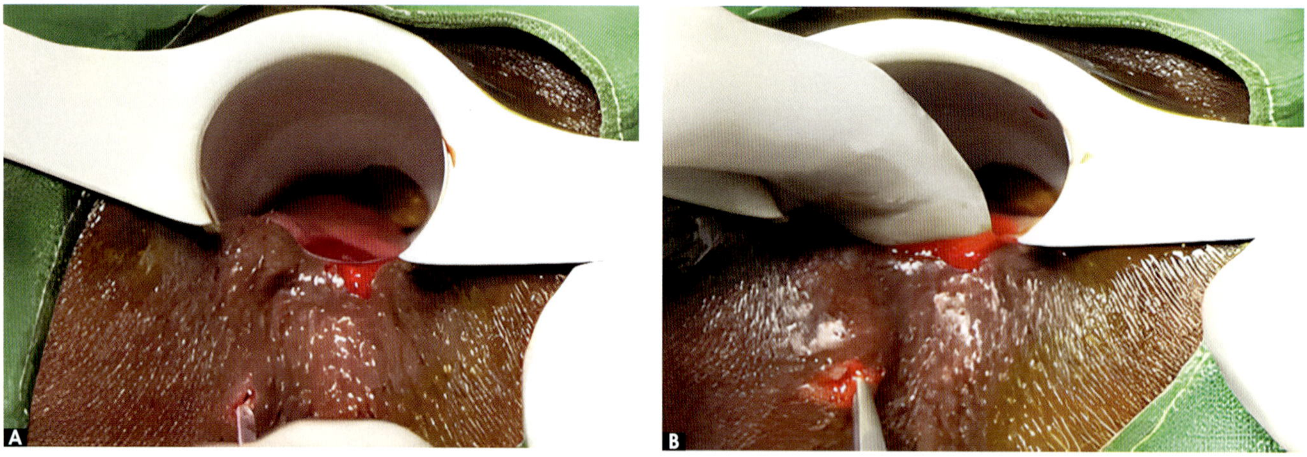

Fig. 6.17(A-B): Fistula laser closure. A) Injecting hydrogen peroxide through the external opening of a tract to identify its internal opening. B) Curetting of a fistula tract

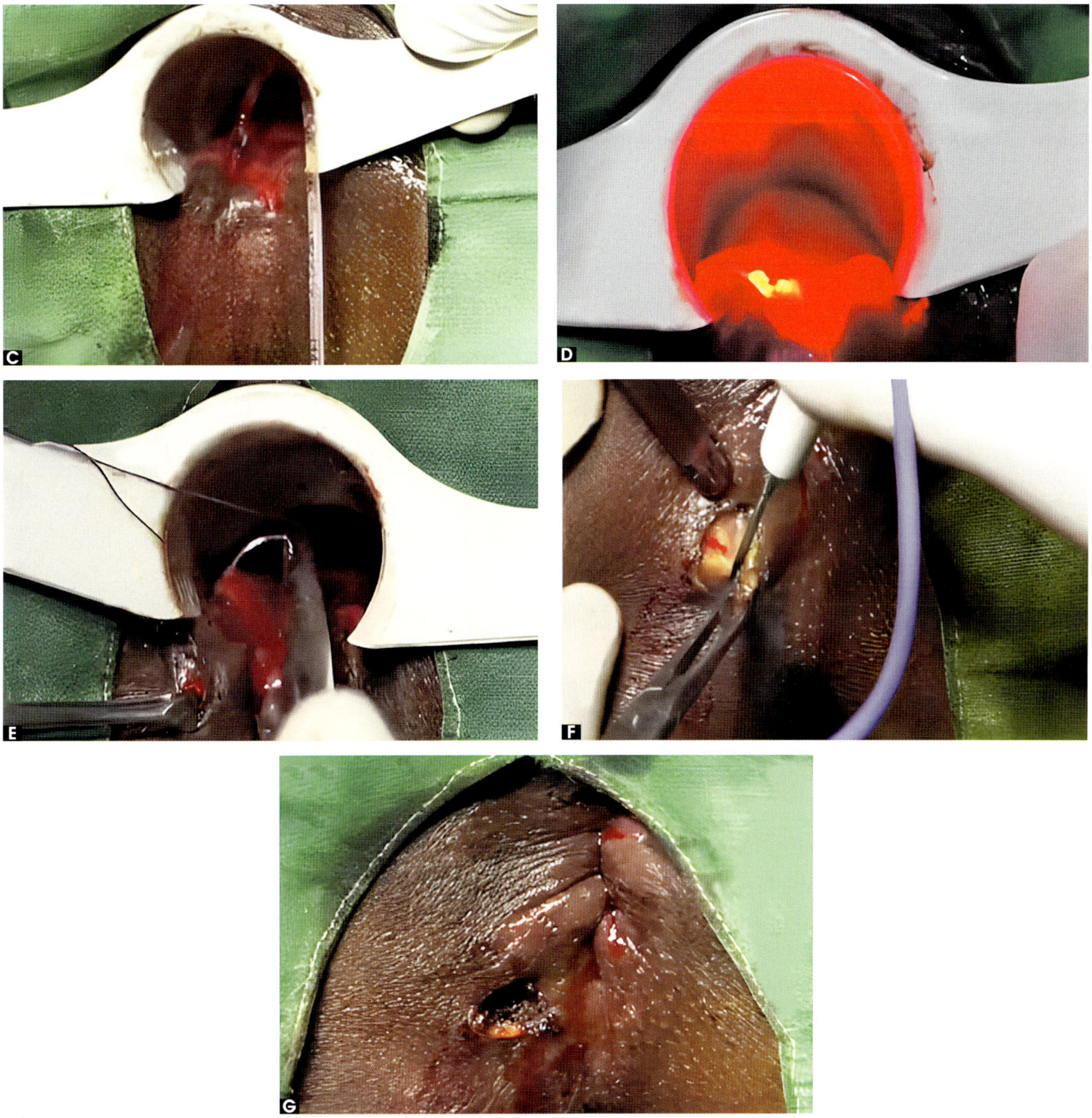

Fig. 6.17(C-G): Fistula laser closure. C) Insertion of laser fiber by railroad method. D) Laser ablation of the fistula tract from internal to external opening. E) Internal opening closure by circumambulation technique using Polyglactin 2-0. F) Widening of the external opening for drainage. G) Final wound as seen at the end of the procedure

Closing the Internal Opening

There are three ways to close the internal opening (Fig. 6.18A–C).

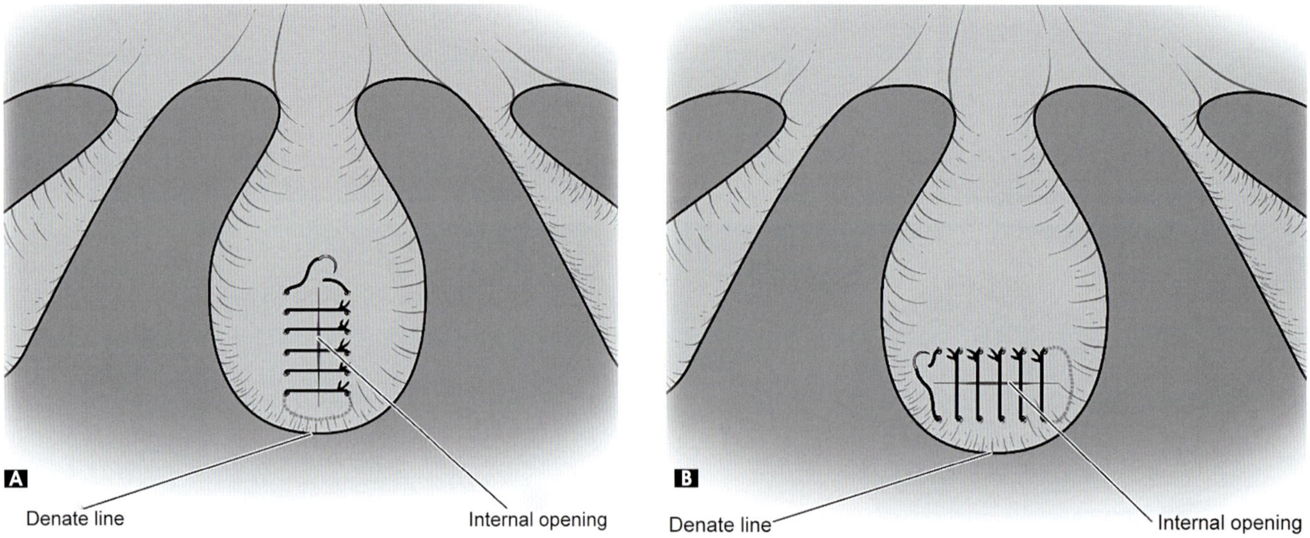

Fig. 6.18(A-B): Closure of the internal opening. A) Closure of internal opening perpendicular to dentate line. B) Closure of internal opening parallel to dentate line

Tips and Tricks

- The energy released for ablation is always given in continuous mode.
- While closing the internal opening, it is advisable to take the stitches parallel to the dentate line to avoid dehiscence of the sutures (Fig. 6.18B).
- Always include some fibres of the internal anal sphincter for proper transfixation. Otherwise, the stitches may give way during defecation due to increased anal canal pressure.
- A purse-string suture may also be used to close the internal opening (Fig. 6.18C).
- Keep on withdrawing the fibre every one mm to avoid skip areas (Fig. 6.19).

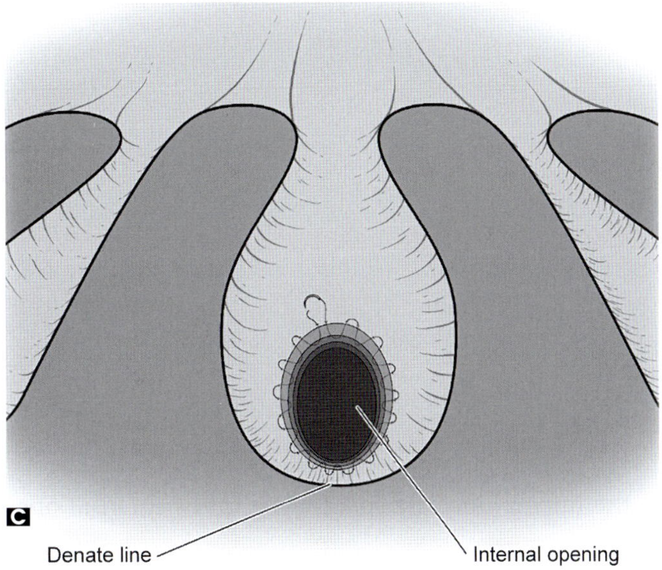

Fig. 6.18(C): Closure of internal opening by purse string suture

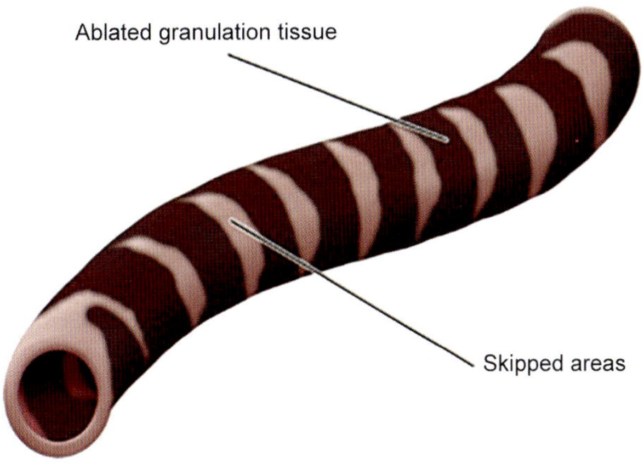

Fig. 6.19: Skip areas. The dark areas show burnt granulation tissue, and the light areas show unburnt skip areas

Scan QR Code for Video on

Fistula Laser Closure (FiLaC)

VIDEO 28

Ligation of Inter-Sphincteric Fistula Tract (LIFT)

Principle

The fistula tract is ligated in the intersphincteric space close to the internal opening with separation of the distal tract.

Instrumentation: Figure 6.10 A-D.

Position of the patient: Lithotomy/Prone

Anaesthesia: Spinal/General/Pudendal nerve block.

Indications

- Trans-sphincteric fistulas

Steps of the Procedure

Step 1: The patient is placed in a prone position, and a metallic half-cut proctoscope is inserted. The external and internal openings are identified by injecting water or a metallic probe from either of the two openings (Fig. 6.20A, B).

Step 2: The intersphincteric groove is palpated, and a curvilinear incision is made at the mucocutaneous junction parallel to the anal canal to enter the intersphincteric space (Fig. 6.20C, D). Dissection is carried out close to the external sphincter to prevent injury to the internal sphincter or breach of the anal mucosa (Fig. 6.20E).

Step 3: The fistula tract is identified, divided, and isolated (Fig. 6.20F). Suture ligations on the distal and proximal ends of the tract are done using 3-0 polyglactin. An additional suture is applied to reinforce tract closure (Fig. 6.20G, H).

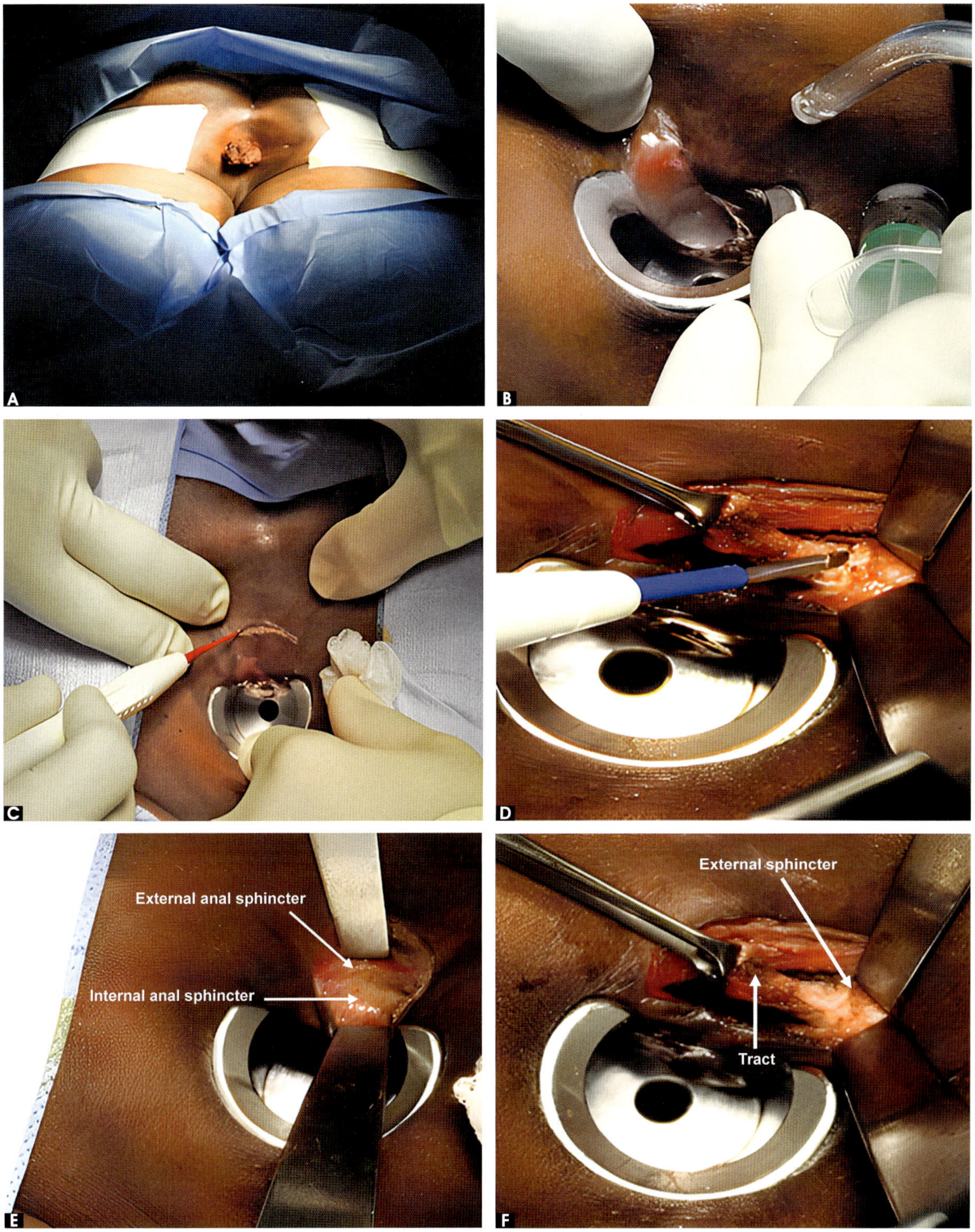

Fig. 6.20(A-F): Ligation of intersphincteric fistula tract. A) Strapping the patient and placing in the prone position. B) Injecting hydrogen peroxide to identify the tract. C) Incision in the intersphincteric space. D) Intersphincteric dissection. E) Dissection of the tract. F) Preparation of the endoloop

Step 4: The fistula tract next to the suture site is divided (Fig. 6.20I). Saline is injected through the external opening after excision of the intersphincteric tract to ensure that the right tract is removed.

Step 5: The internal and external sphincters are approximated again. The surrounding skin is then sutured loosely (Fig. 6.20J, K).

Postoperative images after 2 weeks are shown in Fig. 6.20L, M.

Scan QR Code for Video on
LIFT

VIDEO 29

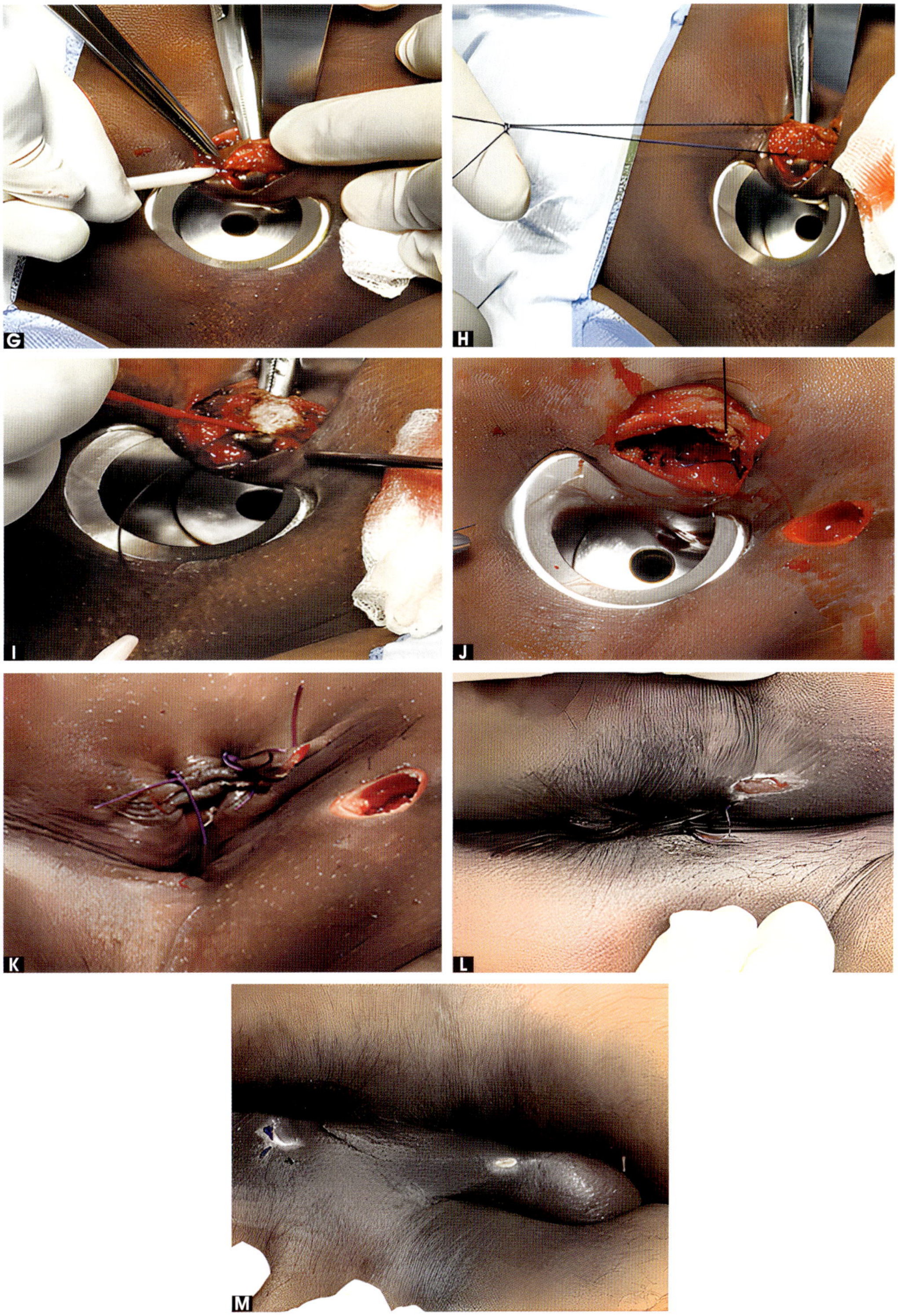

Fig. 6.20(G-M): Ligation of intersphincteric fistula tract. G) Endoloop ligation of the tract. H) Division of the tract. I) Separation of the distal tract. J, K) Approximation of EAS and closure of the LIFT wound. L, M) Postoperative pictures of the patient (procedure, images and video courtesy Dr Parthasarthy, Gem Hospital, Coimbatore)

Submucosal Ligation of Fistula Tract (SLOFT)

Dr D U Pathak from India first described this procedure in 2014.

Principle

To obliterate the internal opening by ligation and separation of the distal tract by disconnecting it near the internal opening (Fig. 6.21).

Indications

- Mature fistula with straight tracts
- In curved and horseshoe tracts, the internal opening can be reached in stages.

Contraindications

- Non -negotiable fistula tract
- High internal opening
- Unable to locate the internal opening
- Friable anorectum secondary to inflammatory bowel disease

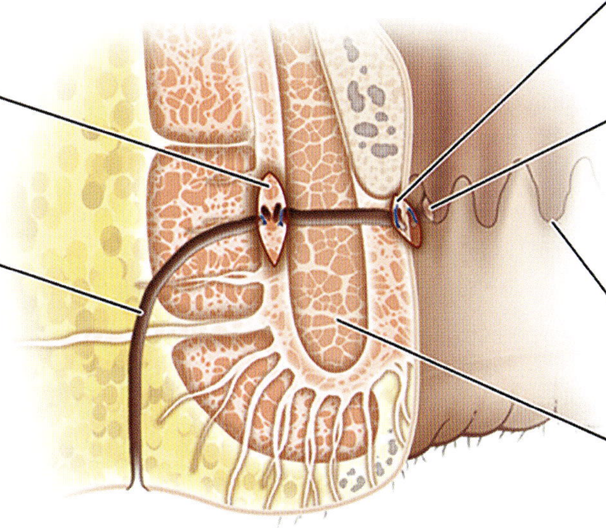

Fig. 6.21: Submucosal ligation of the fistula tract

Steps of the Procedure

Step 1: After identifying the external and internal openings, a malleable metal probe is inserted from the external opening. The probe tip is brought out from the internal opening (Fig. 6.22A).

Step 2: The probe is retained inside the tract, and a circumambulating suture is taken behind the tract to close the internal opening. The stitch is taken as near the internal opening as possible using a 5/8 circle of 27 mm 2-0 polyglactin (Fig. 6.22B).

Step 3: The probe is gently withdrawn before tying the knot. While withdrawing, a sudden jerk indicates that the suture is placed behind the tract (Fig. 6.22C).

Step 4: Normal saline is injected through the external opening to check that the internal opening is duly closed.

Step 4: The probe is re-inserted in the fistula tract, and its tip is palpated nearly 2–3 mm proximal to the internal opening, towards the anal verge. The distal tract is separated at the probe's tip using monopolar cautery, isolating the distal tract containing the cryptoglandular infection (Fig. 6.22D).

Step 5: The normal saline is injected again through the external opening. A free flow of saline indicates the separation of the tract from the internal opening (Fig. 6.22E). One should ensure the tract is completely separated, as a partial separation may lead to recurrence. Finally, the distal tract is curetted, and the external opening is enlarged for drainage. The distal tract may be cored out using FiXcision or laser ablated (Fig. 6.22F, G).

Scan QR Code for Video on
SLOFT

VIDEO 30

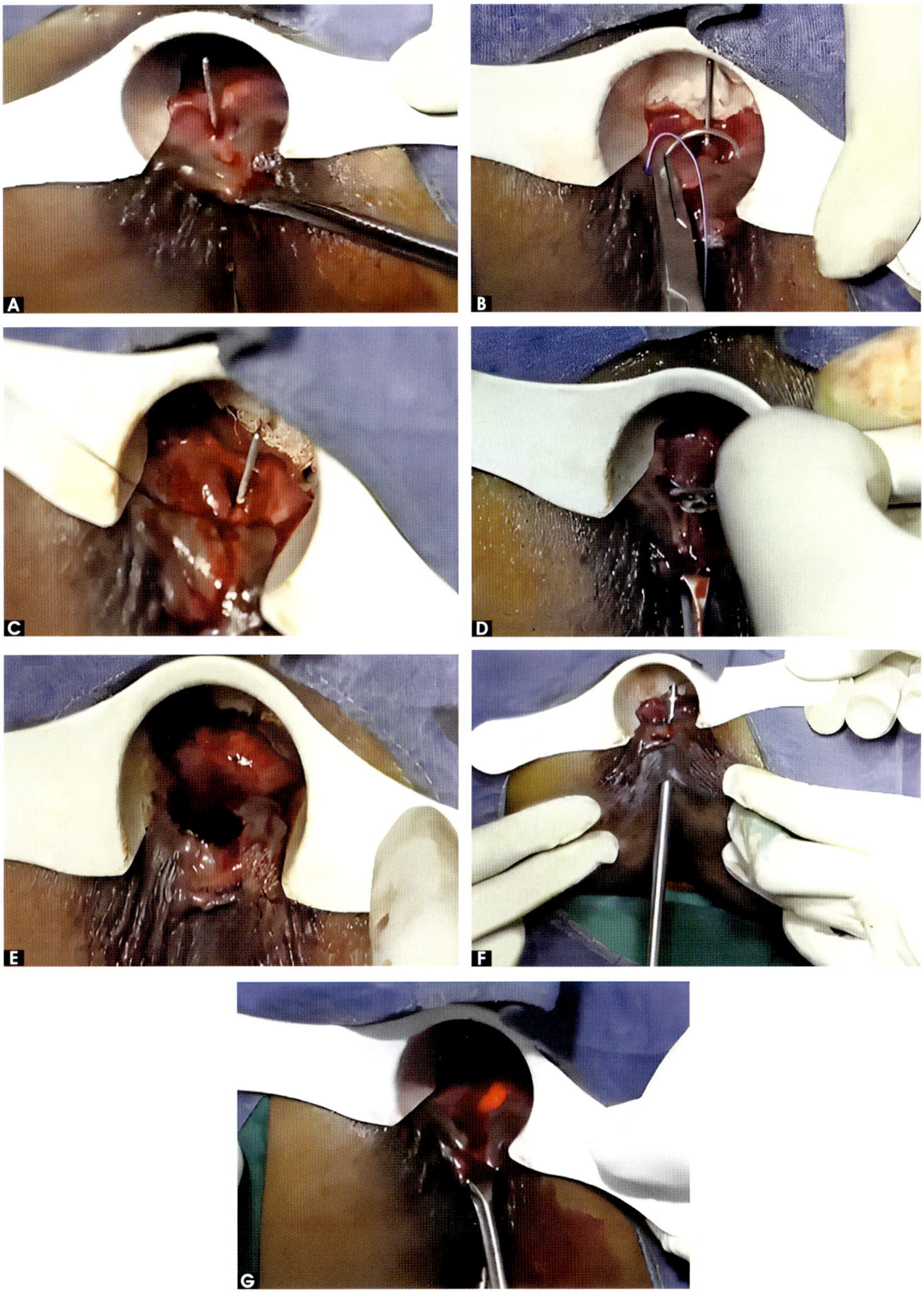

Fig. 6.22(A-G): Submucosal ligation of the fistula tract. A) Insertion of a malleable probe from the external to the internal opening. B) Ligation of the fistula tract near the internal opening. C) Tightening of the knot with gradual withdrawal of the probe. D) Separation of the distal tract. E) Free flow of saline as seen through the separated tract. F) Coring of fistula tract using FiXcision. G) Laser ablation of the distal tract as an alternative

Video-assisted anal Fistula Treatment (VAAFT)

VAAFT was first introduced by P. Meinero in 2006.

Indications

- Acute large anal abscess - ischiorectal, intersphincteric and suprasphincteric
- Superficial and deep postanal abscess
- Anterior abscess
- Mature fistula tract
- Trans-sphincteric high fistula with single or multiple tracts
- Complex fistula (recurrent, horseshoe fistula)
- Fistula extending to retroperitoneum, thigh or anterior abdominal wall
- Diagnostic for fistulas associated with Crohn's, tuberculosis, malignancy and post radiation

Contraindications

- Submucous fistula
- Low perianal fistula
- Immature fistula tract
- Short tract

Instrumentation

Fistuloscope (Fig. 6.23A)

- 8-degree angled eyepiece
- The outer diameter of 3.3 mm at the tip and 4.7 mm at the base.
- Length 18 cm without handle and 14 cm with handle
- The working channel is straight with a diameter of 2.5 mm
- Fibre optic light transmission
- It comes with a handle and is to be inserted with a knob at 9 o'clock; after a click, it is turned to 12 o'clock to lock in place
- The obturator for the endoscope appears as a half-moon at 6 o'clock on the screen. It is used to guide the scope in correct alignment. The fistuloscope should be gripped firmly (Fig. 6.23B)

Grasping forceps (Fig. 6.23C)

Dimensions

- 30 cm length, semi-flexible
- 2 mm diameter

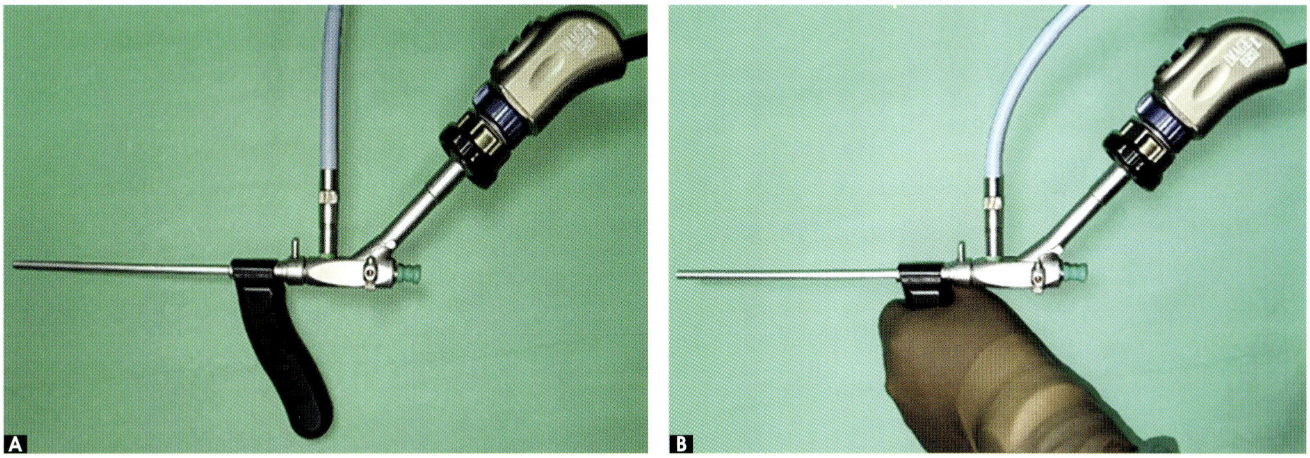

Fig. 6.23A, B: Instrumentation A) Fistuloscope. B) Right way of holding fistuloscope

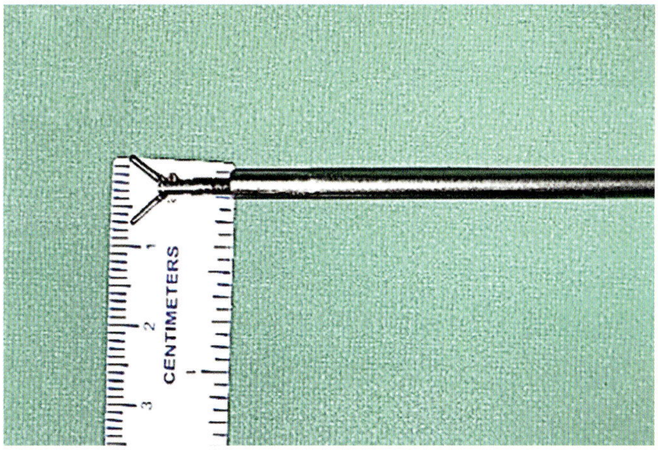

Fig. 6.23C: Grasping forceps

Working of the grasper

- The grasper is inserted through the working channel of the fistuloscope in a closed position (Fig. 6.23D). It is only opened inside the fistula tract when one sees the jaws beyond the scope (Fig. 6.23E). The grasper should never be entered through the fistuloscope with open jaws (Fig. 6.23F).
- Unhealthy tissue is removed from the fistula tract by holding and pulling the tissue with the grasper. The removed necrotic material is dropped inside the lumen of the tract. The irrigation pressure will push out the tissue from the fistula tract.

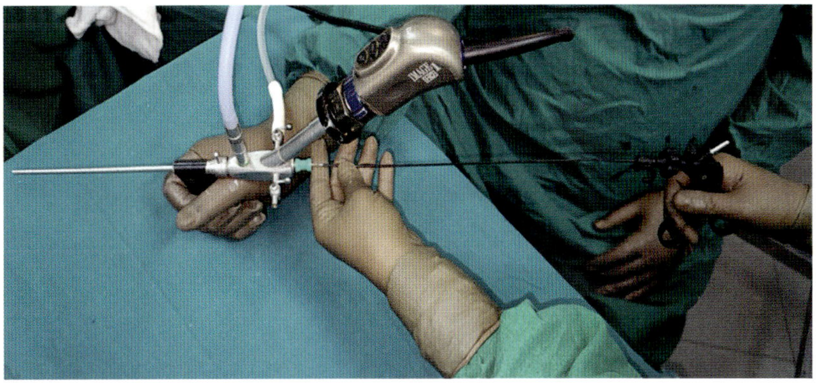

Fig. 6.23D: Insertion of the grasper by an assistant using both hands. One hand guides the tip into the working channel, and the other hand closes the handle, locking the jaw

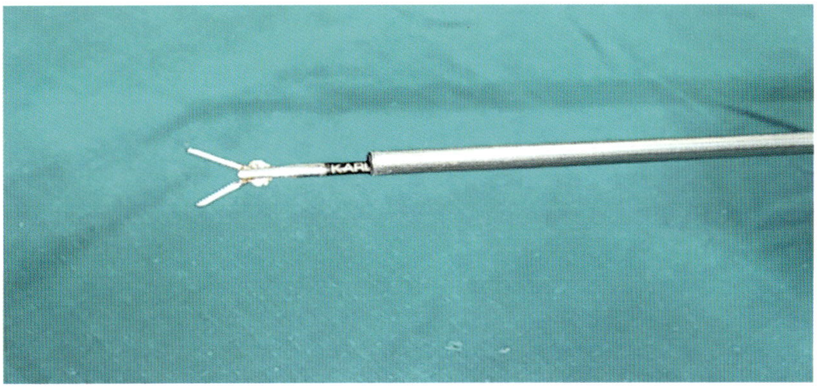

Fig. 6.23E: Opening of the grasper

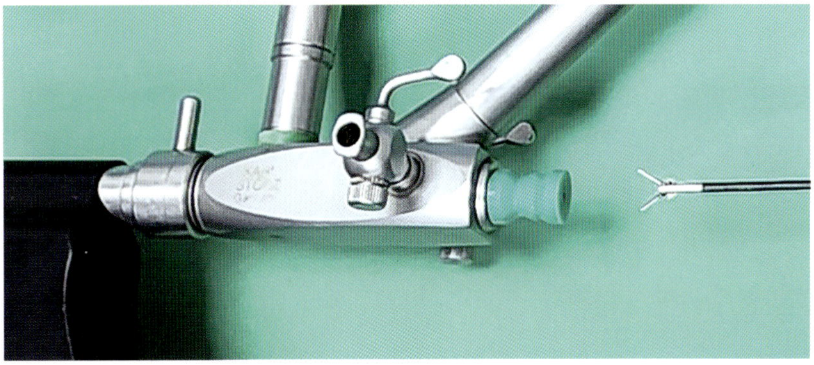

Fig. 6.23F: Do not enter the fistuloscope with an opened grasper

Coagulation Electrode

- 7F with a ball tip for fulguration of the fistula walls
- Insert the coagulation electrode into the working channel of the fistuloscope, and keep pushing till one sees the tip at least 1 cm away from the scope's tip.
- Once the coagulation electrode is activated for fulguration, there should be no in-and-out movement, which can damage the optics (Fig. 6.23G, H, I).

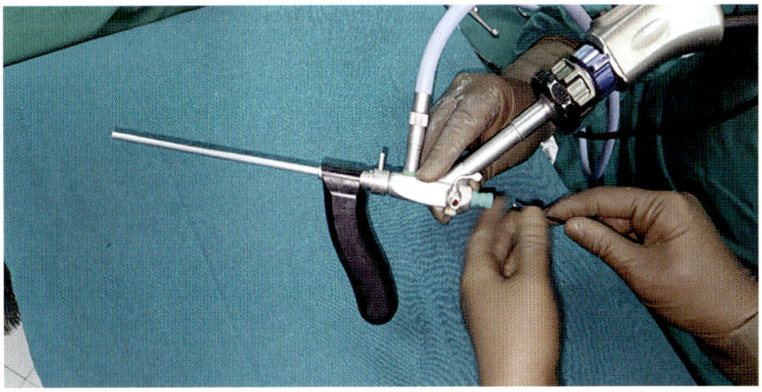

Fig. 6.23G: Insertion of coagulation electrode

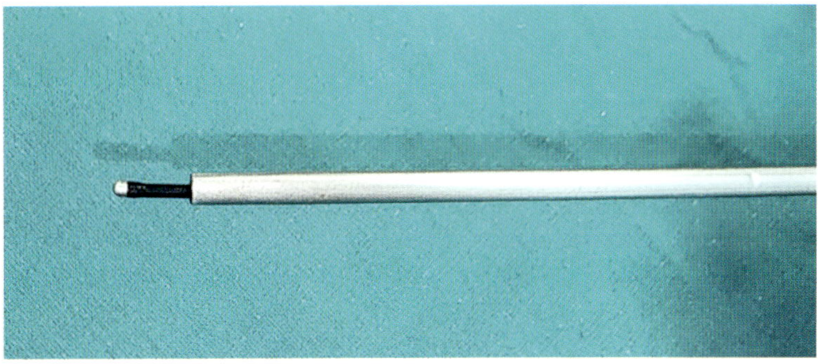

Fig. 6.23H: Electrode tip as seen outside the fistuloscope

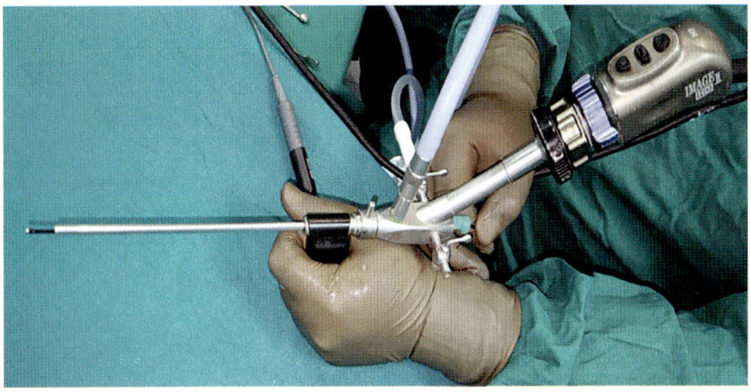

Fig. 6.23.I: Holding the fistuloscope with the electrode inside the working channel

Fistula Brush with Handle

- It has a 3-ring handle with an outer sheath
- 3 brush sizes are available—4 mm, 4.5 mm and 5 mm

Working of the fistula brush

- Insert the brush into the working channel. As the brush assembly is inserted, the outer sheath should not be visible in the tract's field of view.
- With the to and fro movement of the brush, the slough and debris in the tract are cleaned. Progressively increasing brush sizes can be used.

Laser Ablation

Instead of a coagulation electrode, a 360-degree radial fibre can also be used for fulguration (Fig. 6.23J–L). Only the glass part of the fibre tip should be kept outside the fistuloscope. One should be able to see the glass tip from the scope's tip to avoid damage to the optics.

Preoperative Settings of VAAFT Scope

- Laparoscopic camera, fibre optic cable, and light source.
- Fistuloscope (KARL STORZ Tuttingen, Germany).
- Irrigation, 3 litre, 1.5% w/v Glycine plus 100 ml 20% w/v Mannitol.
- Electrocautery, with underwater cutting. The setting of the electrocautery is different for every machine.
- The bucket for the used irrigation fluid is kept on the floor near the surgeon's feet.
- Ideally, surgeons should wear boots and a plastic gown.
- The operation table should be kept with the head side lowered by 15 degrees.
- If the external opening is located far posteriorly, inserting the fistuloscope through the external opening with the patient in the lithotomy position is difficult. It is prudent to place the patient in a prone position and strap the buttocks with a lateral pull.

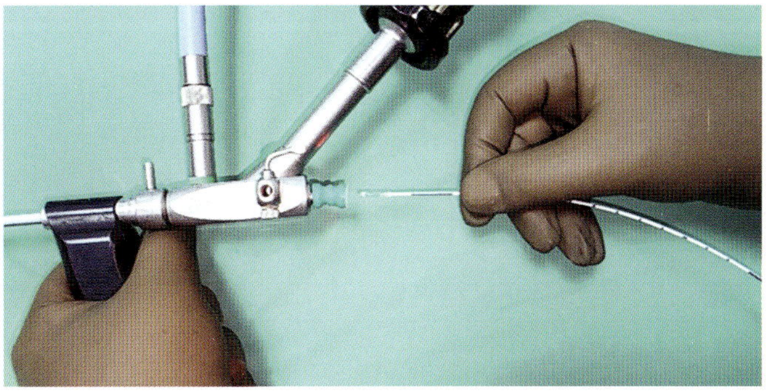

Fig. 6.23J: Entry of laser into the working channel

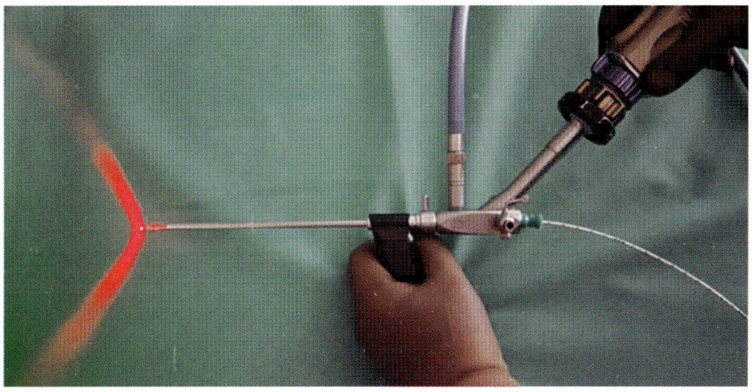

Fig. 6.23K: Laser beam as seen through the fistuloscope tip

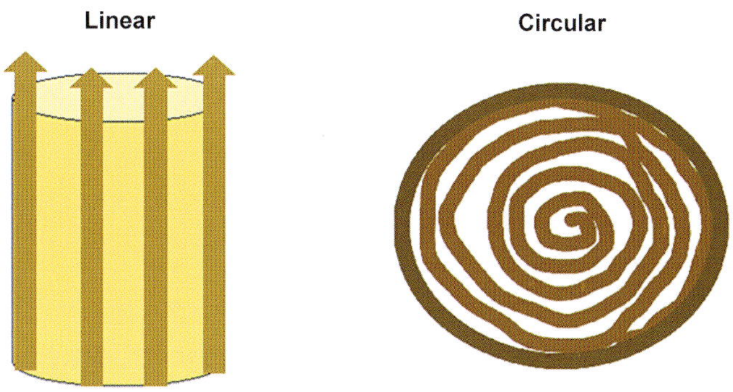

Fig. 6.23L: Burnt pattern of a fistula tract, from internal to external opening. With coagulation electrode, it is linear and with laser fibre, it is radial

Diagnostic Phase

Aim

- Identify the internal opening
- Look for secondary tracts
- Identify the abscess cavity

Step 1: The scope is entered through the external opening and kept at the edge for 5 minutes, with continuous irrigation to dilate the tract (Fig. 6.24A, B). It is then gently advanced. Once the tract is visible, the field is kept in the centre. The scope is directed towards the internal opening, and the secondary tracts or abscess cavities are identified (Fig. 6.24C).

Step 2: On entering the internal opening, one can see the scope's light at the dentate line (Fig. 6.24D). If the fibre optic light is seen higher than the dentate line, it indicates that one is in the wrong plane or a false tract has been created. The debris can be seen in the fistula tract (Fig. 6.24E).

Therapeutic Phase

Step 3: The grasper is inserted through the working channel for debridement. The unhealthy granulation tissue is grasped by pulling and rotating the grasper. If a large piece of tissue is to be removed, it is advisable to remove the whole fistuloscope rather than just the grasper. The tip of the grasper is cleaned with a wet gauze.

Step 4: The coagulation electrode is inserted through the working channel, and the tract is fulgurated (Fig. 6.24F). Alternatively, a 360-degree radial laser fibre can be used. The tract is irrigated to remove the fulgurated tissue. The brush is used to clean the debris (Fig. 6.24G).

Step 5: The internal opening is closed using a fish eye technique (Fig. 6.24H). The mucosa, submucosa and the fibres of the internal anal sphincter are taken, and the internal opening is closed using 2-0 Polyglactin.

Step 6: The external opening is widened up to 5 mm for drainage.

The completely healed wound is shown in Fig. 6.24I.

Scan QR Code for Video on

Ligation of Fistula Tract with Video assisted Laser Ablation of Fistula Tract

VIDEO 31

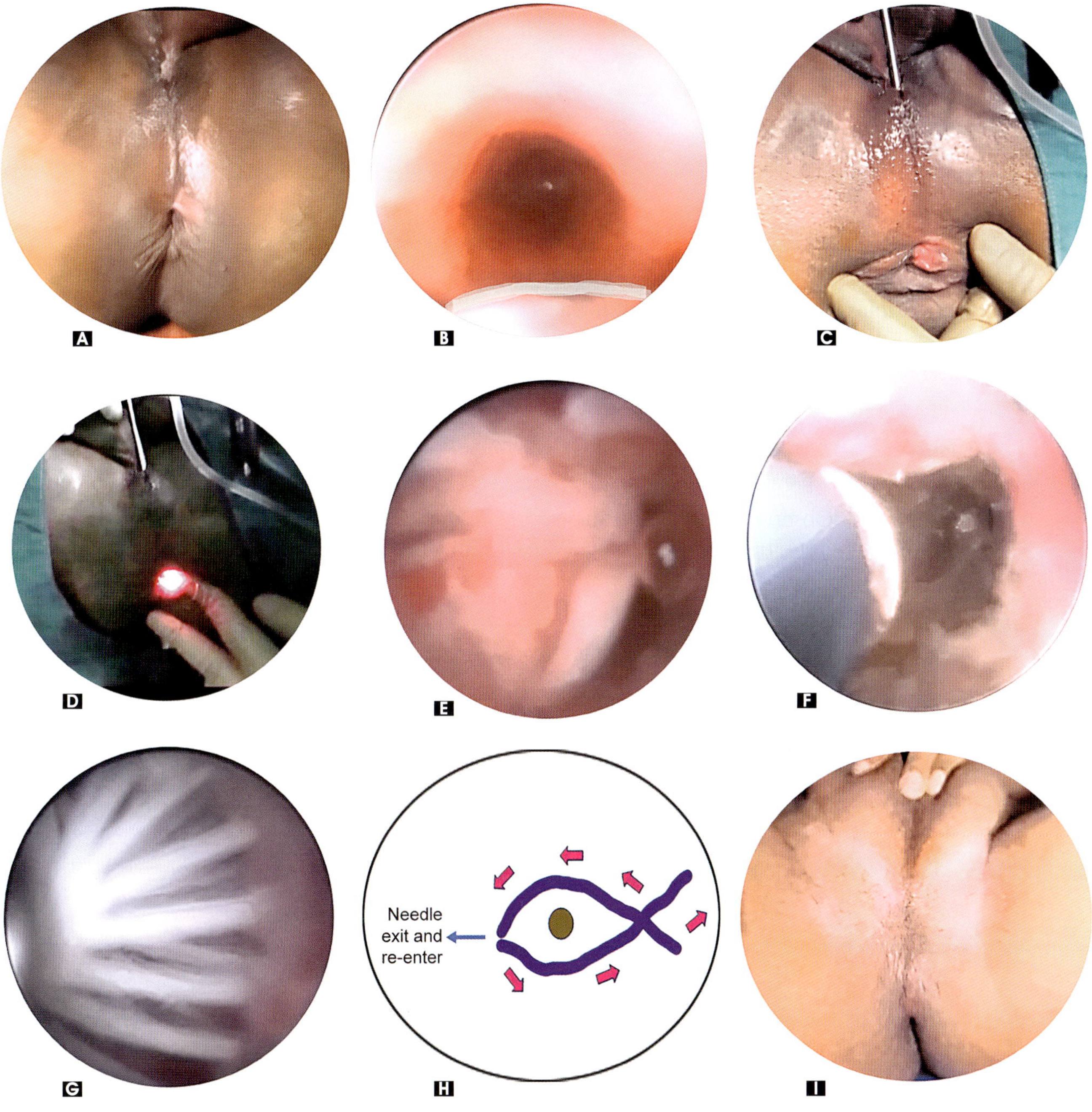

Fig. 6.24(A-I): Technique of VAAFT. A) Preoperative image showing external opening at the base of the scrotum and the internal opening at 12 0'clock. B) Dilated fistula tract after inserting the fistuloscope and irrigating for 5 minutes. C) Scope directed towards the internal opening. D) Illumination of scope as seen at the internal opening at the dentate line. E) Presence of debris in the tract. F) Fulguration of debris with coagulation electrode. G) Removing the debris with a brush. H) Closure of the internal opening with the fish eye technique. I) Final image as seen after complete healing of the wound

Tips and Tricks

1. One finds the fistuloscope in the ischiorectal fossa

It means that the fistula tract has been breached. One sees only fat all around. The irrigant glycine and mannitol have leaked into the ischiorectal fossa. The buttocks become tense and edematous.

This happens when the fistula tract is immature(recently drained abscess).

How to manage?

- If this has happened, then abort the procedure.
- Turn off the irrigation. Observe from the skin surface where the scope tip is located. Withdraw the scope and press out the fluid from the buttocks. Going forward with VAAFT will cause further collection. Do an alternate procedure.

2. One is unable to cauterize the walls

Sometimes the lateral wall seems so distant that cauterizing the walls becomes tedious.

How to manage?

- Stop the irrigation.
- Cauterize or laser ablate while withdrawing.

3. One cannot progress as the tract does not dilate or there is an instrument in the working channel

How to manage?

- Attach a pathfinder to the irrigation line, and pump it when one wants to progress.
- Increase the pressure on the glycine bottle by elevating it or pumping air into it.
- Keeping the working channel empty while progressing.

4. Unable to reach the internal opening

- From within the anal canal, look for the fistuloscope light or the site of irrigation fluid coming into the anus.

5. The probe passes from the external to the internal opening, but the fistuloscope does not

It means that the tract is narrow.

How to manage?

- Allow time and pressure of the irrigant to dilate the tract.
- Alternatively, pass the smallest Hegar from the internal to the external opening to dilate the tract.

FISTULA PLUG

Biological plugs are designed from lyophilized porcine small intestinal submucosa. They act as a strong scaffold for the growth of the fibroblasts and promote the in-growth of native tissues.

Types of Fistula Plugs Available

Currently, there are two commercially fistula plugs which are approved by the FDA. They both vary in design and material.

- Cook Surgisis AFP™ (Cook Surgical Inc., Bloomington, IN).
- Gore Bio-A fistula plug (a product from WL Gore Corporation, Newark, DE).

Indications

- Trans-sphincteric/Suprasphincteric/Extrasphincteric fistula.
- Ano-vaginal fistula.

Contraindications

- Small intersphincteric fistula
- Failure to identify the internal opening
- Acute abscess cavity
- Actively pus draining fistula
- Multiple branching fistula

Position of the patient: Lithotomy

Type of anaesthesia: Spinal/General

Preoperative preparation: Two tablets of bisacodyl one night prior and one dose of antibiotic half an hour before the surgery.

Steps of the Procedure

Step 1: Both the external and the internal openings are identified. The tract is cleaned with a fistula brush or a curette and irrigated with normal saline (Fig. 6.25A, B).

Step 2: A probe is passed from the internal opening and taken out through the external opening (Fig. 6.25C). A thread is tied to the eye of the probe and passed through the tract (Fig. 6.25D).

Step 3: The plug is taken out from the sterile pack and hydrated with sterile saline for 1–3 minutes. The plug is tied with one end of a thread towards the internal opening.

Step 4: The plug is pulled inside the tract with tail-first till resistance is felt (Fig. 6.25E). Once the plug buries in the internal opening (Fig. 6.25F), it is trimmed up to the mucosa level, and fixed with a suture, using 2-0 Polyglactin, taking a figure of 8 stitch.

Step 5: The outer end of the plug is trimmed, leaving the external opening open for drainage (Fig. 6.25G).

A completely healed fistula is shown in Fig. 6.25H.

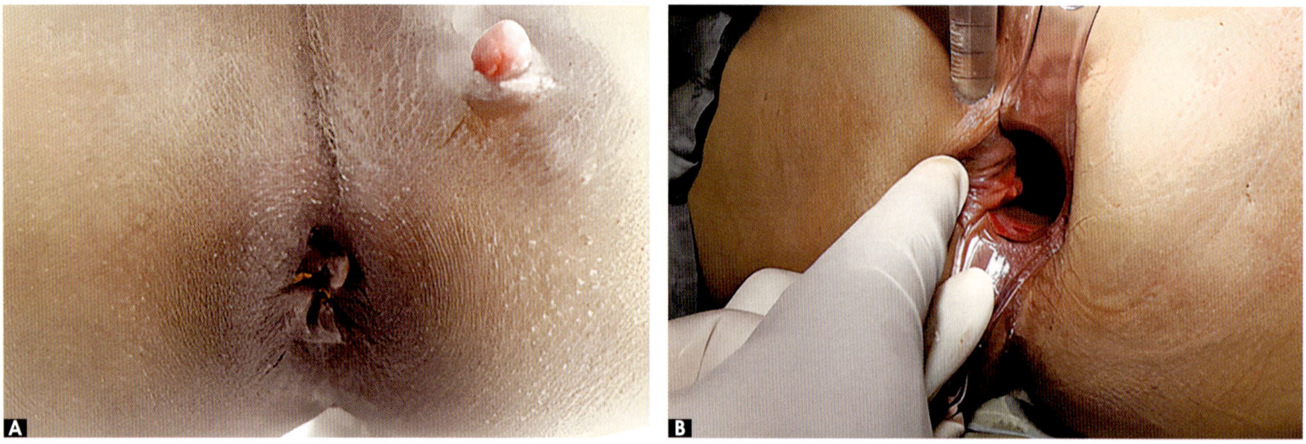

Fig. 6.25A-B: The technique of fistula plug. A) Trans-sphincteric anal fistula. B) Washing of fistula plug after curetting

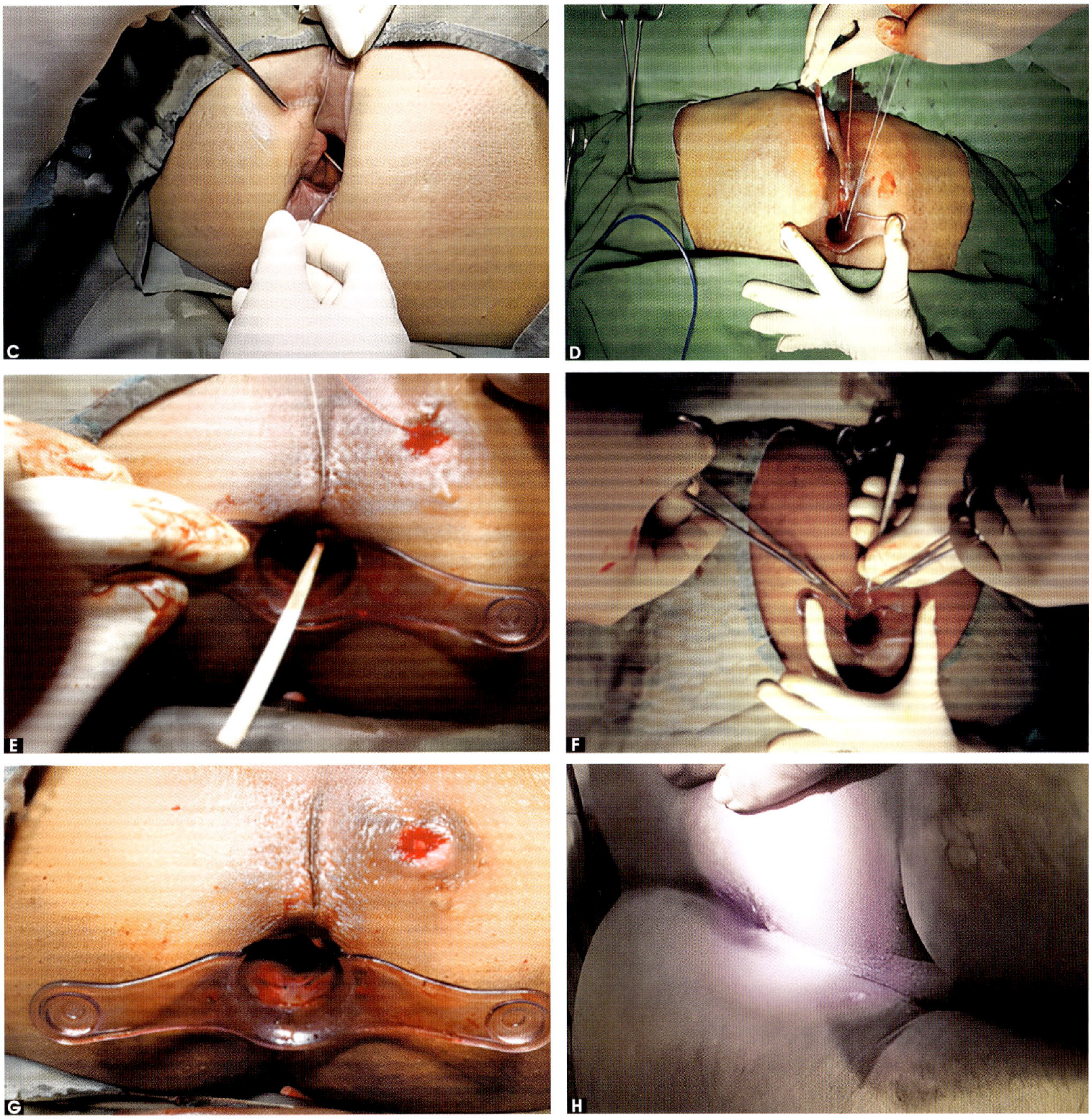

Fig. 6.25C-H: The technique of fistula plug. C) Probing of fistula tract. D) Pulling of thread through fistula probe. E) Pulling of fistula plug inside, after tying with the thread. F) Internal fixation of the plug. G) Flush cutting of fistula plug with the external opening. H) Completely healed fistula. (Procedure, images and video courtesy: Dr Ashish Ganatra, Rajkot)

Tips and Tricks

- Proper anatomical delineation of the tract after a good endorectal USG or MRI fistulogram is necessary.
- Accurate identification of the internal opening.
- If there is acute sepsis or an abscess cavity, a draining seton should be placed for three months for tract maturation.
- Thorough debridement of the tract using a scoop or a fistula brush, and cleaning with normal saline and hydrogen peroxide, is a must before placing the plug.
- Before placing the plug, sending the scrappings from the fistula tract for biopsy and culture to rule out tuberculosis is important.

HYBRID PROCEDURES

Hybrid procedures are minimally invasive tailor-made procedures which combine two or more surgical techniques to yield a better outcome. Although lasers have become popular, the role of lasers in anal fistulas is limited. In our practice, lasers are used mainly for ablating long distal tracts for managing the intersphincteric or trans-sphincteric extensions, where sphincter cutting after a certain level may lead to incontinence.

Although many procedures can be combined with lasers, the most important procedures are:

- Distal coring with proximal fistulotomy (DCPF), where the internal opening is excised by Park's technique and the distal tract is cored out after laser ablation. The role of lasers in this technique is limited to shrinkage of the distal tract. The distal tracts, which are 5 cm long and 5 mm in diameter, are cored out using FiXcision. The tracts which are more than 5 cm in length and 5 mm in diameter are curetted and laser ablated after removal of the primary source of infection (excision of internal opening, opening of intersphincteric and deep intersphincteric spaces). The tracts can be left to heal by secondary intention.
- Distal laser proximal LIFT (DLPL) is a technique where subsequent to LIFT, the distal tract is laser ablated.
- Distal coring or laser ablation following SLOFT (DLPS or DCPS) is another technique where subsequent to SLOFT, the distal tract is laser ablated or cored out.

Similarly, more hybrid procedures can also be attempted. One must know that in all hybrid procedures, the crucial step is to tackle the primary source of infection, and lasers have no significant role.

Hybrid Procedures—When and Why?

When?

- All complex fistulas can be treated with Hybrid procedures

Why?

- To tackle the internal opening more precisely
- To obliterate the fistula tract with the least sphincter cutting
- To create less raw areas, especially in long tracts.

When not to use lasers?

- Fistula associated with an abscess.

Principle of Different Procedures while Using Hybrid Techniques

- *Fistulotomy:* To lay open the fistula tract with the healing of the fistulotomy wound by secondary intention.
- *FiXcision:* To core out the infected distal tract extending from the fistulotomy wound to the external opening (Fig. 6.26).
- *Laser:* To ablate the unhealthy granulation tissue and shrinkage of the tract. The diameter of the tract is reduced, making it easier to core out without creating large raw areas.

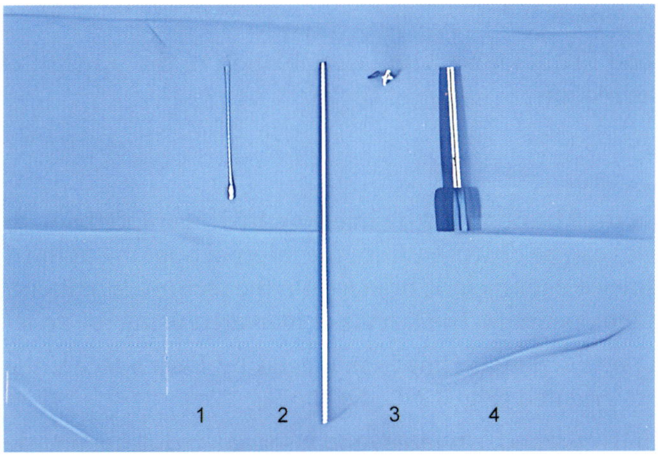

Fig. 6.26: Parts of FiXcision. 1) Malleable probe. 2) Shaft. 3) Button. 4) Cutter

Based on the classification of fistulas, a few cases commonly seen in practice are discussed.

Managing A3 Intersphincteric Fistula in Ano

A3 type of intersphincteric fistula with the internal opening at the dentate line and an upward extension opening into the rectum.

Instrumentation: Figure 6.10 A-D

Preoperative preparation: Two bisacodyl tablets one night prior and intravenous antibiotics 30 minutes before surgery.

Position of the patient: Lithotomy

Type of anaesthesia: Spinal/General.

Procedure performed: Low-end fistulolotmy with laser ablation of the upward extension and closure of the upper internal opening in the rectum.

Steps of the Procedures

Step 1: The path of the fistula tract is identified by injecting hydrogen peroxide through the external opening of the fistula tract. The bubbles can be observed from the internal opening at the dentate line and the opening of the upward extension of the intersphincteric branch into the rectum. A half-cut proctoscope is inserted into the anal canal to locate both the openings. The tract is demarcated using methylene blue (Fig. 6.27A, B).

Step 2: The internal opening at the dentate line is managed by Park's technique. The deep intersphincteric space is opened, curetted and irrigated (Fig. 6.27C, D).

Step 3: The upward extension is curetted, irrigated, and laser ablated using 360-degree radial fibre (Fig. 6.27E, F, G). The laser energy is given upto 12 watts per second per mm. The mode set is continuous to ensure efficient ablation and destruction of the unhealthy granulation tissue.

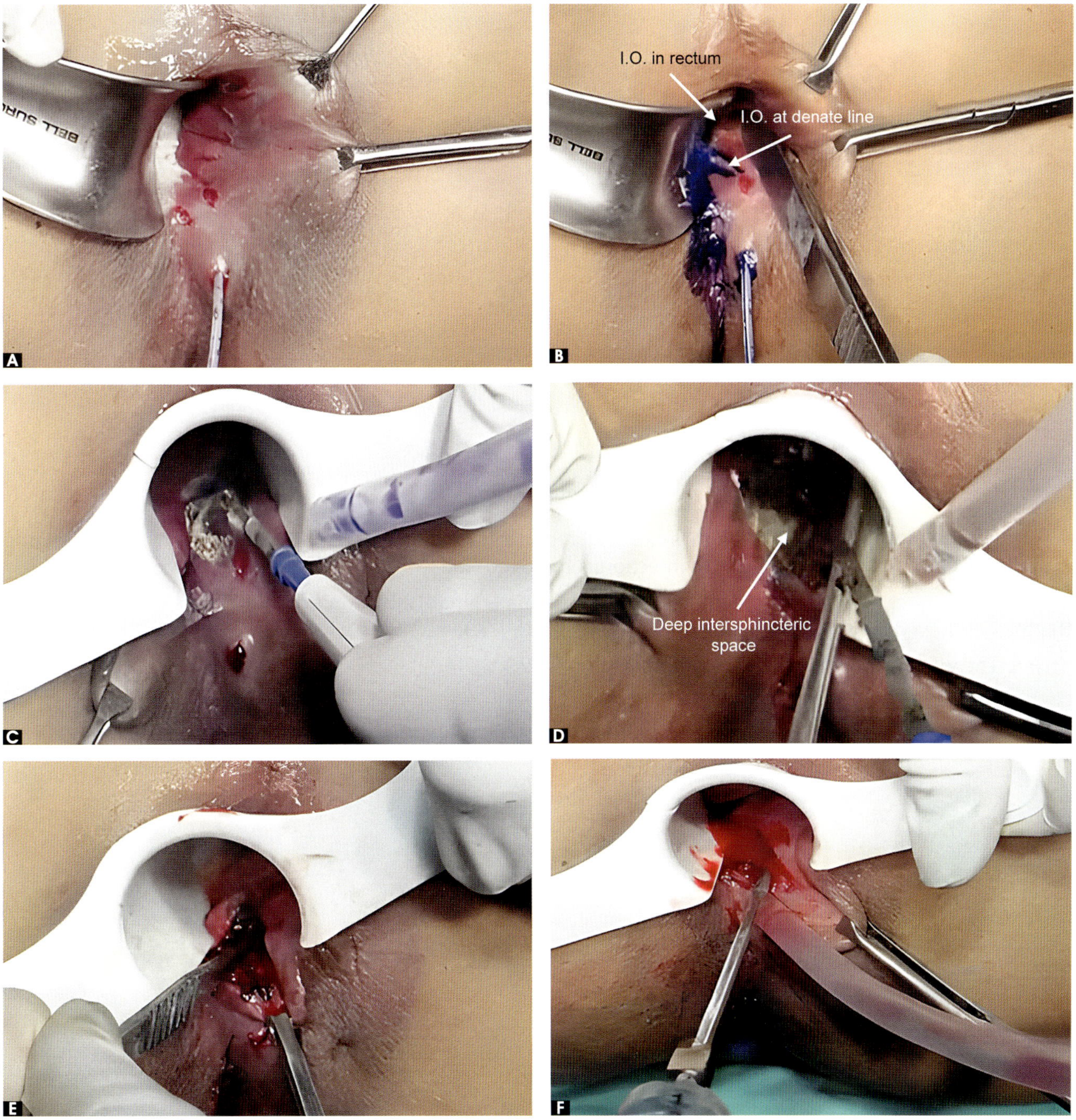

Fig. 6.27(A-F): Managing A3 type of fistula. A, B) Injecting hydrogen peroxide and methylene blue to identify the internal opening and course of fistula tract. C) Excision of the internal opening using Park's technique D) Opening, curetting and irrigation of deep intersphincteric space. E, F) Curetting, irrigation, and laser ablation of intersphincteric extension

Step 4: The opening in the distal rectum is closed using Vicryl 2-0 (Fig. 6.27H). The closure of the rectal opening is optional. Once the primary source of infection is removed, the extensions heal on their own.

Step 5: As the tract associated with intersphincteric fistula is small, a low-end fistulotomy is done to lay open the tract, followed by curretting and irrigation (Fig. 6.27I, J, K).

Step 6: The wound margins are marsupialized (Fig. 6.27L).

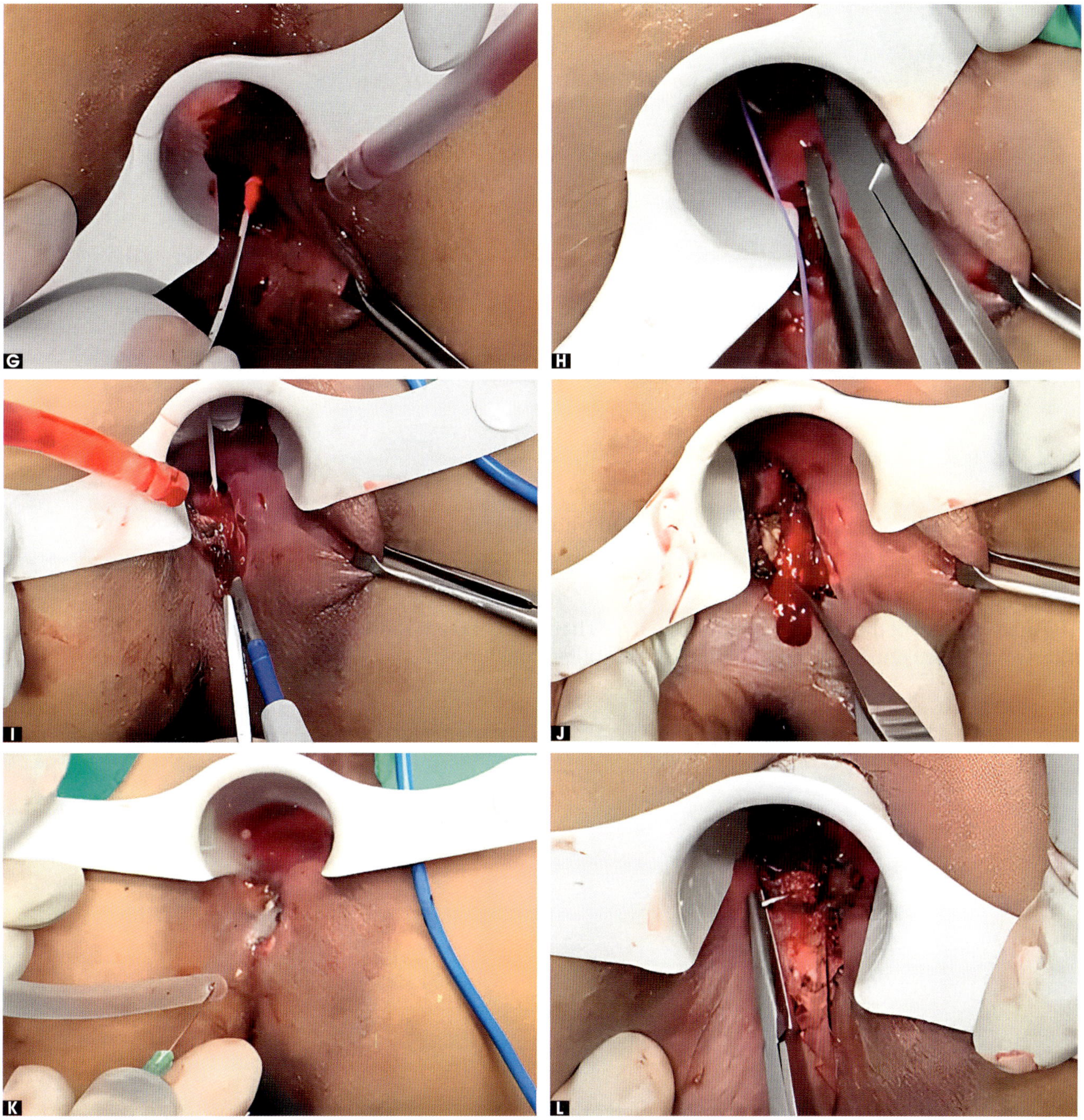

Fig. 6.27(G-L): Managing A3 type of fistula. G) Curetting, irrigation, and laser ablation of intersphinctric extension. H) Closure of internal opening with Vicryl 2-0. I, J, K) Low-end fistulotomy followed by curetting and irrigation. L) Marsupialization of the wound

Step 7: Local infiltration of bupivacaine 0.5% and pudendal nerve block is given (Fig. 6.27M, N, O).

Management of A4 Fistula

The management of the A4 has been covered in the chapter of paraanal and pararectal spaces, under the heading, intersphincteric fistula with communicating A4 intersphincteric fistula.

Scan QR Code for Video on
Intersphincteric Fistula Type A3
VIDEO 32

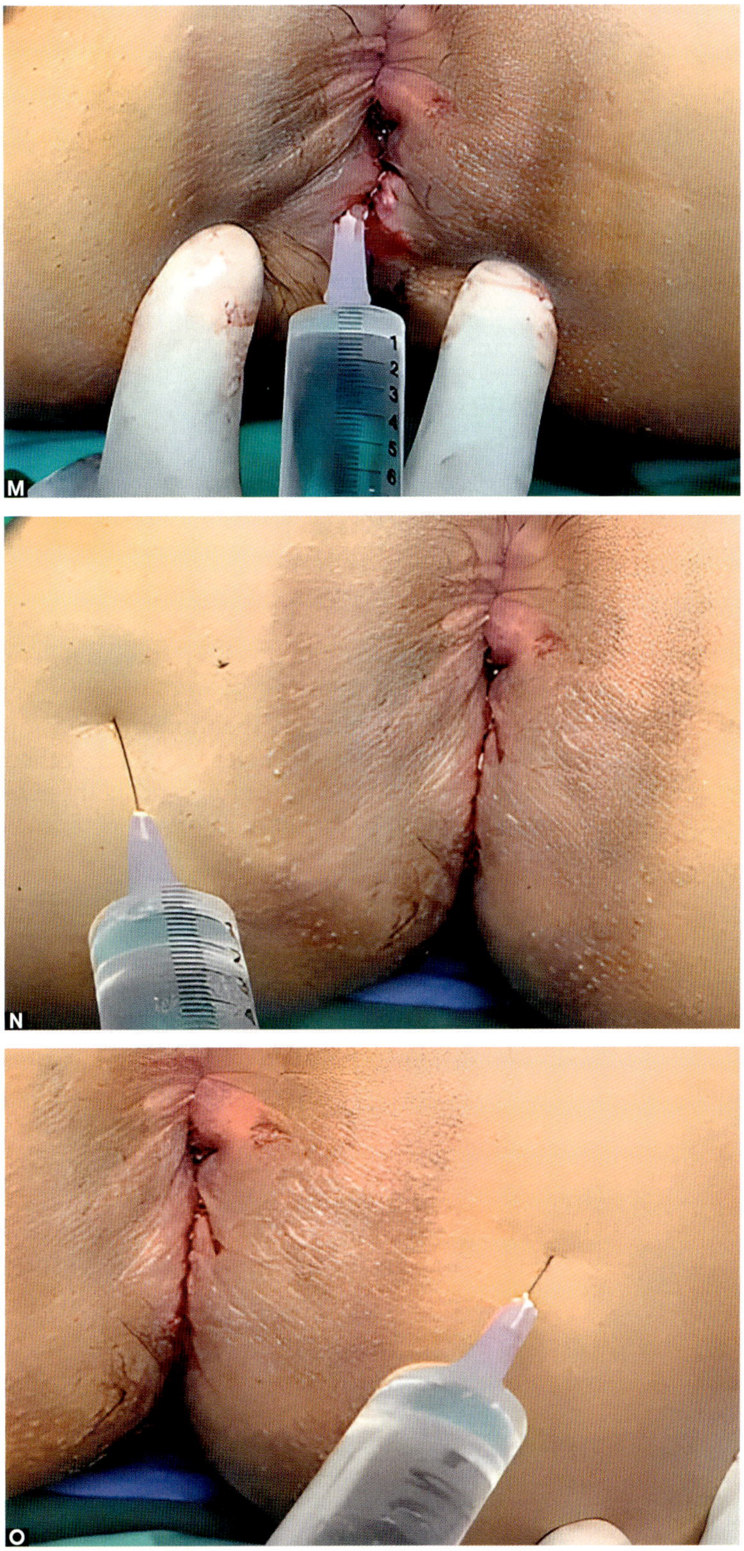

Fig. 6.27(M-O): Managing A3 type of fistula. M, N, O) Local infiltration of bupivacaine 0.5% and pudendal nerve block

Managing Trans-sphincteric Fistula (B2)

The trans-sphincteric fistula is associated with an extension.

Instrumentation: Figure 6.10A-D

Preoperative preparation: Two bisacodyl tablets one night prior and intravenous antibiotics 30 minutes before surgery.

Position of the patient: Lithotomy

Type of anaesthesia: Spinal/General.

Procedure performed: Proximal fistulotomy (from the dentate line up to the anal verge) with laser ablation of the trans-sphincteric fistula tract and intersphincteric extension.

The principle of combining both techniques is the same as mentioned in A3 intersphincteric fistula. As mentioned earlier, it is important to assess the amount of sphincter involved in the trans-sphincteric fistula. Although no clear-cut method can estimate the exact amount of sphincter involved, with experience and preoperative MRI evaluation, one can assess and decide the amount of sphincter to be cut.

Steps of the Procedures

Step 1: The path of the fistula tract is identified by injecting hydrogen peroxide through the external opening. Bubbles can be observed from the internal opening. A half-cut proctoscope is inserted into the anal canal. The tract is demarcated using methylene blue (Fig. 6.28A, B).

Step 2: The internal opening is excised by Park's technique (Fig. 6.28C). The wound is thoroughly irrigated (Fig. 6.28D). The deep intersphincteric space is opened, and methylene blue-stained extensions, if any, are identified and excised (Fig. 6.28E).

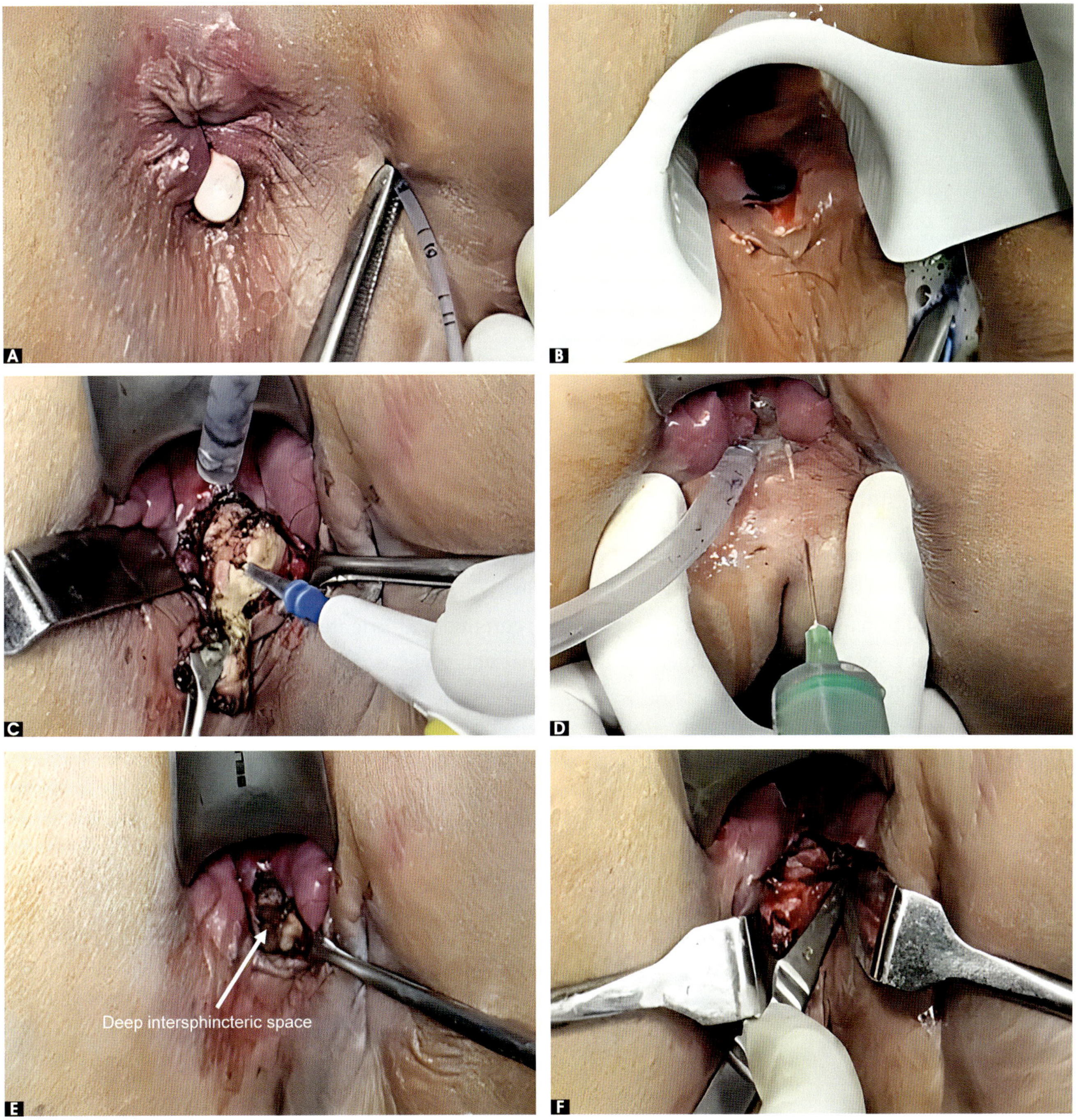

Fig. 6.28A-F: Managing trans-sphincteric fistula (B2). A, B) Injecting hydrogen peroxide and methylene blue to identify the internal opening and course of the fistula tract. C) Excision of the internal opening using Park's technique. D) Thorough irrigation of the wound. E) Opening of the deep intersphincteric space and excision of methylene blue-stained extensions, if any. F) Curetting, irrigation and laser ablation of the intersphincteric extension

Step 3: The trans-sphincteric fistula mentioned here has an intersphincteric extension which can easily be identified by methylene blue stained unhealthy granulation tissue. The extension is curetted, irrigated, and laser ablated (Fig. 6.28F, G, H). After laser ablation, the extension is again curetted and irrigated to remove the ablated necrotic material (Fig. 6.28I). Alternatively, the intersphincteric space can be opened up to the anorectal ring.

Step 4: The distal trans-sphincteric tract is laser ablated, curetted and irrigated (Fig. 6.28J).

Step 5: Proximal fistulotomy is performed up to the anal verge Fig. 6.28K). The margins of the wound are marsupialized (Fig. 6.28L).

Scan QR Code for Video on

Type B2 Trans-sphincteric Fistula with Underlying Abscess

VIDEO 33

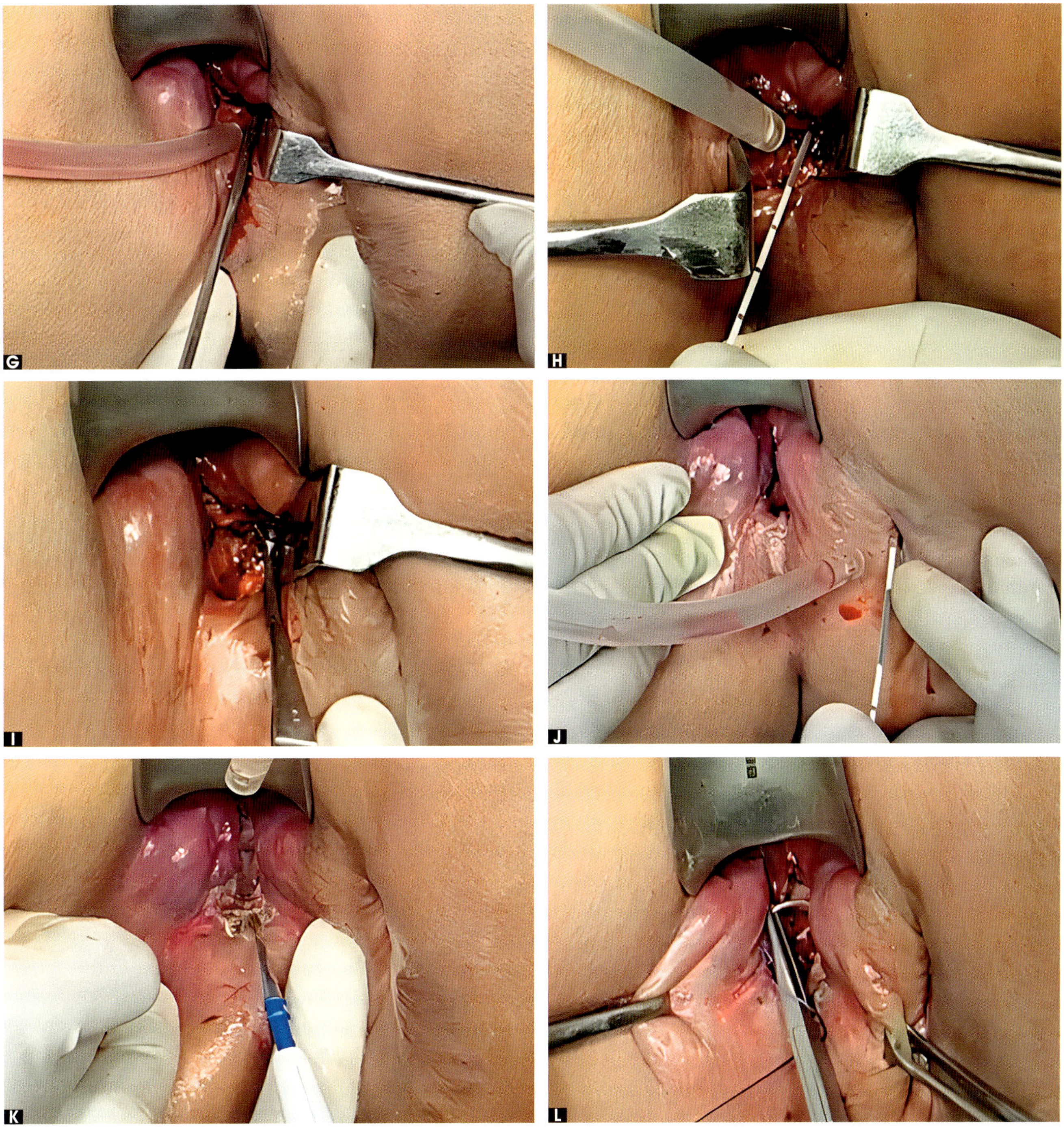

Fig. 6.28G-L: Managing trans-sphincteric fistula (B2). G, H) Curetting, irrigation and laser ablation of the intersphincteric extension. I) Curetting and irrigation of the extension after laser ablation to remove the ablated necrotic material. J) Laser ablation, curetting, and irrigation of the distal trans-sphincteric tract. K) Proximal fistulotomy up to the anal verge. L) Marsupialization of the margins of the wound

Step 6: Local infiltration of bupivacaine 0.5% and pudendal nerve block is given (Fig. 6.28M, N, O, P).

Managing Anterior Fistula in Females

The anterior fistula in females is complex and should be operated on carefully because of the presence of the perineal body. The integrity of the perineal body is important for maintaining continence and preventing pelvic organ prolapse (Fig. 6.29).

Instrumentation: Figure 6.10A-D

Preoperative preparation: Two bisacodyl tablets one night prior and intravenous antibiotics 30 minutes before surgery.

Position of the patient: Lithotomy

Type of anaesthesia: Spinal/General.

Procedure performed: Distal coring with proximal fistulotomy and laser ablation (DCPF).

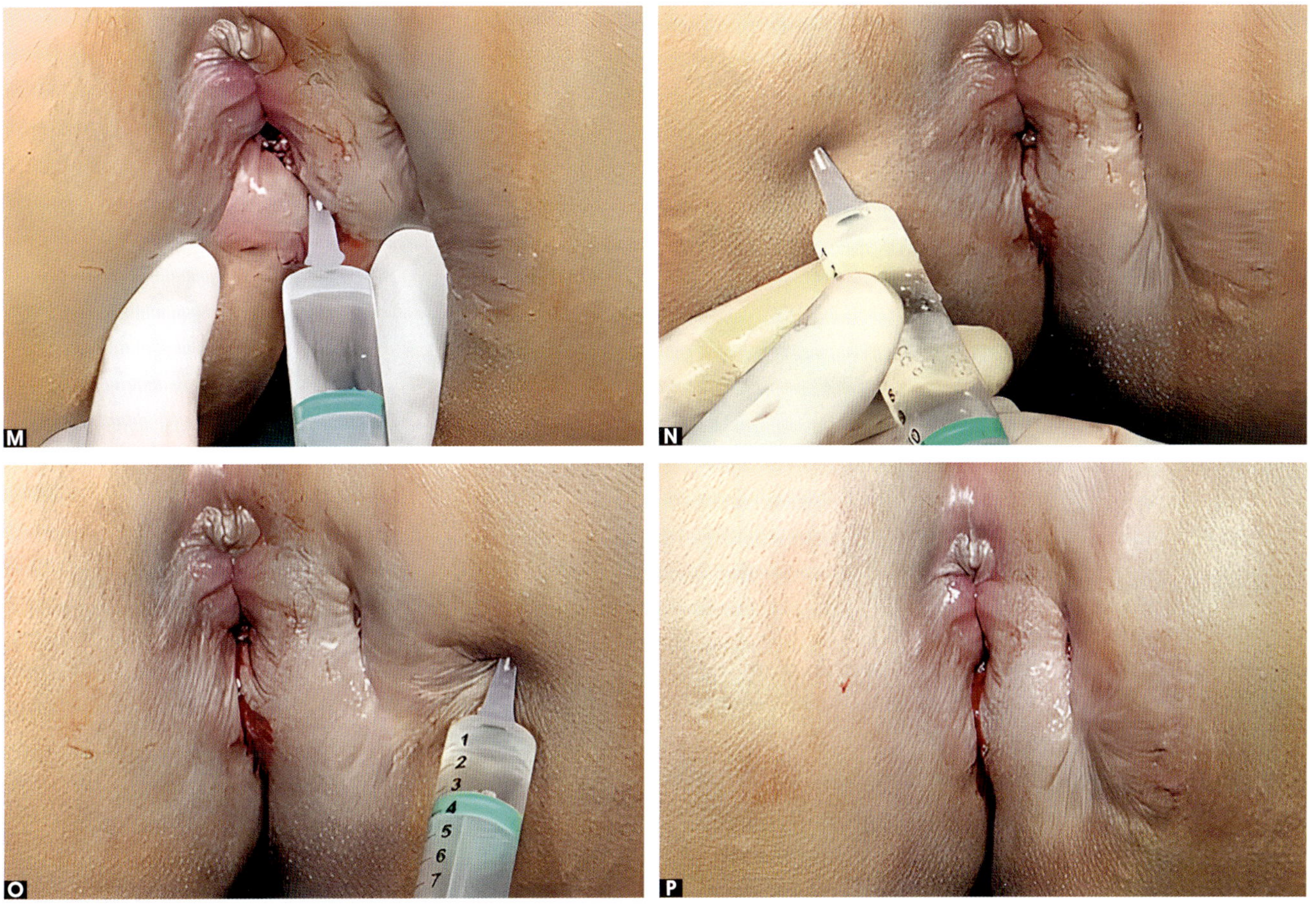

Fig. 6.28M-P: Managing trans-sphincteric fistula (B2). M, N, O) Local infiltration of bupivacaine 0.5% and pudendal nerve block. P) Final wound picture

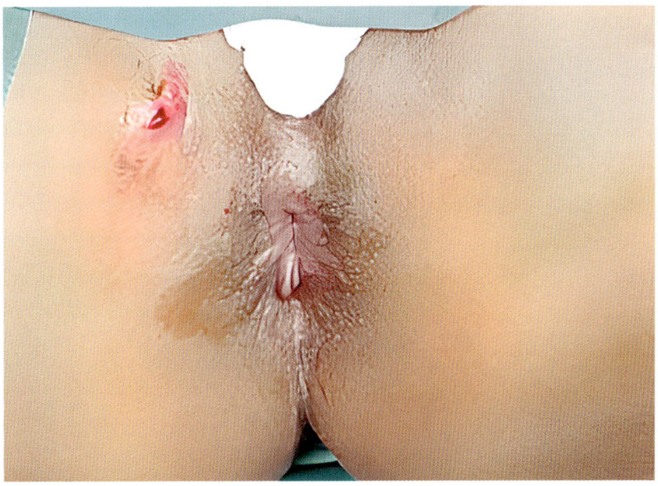

Fig. 6.29: Anterior fistula in females

Steps of the Procedure

Step 1: The course of the fistula tract is identified by injecting hydrogen peroxide through the external opening of the fistula tract. Bubbles can be observed from the internal opening. The tract is demarcated using methylene blue. A half-cut proctoscope is inserted into the anal canal to know the exact location of the internal opening (Fig. 6.29A, B).

Step 2: Internal opening is excised by Park's technique (Fig. 6.29C). The deep intersphincteric space is opened, curetted and irrigated.

Step 3: A 360-degree radial fibre is inserted into the fistula tract, and the tract is laser-ablated (Fig. 6.29D).

Step 4: After the laser ablation, the tract is curetted to remove ablated unhealthy tissue. Irrigation is done with normal saline. This step aims to cleanse the tract by removing debris of ablated tissue.

Step 5: The distal tract is cored out using fixcision (Fig. 6.29E). The cored-out fistula tract is shown in Fig. 6.29F.

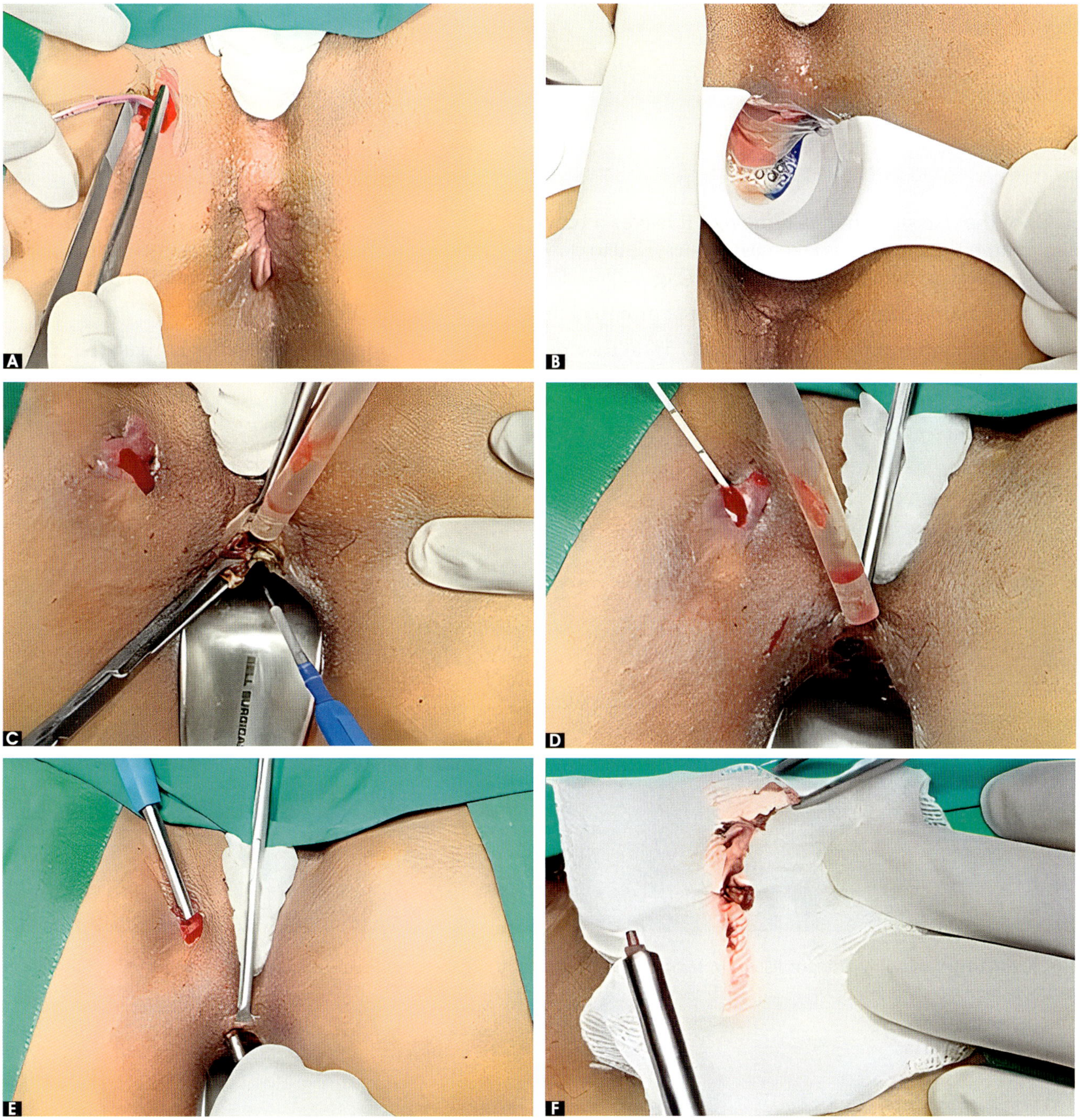

Fig. 6.29(A-F): Managing anterior fistula in females. A, B) Injecting hydrogen peroxide and methylene blue to identify the internal opening and course of the fistula tract. C) Excision of the internal opening using Park's technique. D) Laser ablation of the fistula tract using a 360-degree radial fibre. E) Coring of the distal tract using fixcision. F) Cored out fistula tract

Once the fixcision shaft is removed, it leaves a tunnel behind. The shaft is re-inserted into the tract, and a circumambulation stitch is taken using Vicryl 2-0 to close the tunnel. Closing the tunnel with a stitch is important to avoid fecal matter entering the tunnel (Fig. 6.29G). The external opening is widened for irrigation (Fig. 6.29H).

Step 6: Marsupialization of the margins of proximal fistulotomy is done (Fig. 6.29I).

Step 7: Local infiltration of bupivacaine 0.5% at the operated site and pudendal nerve block is given (Fig. 6.29J, K, L).

The final postoperative image is shown in Fig. 6.29M.

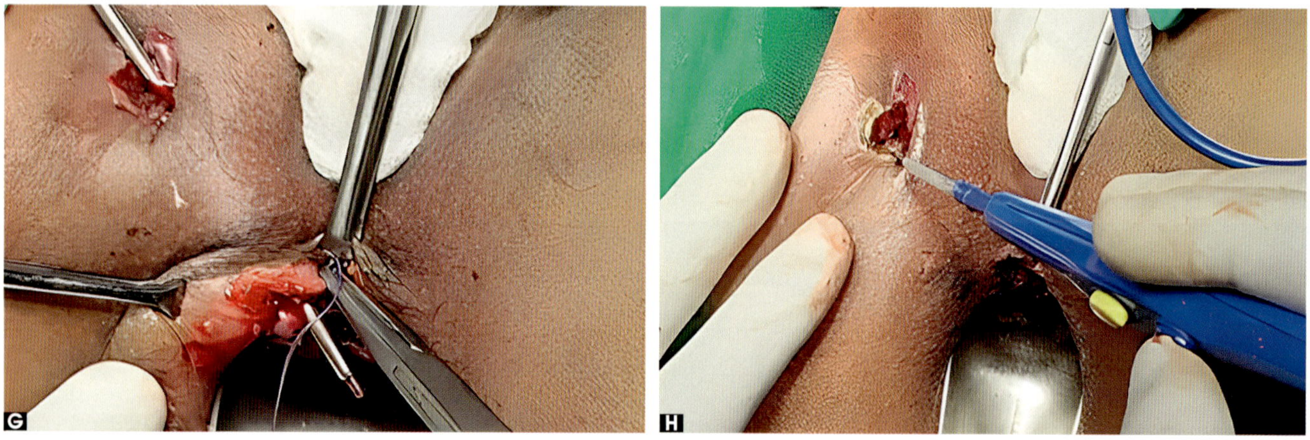

Fig. 6.29(G-H): Managing anterior fistula in females. G) Closure of the tunnel by circumambulation stitch. H) Widening of the external opening

Scan QR Code for Video on

Anterior Fistula in Females

VIDEO 34

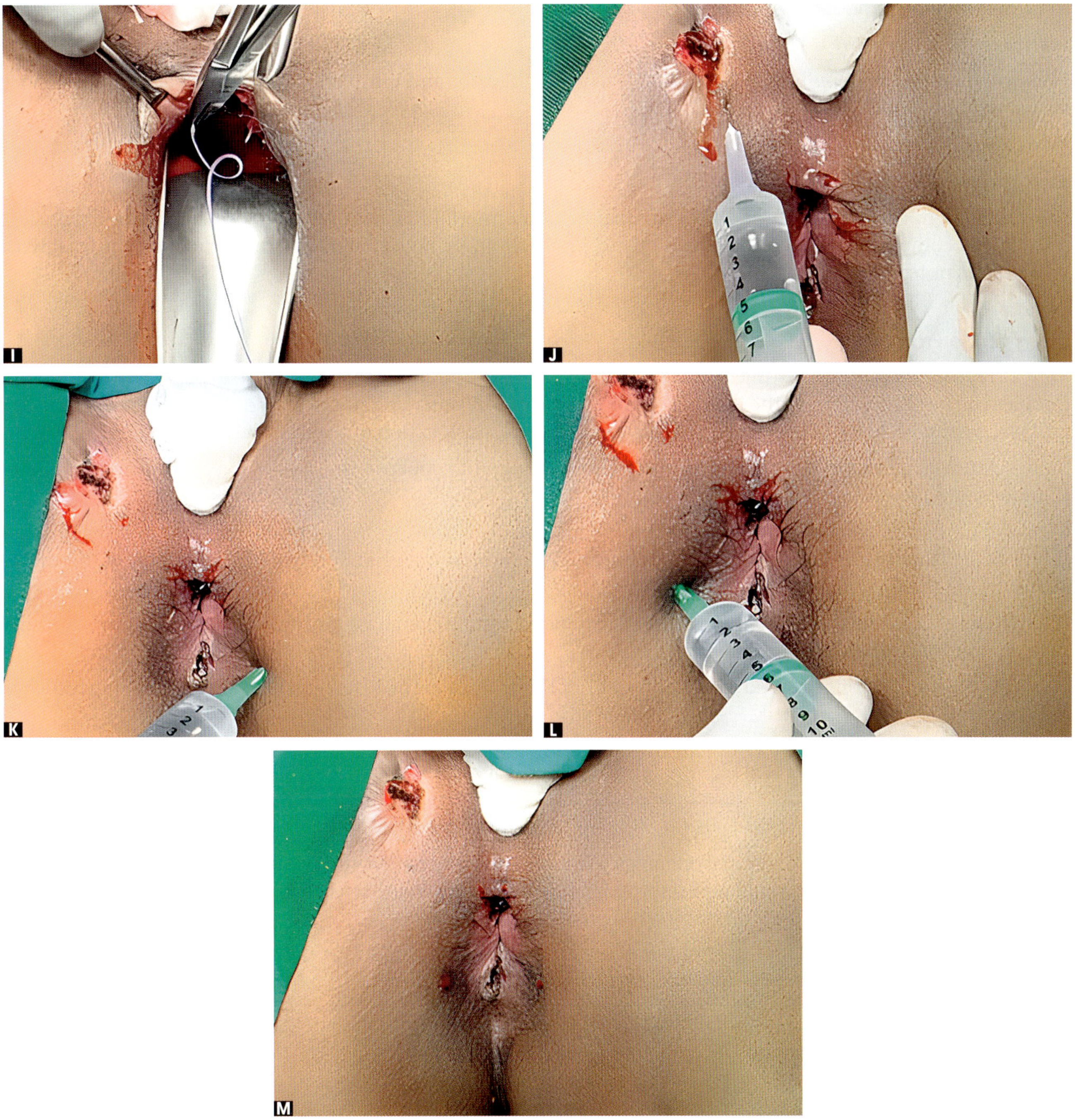

Fig. 6.29(I-L): Managing anterior fistula in females. I) Marsupialization of the margins. J, K, L) Local infiltration of bupivacaine 0.5% at the operated site and pudendal nerve block. M) Final postoperative picture

Managing Anterior Fistula in Males

The anterior fistula in males involves the root of the scrotum or penoscrotal junction. Therefore, it is advisable to catheterize the patient before surgery.

Instrumentation: Figure 6.10 A-D

Preoperative preparation: Two bisacodyl tablets one night prior and intravenous antibiotics 30 minutes before surgery.

Position of the patient: Lithotomy

Type of anaesthesia: Spinal/General.

Procedure performed: Distal laser with Proximal Fistulotomy (DLPF) with seton placement for drainage. The principle of combining the techniques has been discussed earlier. Since the tracts are long, coring the tract with FiXcision is not possible.

Steps of the Procedure

Step 1: Hydrogen peroxide is injected through the external opening at the base of the penoscrotal junction. Bubbles can be observed from the internal opening present anteriorly at 12 o'clock. The tract is demarcated using methylene blue. A half-cut proctoscope is inserted to check the location of the internal opening (Fig. 6.30A, B).

Step 2: Internal opening is demarcated and excised along with mucosa, submucosa and surrounding tissue (Park's technique—Fig. 6.30C).

Step 3: The fistula tract extending from the penoscrotal junction to the internal opening is laser ablated (Fig. 6.30D). The tract is curetted to remove the ablated necrotic material, followed by irrigation with normal saline.

Step 4: The excised internal opening wound is extended upto the anal verge (proximal fistulotomy), and the margins are marsupialized (Fig. 6.30E).

Step 5: A draining seton is placed in the anterior tract (Fig. 6.30F). The seton can be changed or removed after 7 days.

Step 6: Local infiltration of 0.5% bupivacaine and pudendal nerve block is given.

Tips and Tricks

- In the presence of multiple external openings, invariably, the internal opening is single. All the communicating external tracts can be curetted and laser ablated without creating extensive raw areas. Once the internal opening is excised, all the distal tracts are separated.
- Since only the subcutaneous part of the external sphincter and the lower part of the internal sphincter is divided in fistulotomy, there is no chance of anal incontinence.

Scan QR Code for Video on

Anterior Fistula in Males

VIDEO 35

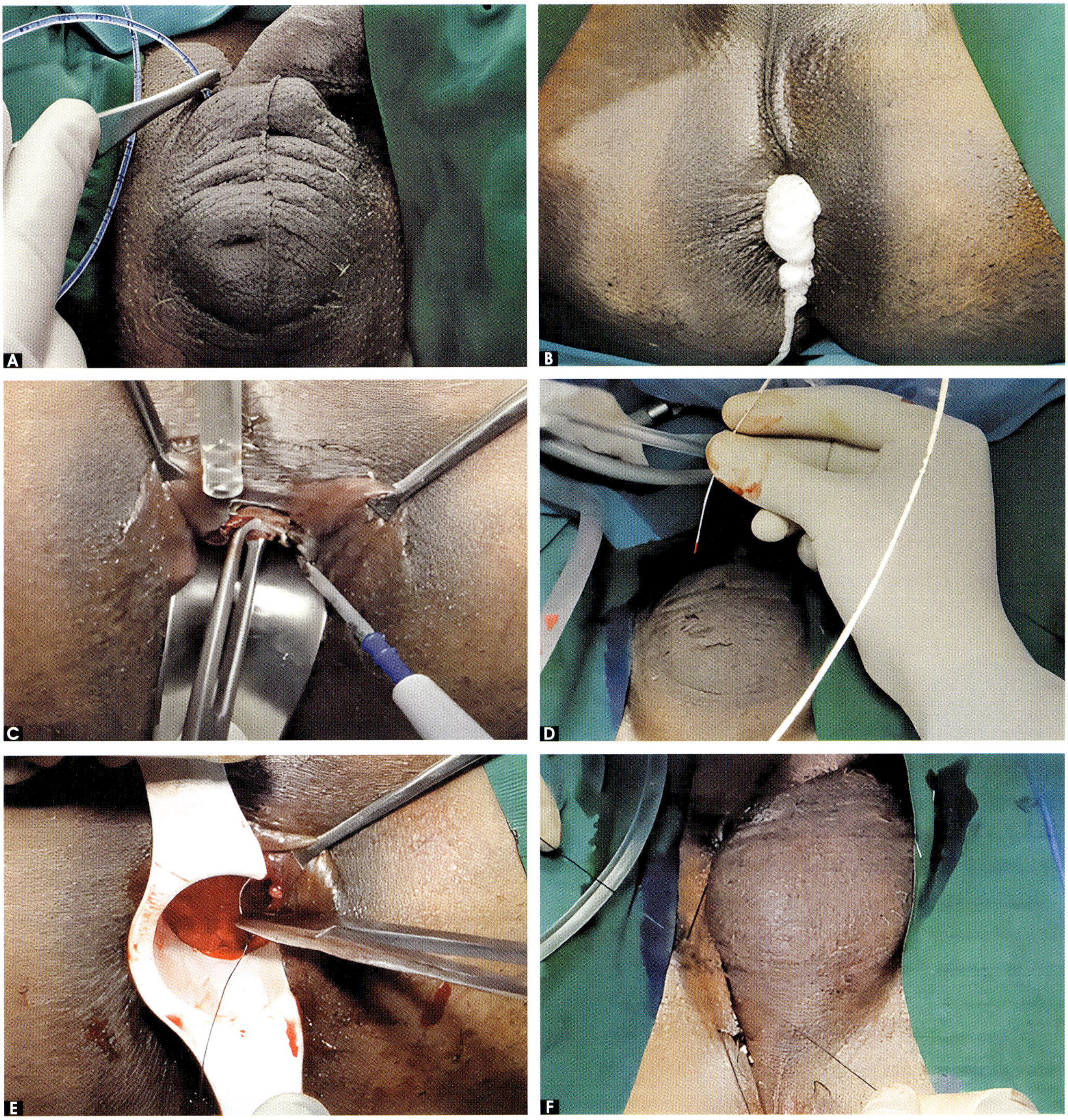

Fig. 6.30A-F: Managing anterior fistula in males. A, B) Injecting hydrogen peroxide and methylene blue to identify the internal opening and course of tract. C) Excision of the internal opening using Park's technique. D) Laser ablation of the fistula tract extending from the penoscrotal junction to the internal opening. E) Proximal fistulotomy with marsupialization of the margins. F) Placement of the draining seton in the anterior tract

Synchronous Fistula

Synchronous fistula means the simultaneous presence of two separate fistula tracts. The tracts have two external openings with two separate internal openings. One should differentiate a synchronous fistula from a branching fistula, where irrespective of the number of multiple external openings, a single internal opening is present.

These fistulas are not difficult to operate; however, the choice of procedure for different types of tracts may vary.

Procedures for Synchronous Fistula

- One can lay open the tracts if both the fistulas are small and sphincter involvement is less than 30%.
- If both fistula tracts are complex, minimally invasive hybrid techniques are advised.
- Sometimes the smaller tract can be dealt with fistulotomy, and the other tract is dealt with a hybrid technique.

Instrumentation: Figure 6.10A–D. Additional equipment like a diode laser and FiXcision may be required.

Position of the patient: Lithotomy

Type of anaesthesia: Spinal/General

Steps of the Procedure

The case discussed is of a patient with two separate fistula tracts, one having the external opening at 3 o'clock with the internal opening at 12 o'clock and the other tract with the external opening at 6 o'clock with the internal opening at 6 o'clock.

Step 1: Hydrogen peroxide was injected from the external opening at 3 o'clock. The bubbles could be seen coming out at 12 o'clock, indicating the course of the fistula tract (Fig. 6.31A).

Step 2: Hydrogen peroxide was injected from the external opening at 6 o'clock, but bubbles could not be seen coming out of the internal opening. However, the internal opening could be palpated on DRE at 6 o'clock (Fig. 6.31B).

Step 3: Demarcation of the fistula tract was done from 3 o'clock to 12 o'clock using methylene blue (Fig. 6.31C).

Step 4: The internal opening at 12 o'clock was excised by Park's technique (Fig. 6.31D). The deep intersphincteric space was opened and curetted.

Step 5: The distal tract was curetted and laser ablated, followed by a repeat curetting to remove the ablated tissue (Fig. 6.31E, F).

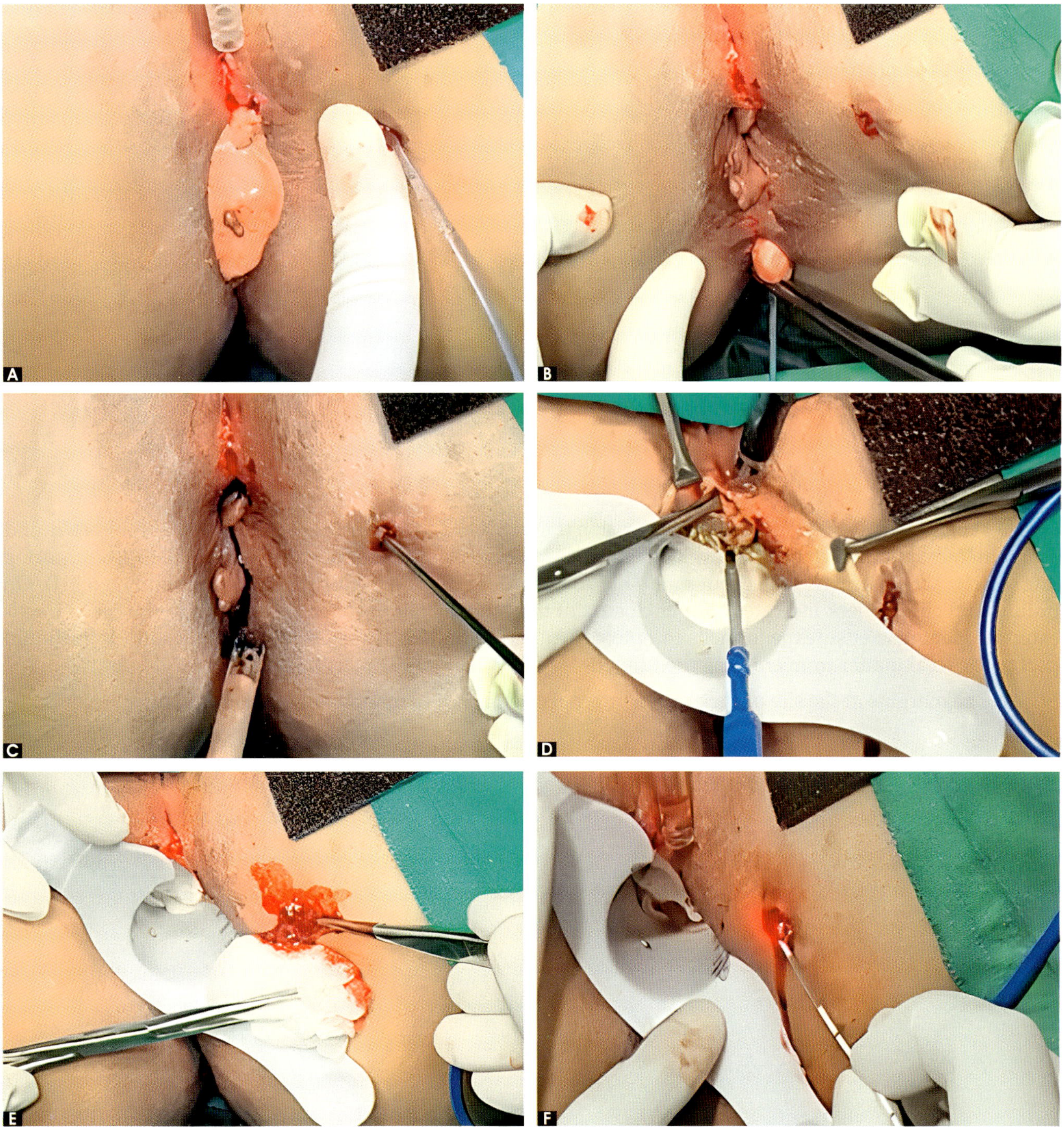

Fig. 6.31A-F: Managing synchronous fistula. A) Hydrogen peroxide injected from the external opening at 3 o'clock. B) Hydrogen peroxide injected from the external opening at 6 o'clock. No bubbles are present at the internal opening at 6 o'clock. C) Demarcation of the tract from 3 to 12 o'clock. D) Excision of internal opening at 12 o'clock (Park's technique). E, F) Curetting and laser ablation of the tract

Step 6: The distal tract was cored out using fixcision (Fig. 6.31G, H). The shaft of the fixcision was reinserted, and a circumambulation stitch using Polyglactin 2-0 was taken to close the tunnel formed after fistula tract coring (Fig. 6.31I). The shaft was pulled out gradually to ensure the complete closure of the tunnel (Fig. 6.31J). On pulling, a feeling of jerk indicated proper closure of the tunnel. Saline was injected through the cored tract's external opening to ensure the tunnel's complete closure (Fig. 6.31K). This step is crucial as it forbids the liquid part of the fecal matter from entering the tunnel.

Step 7: The margins at the site of the excised internal opening were marsupialized (Fig. 6.31L).

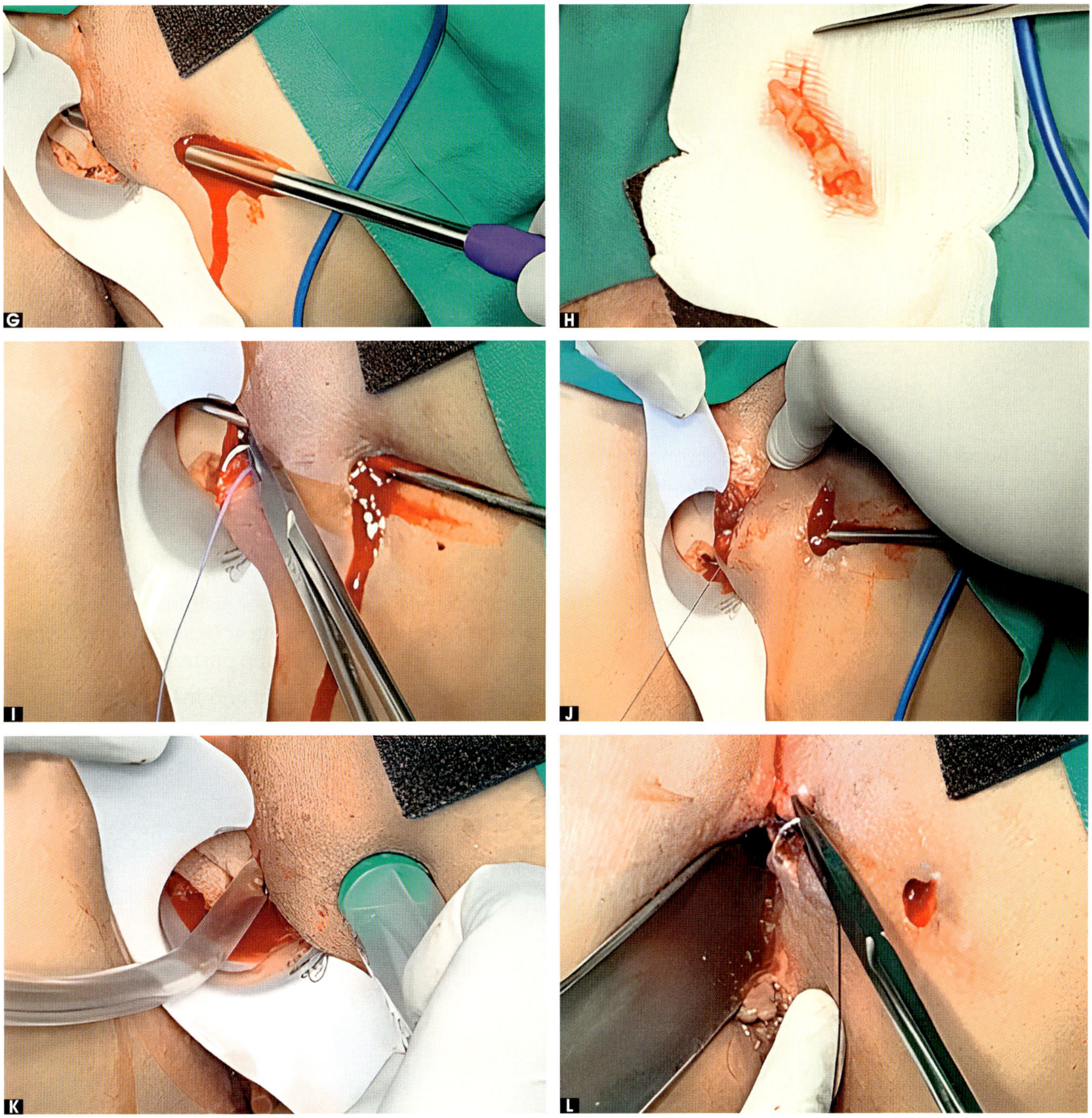

Fig. 6.31G-L: Managing synchronous fistula. G, H) Coring of the tract using FiXcision and cored out fistula tract. I, J) Closure of tunnel after coring. K) Injecting saline through the external opening. L) Marsupialization of the margins of the excised internal opening

Step 8: The next step is to deal with the second tract. Hydrogen peroxide was injected again through the external opening at 6 o'clock (Fig. 6.31M). In some cases, the bubbles can be seen coming from the internal opening, but in the case presented here, the bubbles could not be seen coming out from the internal opening. Therefore, at the site of induration at 6 o'clock, the internal opening was excised (Fig. 6.31N).

Step 9: A probe is inserted from the external opening at 6 o'clock and could be seen coming out freely at the site of excised internal opening, indicating a communicating fistula tract. Posterior fistulotomy was done (Fig. 6.31O). As the tract passed through the deep postanal space, the anal coccygeal ligament was incised vertically, and the deep postanal space was opened by extending the fistulotomy wound posteriorly (Fig. 6.31 P).

Step 10: Curetting was done to remove the necrotic material, followed by irrigation and marsupialization of the margins (Fig. 6.31Q, R).

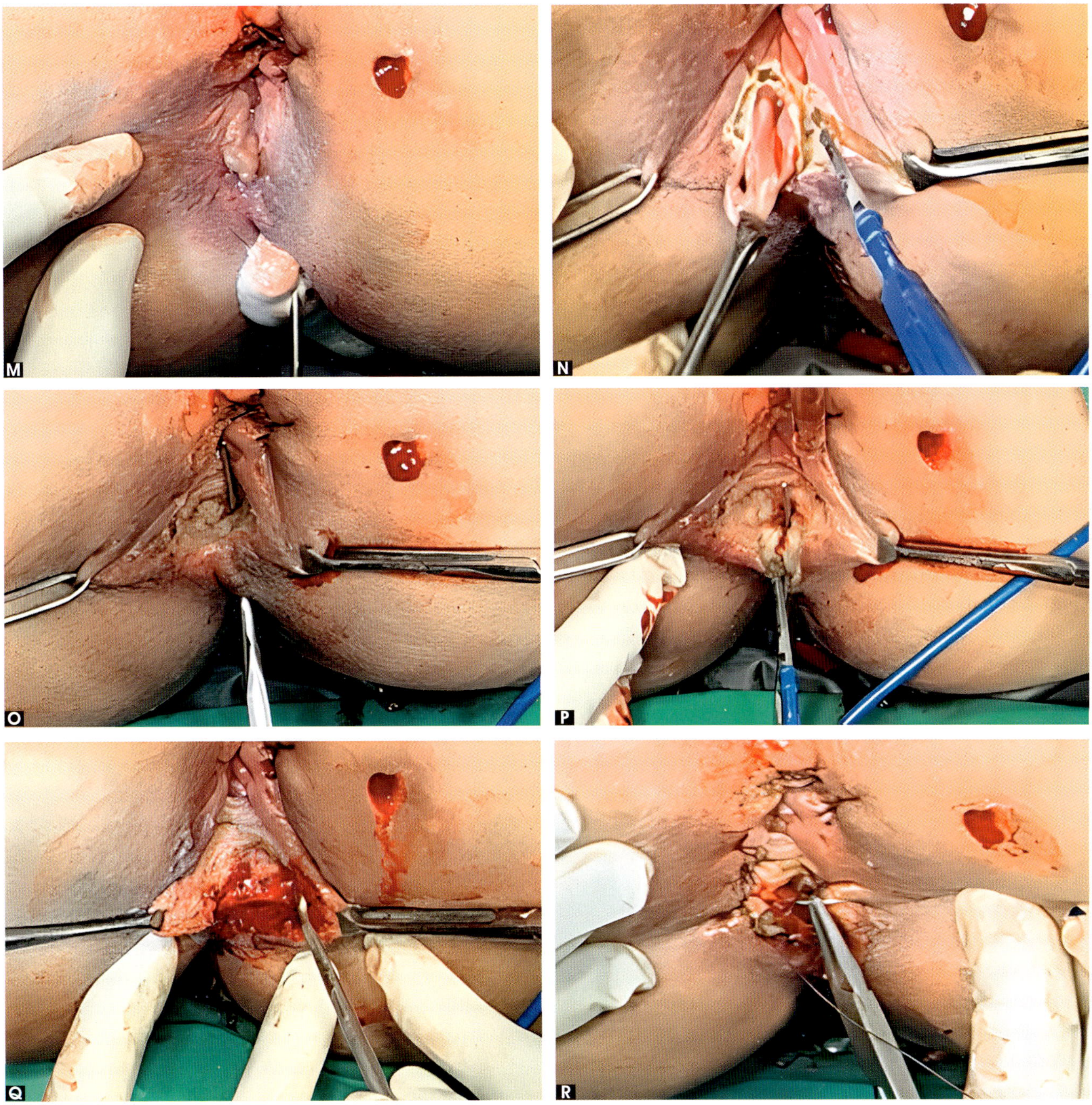

Fig. 6.31M-R: Managing synchronous fistula. M) Injecting hydrogen peroxide in the second tract at 6 o'clock. N) Excision of the internal opening at 6 o'clock. O) Posterior fistulotomy at 6 o'clock. P) Opening of the deep postanal space. Q, R) Curetting, irrigation and marsupialization of the posterior fistulotomy wound

Step 11: Local infiltration of 0.5% bupivacaine at the incision site followed by pudendal nerve block is given (Fig. 6.31S, T, U). The final wound picture is shown in Fig. 6.31V.

Scan QR Code for Video on
Synchronous Fistula
VIDEO 36

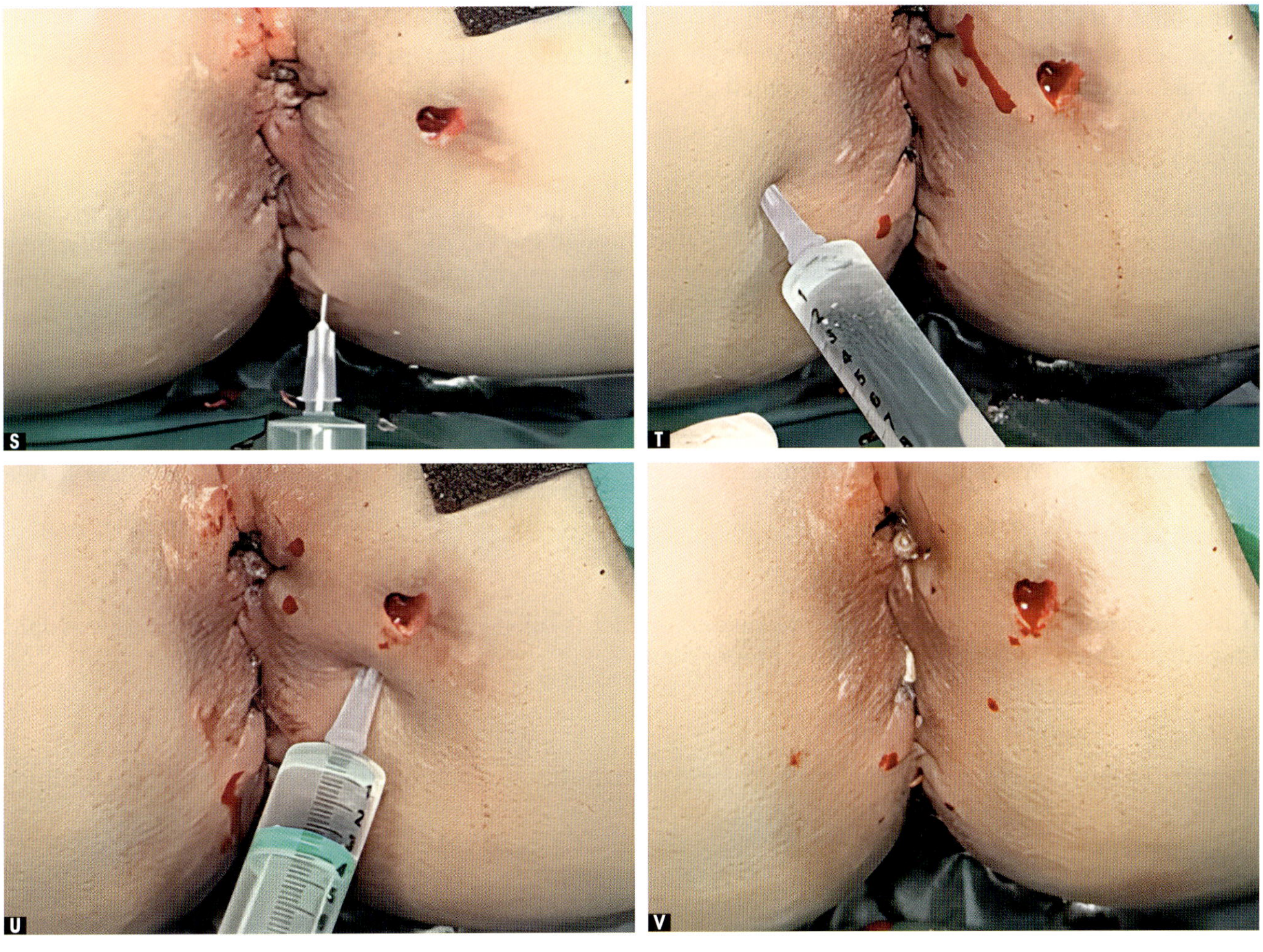

Fig. 6.31S-V: Managing synchronous fistula. S, T, U) Local infiltration of bupivacaine and pudendal nerve block. V) Final wound at the end of the procedure

Dealing with Tricky Situations while Operating a Fistula

No Internal Opening

- In such cases, gently insert the probe from the external opening and observe if it goes smoothly.
- Palpate the tip of the probe and give a nick over the tip and bring it out.
- Apply Allis forceps towards the medial part of the opened tract and give traction outwards.
- If one can see the pull over the mucosa inside, it invariably indicates the internal opening site.
- Alternatively, one can inject saline into the mucosa at the dentate line posteriorly. The part of mucosa which does not lift indicates the fibrotic part of the tract (Fig. 6.32).
- Still, if the internal opening cannot be identified, leave the incised distal part of the tract as such. If the fistula forms subsequently, the tract will be a small one.

Difficult to Probe!

Sometimes, the fistula tract has an hourglass deformity in the intersphincteric space, making probing impossible. Even when hydrogen peroxide is injected through the external opening, the internal opening may not be identified. It is better to take a lacrimal probe used by ophthalmologists to probe the tract. One should remember that necrotic material in the fistula tract can also lead to clogging. Sometimes after curetting, if hydrogen peroxide is injected, the course of the fistula tract may be identified.

Alternatively, such tracts can be dealt with by fistulectomy. One can probe the tract under vision using the VAAFT scope.

If the probing from an external opening fails, one can inject hydrogen peroxide using a 6F infant feeding tube through the internal opening. The emergence of bubbles from the external opening indicate a patent fistula tract.

Identification of the Correct Plane during Fistulectomy?

If the dissection is done in the wrong plane and a tract is opened, the presence of necrotic tissue would immediately alert the surgeon to find the proper plane.

No External Opening

One may be dealing with A 4 type of fistula. Probing from the internal opening may help in identifying the tract.

Conclusion

For the management of anal fistulas, three techniques are commonly used, sphincter cutting, sphincter sparing and hybrid procedures. Fistulotomy and fistulectomy are sphincter-cutting procedures, and their use has been undisputed over the years. Two techniques, Park's procedure and Eisenhammer's, aim to remove the primary source of infection. Primary sphincter repair is an excellent technique that prevents anal incontinence. Setons can be placed in the tract to drain the pus. FilaC, LIFT, Submucosal ligation of the fistula tract, and VAAFT are minimally invasive techniques that have become popular as sphincter-saving procedures. Hybrid techniques involve a combination of different procedures to treat fistula effectively. Anatomically high anal fistulas are a challenge to treat.

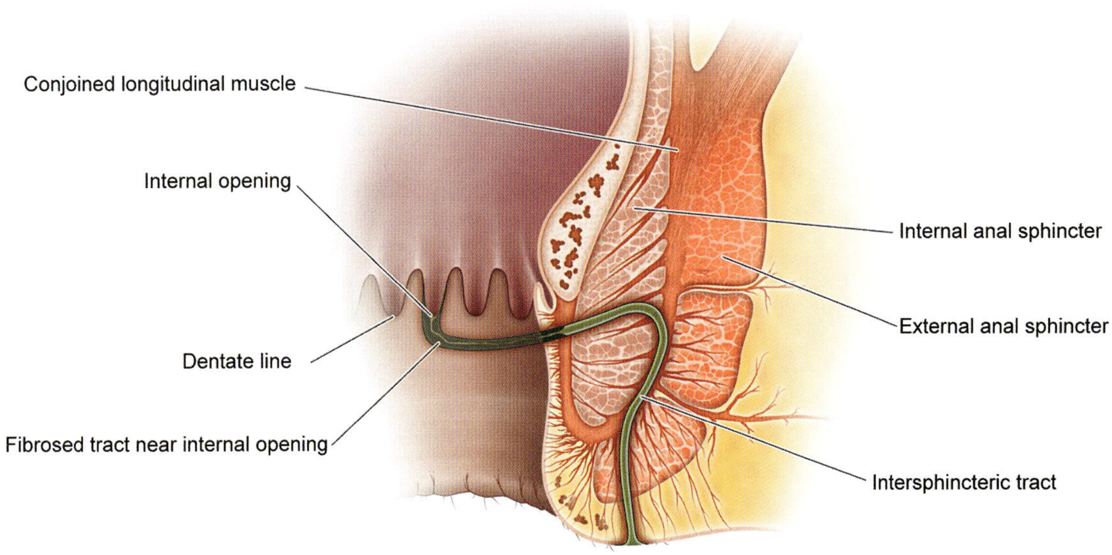

Fig. 6.32: Fibrotic fistula tract near the internal opening

FURTHER READING

- Abou-Zeid AA. Anal Fistula: intraoperative difficulties and unexpected findings. World J Gastroenterol. 2011 Jul 28;17(28):3272–6. doi: 10.3748/wjg.v17.i28.3272. PMID: 21876613; PMCID: PMC3160529.
- Aho Fält U, Zawadzki A, Starck M, Bohe M, Johnson LB. Long-term outcome of the Surgisis® (Biodesign®) anal fistula plug for complex cryptoglandular and Crohn's fistulas. Colorectal Dis. 2021 Jan;23(1):178–185. doi: 10.1111/codi.15429. Epub 2020 Dec 26. PMID: 33155391; PMCID: PMC7898619.[PubMed]
- Al Sebai OI, Ammar MS, Mohamed SH, & El Balshy MA. (2021). Comparative study between inter sphincteric ligation of perianal Fistula versus conventional fistulotomy with or without seton in the treatment of perianal Fistula: a prospective randomized controlled trial. Annals of Medicine and Surgery, 61, 180–184. [Google Scholar]
- Cantero Cid R, Salinas Gómez J, García Olmo D. How to place a seton and prevent it slipping: mission impossible? Tech Coloproctol. 2014 Jun;18(6):603. doi: 10.1007/s10151-013-1118-4. Epub 2014 Feb 14. PMID: 24526396.
- Christoforidis D, Pieh MC, Madoff RD, Mellgren AF. A comparative study is the treatment of transsphincteric anal fistulas by endorectal advancement flap or collagen fistula plug. Dis Colon Rectum. 2009 Jan;52(1):18–22. doi: 10.1007/DCR.0b013e31819756ac. PMID: 19273951.[PubMed]
- Corman ML, Bergamaschi RC, Nicholls RJ & Fazio VW (2017). Corman–Cirurgia Colorretal. Thieme Revinter Publicações LTDA.[PubMed]
- Donmez T, & Hatipoglu E. (2017). Closure of Fistula Tract with FiLaC [TM] Laser as a Sphincter-Preserving Method in Anal Fistula Treatment/Anal Fistul Tedavisinde Sfinkter Koruyucu Yontem Olarak FiLaC [TM] Lazer Yontemiyle Fistula Traktinin Kapatilmasi. Turkish Journal of Colorectal Disease, 27(4), 142–148. [PubMed]
- Eisenhammer S. The final evaluation and classification of the surgical treatment of the primary anorectal cryptoglandular intermuscular (inter-sphincteric) fistulous abscess and Fistula. DisColon Rectum. 1978 May-Jun;21(4):237–54. Doi 10.1007/BF02586698. PMID: 657933. [PubMed]
- Ellis CN, Rostas JW, Greiner FG. Long-term outcomes with the use of bioprosthetic plugs to manage complex anal fistulas. Dis Colon Rectum. 2010 May;53(5):798–802. doi: 10.1007/DCR.0b013e3181d43b7d. PMID: 20389214.
- Emile SH, Khan SM, Adejumo A, Koroye O. Ligation of intersphincteric fistula tract (LIFT) in treatment of anal Fistula: An updated systematic review, meta-analysis, and meta-regression of the predictors of failure. Surgery. 2020 Feb;167(2):484–492. doi: 10.1016/j.surg.2019.09.012. Epub 2019 Oct 21. PMID: 31648932.[PubMed]
- Fakhrosadat Anaraki, Gholamreza Bagherzade, Roubik Behboo, Omid Etemad, Long-term results of ligation of intersphincteric fistula tract (LIFT) for management of anal Fistula, Journal of Coloproctology, Volume 36, Issue 4,2016, Pages 227–230.
- Farag AFA, Elbarmelgi MY, Mostafa M, & Mashhour AN. (2019). One stage fistulectomy for high anal Fistula with the reconstruction of an anal sphincter without fecal diversion. Asian Journal of Surgery, 42(8), 792–796.[Google Scholar].
- FiXcision AMI https://www.ami.at/en/produkt/fixcision.
- Garcés-Albir M, García-Botello SA, Esclapez-Valero P, Sanahuja-Santafé A, Raga-Vázquez J, Espi-Macías A, Ortega-Serrano J. Quantifying the extent of fistulotomy. How much sphincter can we safely divide? A three-dimensional endosonographic study. Int J Colorectal Dis. 2012 Aug;27(8):1109–16. [PubMed] [Reference list]
- García-Aguilar, J, Belmonte, C, Wong, DW, Goldberg, SM, Madoff RD. Cutting seton versus two-stage seton fistulotomy in the surgical management of high anal Fistula. Br J Surg. 1998 Feb;85(2):243–5. doi: 10.1046/j.1365-2168.1998.02877.x. PMID: 9501826.
- Garg P. Is fistulotomy still the gold standard in the present era, and is it highly underutilized? An audit of 675 operated cases. Int J Surg. 2018 Aug; 56:26–30. doi: 10.1016/j.ijsu.2018.06.009. Epub 2018 Jun 8. PMID: 29886281.
- Giamundo P, Geraci M, Tibaldi L, Valente M. Closure of fistula-in-ano with a laser--FiLaC™: an effective novel sphincter-saving procedure for complex disease. Colorectal Dis. 2014 Feb;16(2):110–5. DOI: 10.1111/codi.12440. PMID: 24119103. [PubMed]
- Gupta K, Mital K, Gupta R and Bakshi T (2020). Distal Laser Proximal Fistulotomy-A new sphincter-saving technique. A comparative study with other sphincter saving procedures.[Google Scholar]
- Hall JF, Bordeianou L, Hyman N, Read T, Bartus C, Schoetz D, & Marcello PW. (2014). Outcomes after operations for anal Fistula: results of a prospective, multicenter, regional study. Diseases of the Colon & Rectum, 57(11), 1304–1308.
- Hammond TM, Knowles CH, Porrett T, Lunniss PJ. The Snug Seton: short and medium-term results of slow fistulotomy for idiopathic anal fistulae. Colorectal Dis. 2006 May;8(4):328–37. doi: 10.1111/j.1463-1318.2005.00926.x. PMID: 16630239.
- Hill MR, Sheryock, ReBell FG: Role of anal glands in the pathogenesis of the anorectal disease.JAMA 121:742,1943
- Hirschburger M, Schwandner T, Hecker A, Kierer W, Weinel R, Padberg W. Fistulectomy with primary sphincter reconstruction in treating high trans-sphincteric anal fistulas. Int J Colorectal Dis. 2014 Feb;29(2):247–52. doi: 10.1007/s00384-013-1788-4. Epub 2013 Dec 15. PMID: 24337835.[PubMed]

- Ho YH, Tan M, Leong AF, Seow-Choen F. Marsupialization Ho YH, Tan M, Leong AF, Seow-Choen F. Marsupialization of fistulotomy wounds improves healing: a randomized controlled trial. Br J Surg. 1998 Jan;85(1):105–7. doi: 1046/j.1365-2168.1998.00529.x. PMID: 9462396 [PubMed]
- Hyman N, O'Brien S, Osler T. Outcomes after fistulotomy: results of a prospective, multicenter regional study. Dis Colon Rectum. 2009 Dec;52(12):2022–7. doi: 10.1007/DCR.0b013e3181b72378. PMID: 19934925. [pubmed]
- Jimenez M, Mandava N. Anorectal Fistula. 2021 Sep 27. In: StatPearls [Internet]. Treasure Island (FL): StatPearls Publishing; 2022 Jan. PMID: 32809492.
- Jivapaisarnpong P. Core out fistulectomy, anal sphincter reconstruction, and primary repair of internal opening in treating complex anal Fistula. J Med Assoc Thai. 2009 May;92(5):638–42. PMID: 19459524.[Pu Med]
- Kasiri MM, Riss S, Stift A, Binder AD, Kogovšek U, Huth M & Kronberger IE. (2019). Optimized fistulectomy using the novel FiXcision® device: a technical feasibility study and evaluation of short-term healing rates. Techniques in coloproctology, 23(6), 579–582.[Google Scholar]
- Kelly ME, Heneghan HM, McDermott FD, Nason GJ, Freeman C, Martin ST, & Winter DC. (2014). The role of loose seton in the management of anal Fistula: a multicenter study of 200 patients. Techniques in coloproctology, 18(10), 915-919.[Google Scholar]
- Lauretta A, Falco N, Stocco E, Bellomo R, Infantino A. Anal Fistula Laser Closure: the length of the Fistula is the Achilles' heel. Tech Coloproctol. 2018 Dec;22(12):933–939. DOI: 10.1007/s10151-018-1885-z. Epub 2018 Dec 8. PMID: 30535666. [PubMed]
- Lockhart-Mummery, J. P. (1929). Discussion on fistula-in-ano [Google Scholar]
- Marref I, Spindler L, Aubert M, Lemarchand N, Fathallah N, Pommaret E, Soudan D, Pillant-le Moult H, Safa Far E, Fellous K, Crochet E, Mory B, Benfredj P, de Parades V. The optimal indication for FiLaC® is high trans-sphincteric fistula-in-ano: a prospective cohort of 69 consecutive patients. Tech Coloproctol. 2019 Sep;23(9):893–897. DOI: 10.1007/s10151-019-02077-9. Epub 2019 Sep 26. PMID: 31559547. [PubMed]
- Mascagni D, Pironi D, Pontone S, Tonda M, Eberspacher C, Panarese A, Miscusi G, Grimaldi G, Catania A, Santoro A, Filippini A, Sorrenti S. Total fistulectomy, sphincteroplasty and closure of the residual cavity for trans-sphincteric perianal Fistula in the elderly patient. Aging Clin Exp Res. 2017 Feb;29(Suppl 1):101–108. doi 10.1007/s40520-016-0652-0. Epub 2016 Nov 9. PMID: 27830517.[PubMed]
- Meinero P, Mori L, Gasloli G. Video-assisted anal fistula treatment: a new concept of treating anal fistulas. Dis Colon Rectum. 2014 Mar;57(3):354–9. doi: 10.1097/DCR.0000000000000082. PMID: 24509459.[PubMed]
- Meinero P, Mori L. Video-assisted anal fistula treatment (VAAFT): a novel sphincter-saving procedure for treating complex anal fistulas. Tech Coloproctol. 2011 Dec;15(4):417–22. doi: 10.1007/s10151-011-0769-2. Epub 2011 Oct 15. Erratum in: Tech Coloproctol. 2012 Feb;16(1):111. PMID: 22002535; PMCID: PMC3226694.[PubMed]
- Nottingham JM & Rentea RM (2020). Anal Fistulotomy (Seton Placement).[Google Scholar].
- Oztürk E, Gülcü B. Laser ablation of fistula tract: a sphincter-preserving method for treating fistula-in-ano. Dis Colon Rectum. 2014 Mar;57(3):360–4. DOI: 10.1097/DCR.67. PMID: 24509460. [PubMed]
- Panigrahi HK, Rani MR & Padhi MM. (2009). Clinical Evaluation of Kshara sutra Therapy in the management of Bhagandara (Fistula-in-Ano)-A prospective study. The ancient science of life, 28(3), 29.[PubMed]
- Parks AG, Gordon PH, Hardcastle JD. A classification of fistula-in-ano. Br J Surg. 1976 Jan;63(1):1–12. doi: 10.1002/bjs.1800630102. PMID: 1267867.[PubMed]
- PARKS AG. Pathogenesis and treatment of fistula-in-ano. Br Med J. 1961 Feb 18;1(5224):463–9. doi: 10.1136/bmj.1.5224.463. PMID: 13732880; PMCID: PMC1953161.[PubMed]
- Pathak DU, Agrawal V, & Taneja VK. (2014). Submucosal Ligation Of Fistula Tract (SLOFT) for anorectal Fistula: An effective and easy technique. Ambulatory Surg, 20(3), 42–43.[Google Scholar]
- Pescatori M. (2021). Surgery for anal fistulae: state of the art. International Journal of Colorectal Disease, 36(10), 2071–2079. [Google Scholar]
- Pescatori M, Ayabaca SM, Cafaro D, Iannello A, Magrini S. Marsupialization of fistulotomy and fistulectomy wounds improves healing and decreases bleeding: a randomized controlled trial. Colorectal Dis. 2006 Jan;8(1):11-4. doi: 10.1111/j.1463-1318.2005.00835.x. PMID: 16519632.[PubMed]
- Practice Parameters for the Management of Perianal Abscess and Fistula-in-Ano Scott R. Steele, MD, Ravin Kumar, MD, Daniel L Feingold, MD Janice L Rafferty, MD W Donald Buie, MD Prepared by the Standards Practice Task Force of the American Society of Colon and Rectal Surgeon
- Raja Ram NK, Chan KK, Md Nor SF, Sagap I. A prospective evaluation of the outcome of submucosal ligation of the fistula tract. Colorectal Dis. 2020 Dec;22(12):2199–2203. doi: 10.1111/codi.15305. Epub 2020 Oct 6. PMID: 32780561.[PubMed]

- Raslan SM, Aladwani M, Alsanea N. Evaluation of the cutting seton as a treatment method for perianal Fistula. Ann Saudi Med. 2016 May-Jun;36(3):210–5. doi: 10.5144/0256-4947.2016.210. PMID: 27236393; PMCID: PMC6074548.[PubMed]
- Regusci L, Fasolini F, Meinero P, Caccia G, Ruggeri G, Serati M, Braga A. Video-Assisted Anal Fistula Treatment (VAAFT) for complex anorectal Fistula: efficacy and risk factors for failure at 3-year follow-up. Tech Coloproctol. 2020 Jul;24(7):741–746. doi: 10.1007/s10151-020-02213-w. Epub 2020 Apr 21. PMID: 32318991. [PubMed]
- Rojanasakul, A. (2009). LIFT procedure: A simplified technique for fistula-in-ano. Techniques in coloproctology, 13(3), 237–240. [Google Scholar]
- Romaniszyn M, Walega P. Video-Assisted Anal Fistula Treatment: Pros and Cons of This Minimally Invasive Method for Treatment of Perianal Fistulas. Gastroenterol Res Pract. 2017;2017:9518310. Doi: 10.1155/2017/9518310. Epub 2017 Jun 7. PMID: 28680443; PMCID: PMC5478827.[PubMed]
- S. Eisenstein and AJ Ky Biologic fistula plugs H. Abcarian Anal Fistula: Principles and management, DOI:10.1007/978-1-4614-9014-2_12
- Saba RB, Tizmaghz A, Ajeka S, Karami M. Treating anal Fistula with the anal fistula plug: case series report of 12 patients. Electron Physician. 2016 Apr 25;8(4):2304–7. doi: 10.19082/2303. PMID: 27280009; PMCID: PMC4886575.[PubMed]
- Schwandner O. Video-assisted anal fistula treatment (VAAFT) combined with advancement flap repair in Crohn's disease. Tech Coloproctol. 2013 Apr;17(2):221–5. doi: 10.1007/s10151-012-0921-7. Epub 2012 Nov 23. PMID: 23179892.[PubMed]
- Serin KR, Hacim NA, Karabay O, Terzi MC. Retrospective Analysis of Primary Suturing of the Internal Orifice of Perianal Fistula During FiLaC Procedure. Surg Laparosc Endosc Percutan Tech. 2020 Jun;30(3):266–269. DOI: 10.1097/SLE.0000000000000774. PMID: 32080021. [PubMed]
- Seyfried S, Bussen D, Joos A, Galata C, Weiss C, Herold A. Fistulectomy with primary sphincter reconstruction. Int J Colorectal Dis. 2018 Jul;33(7):911–918. doi: 10.1007/s00384-018-3042-6. Epub 2018 Apr 12. PMID: 29651553.[PubMed]
- Sheikh P, Baakza A. Management of Fistula-in-Ano-The Current Evidence. Indian J Surg. 2014 Dec;76(6):482–6. doi: 10.1007/s12262-014-1150-2. Epub 2014 Aug 15. PMID: 25614724; PMCID: PMC4297991.[PubMed]
- Simple clinical examination predicts complexity of perianal fistula Becker A, Koltun L, Sayfan J Colorectal Dis. 2006 Sep; 8(7):601–4. [PubMed]
- Singh M & Godse S. (2018). Simple New Approach for Anorectal Fistula: Submucosal Ligation of Fistula Tract. IJSS Journal of Surgery, 4(2), 47–48.[Google Scholar]
- Springer. Abcarian, H. (2014). Classification and management strategies. In Anal Fistula (pp. 39-44). Springer, New York, NY.
- Stijns J, van Loon YT, Clermonts SHEM, Göttgens KW, Wasowicz DK, Zimmerman DDE. Implementation of laser ablation of fistula tract (LAFT) for perianal fistulas: do the results warrant continued application of this technique? Tech Coloproctol. 2019 Dec;23(12):1127–1132. DOI: 10.1007/s10151-019-02112-9. E-pub 2019 Nov 28. PMID: 31781883. [PubMed]
- Subhas G, Singh Bhullar J, Al-Omari A, Unawane A, Mittal VK, Pearlman R. Setons in the treatment of anal Fistula: a review of variations in materials and techniques. Dig Surg. 2012;29(4):292–300. doi: 10.1159/000342398. Epub 2012 Aug 31. PMID: 22948115.[PubMed]
- Van Onkelen RS, Gosselink MP, van Rosmalen J, Thijsse S, Schouten WR. Different characteristics of high and low trans-sphincteric fistulae. Colorectal Dis. 2014 Jun;16(6):471–5. doi: 10.1111/codi.12578. PMID: 24471695.[PubMed]
- Van Onkelen RS, Gosselink MP, Schouten WR. Treatment of anal fistulas with high inter-sphincteric extension. DisColon Rectum. 2013 Aug;56(8):987–91. DOI: 10.1097/DCR.0b013e3182908be6. PMID: 23838868.[PubMed]
- Velchuru VR (2014). Seton (Loose, Cutting, Chemical). In Anal Fistula (pp. 45-52). Springer, New York, NY.[Google Scholar]
- Walfisch S, Menachem Y, Koretz M. Double seton--a new modified approach to high transsphincteric anal Fistula. Dis Colon Rectum. 1997 Jun;40(6):731–2. doi: 10.1007/BF02140905. PMID: 9194470.
- Wilhelm A, Fiebig A, Krawczak M. Five years of experience with the FiLaC™ laser for fistula-in-ano management: long-term follow-up from a single institution. Tech Coloproctol. 2017 Apr;21(4):269–276. DOI: 10.1007/s10151-017-1599-7. Epub 2017 Mar 7. PMID: 28271331; PMCID: PMC5423928. [PubMed]
- Wilhelm A. A new technique for sphincter-preserving anal fistula repair using a novel radial emitting laser probe. Tech Coloproctol. 2011 Dec;15(4):445–9. DOI: 10.1007/s10151-011-0726-0. E-pub 2011 Aug 16. PMID: 21845480. [PubMed]
- Zheng L, Shi Y, Zhi C, Yu Q, Li X, Wu S, Zhang W, Liu Y, Huang Z. Loose combined cutting seton for patients with high intersphincteric Fistula: a retrospective study. Ann Transl Med. 2020 Oct;8(19):1236. doi: 10.21037/atm-20-6123. PMID: 33178768; PMCID: PMC7607110.[PubMed]

Chapter

7

Surgical Management of Pilonidal Sinus

Pilonidal Sinus is one of the commonest disorders affecting people between the age groups of 15 to 29 years. It is derived from the words Pilus and Nidus, meaning "hair" and "nest". Pilonidal sinus disease (PSD) is characterized by a sacrococcygeal cavity or a tract created by recurring infection and chronic inflammation (Fig. 7.1). The primary openings in the midline are called pits (Fig. 7.2).

This chapter provides insight into surgical techniques like Karydaykis, Bascom, Rhomboid flap, Z Plasty and minimally invasive procedures like Video-assisted laser ablation of the pilonidal sinus (VALAPS).

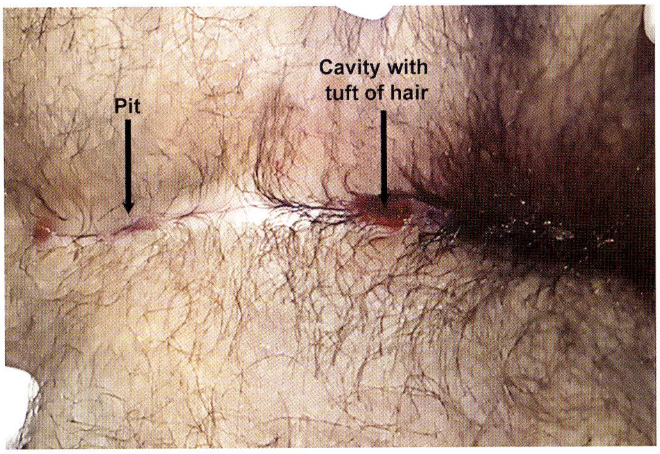

Fig. 7.1: Pilonidal sinus cavity with pit and tuft of hair.

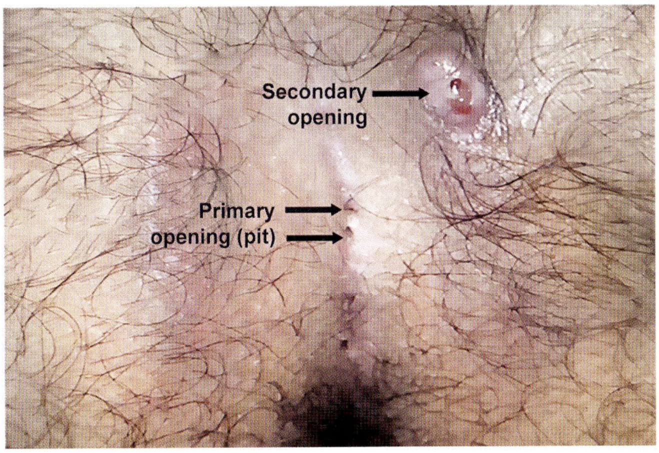

Fig. 7.2: Pilonidal Sinus with multiple primary pits and a secondary opening.

THE NAVICULAR AREA

The navicular area is located between the lateral edges of the natal cleft (the groove between the buttocks) and their posterior extensions. The posterior border of the anal triangle marks the posterior boundary.

The patient is made to stand to mark the navicular area. The buttocks are drawn together, and as they are brought closer, the lateral edges of the natal cleft become apparent. These edges are marked with a pen before releasing the buttocks.

The resultant marked area resembles the shape of a ship, hence the term navicular area. The marking indicates a specific region for surgical intervention (Fig. 7.3A-D).

It is imperative to know about the navicular area to understand the classification of the pilonidal sinus.

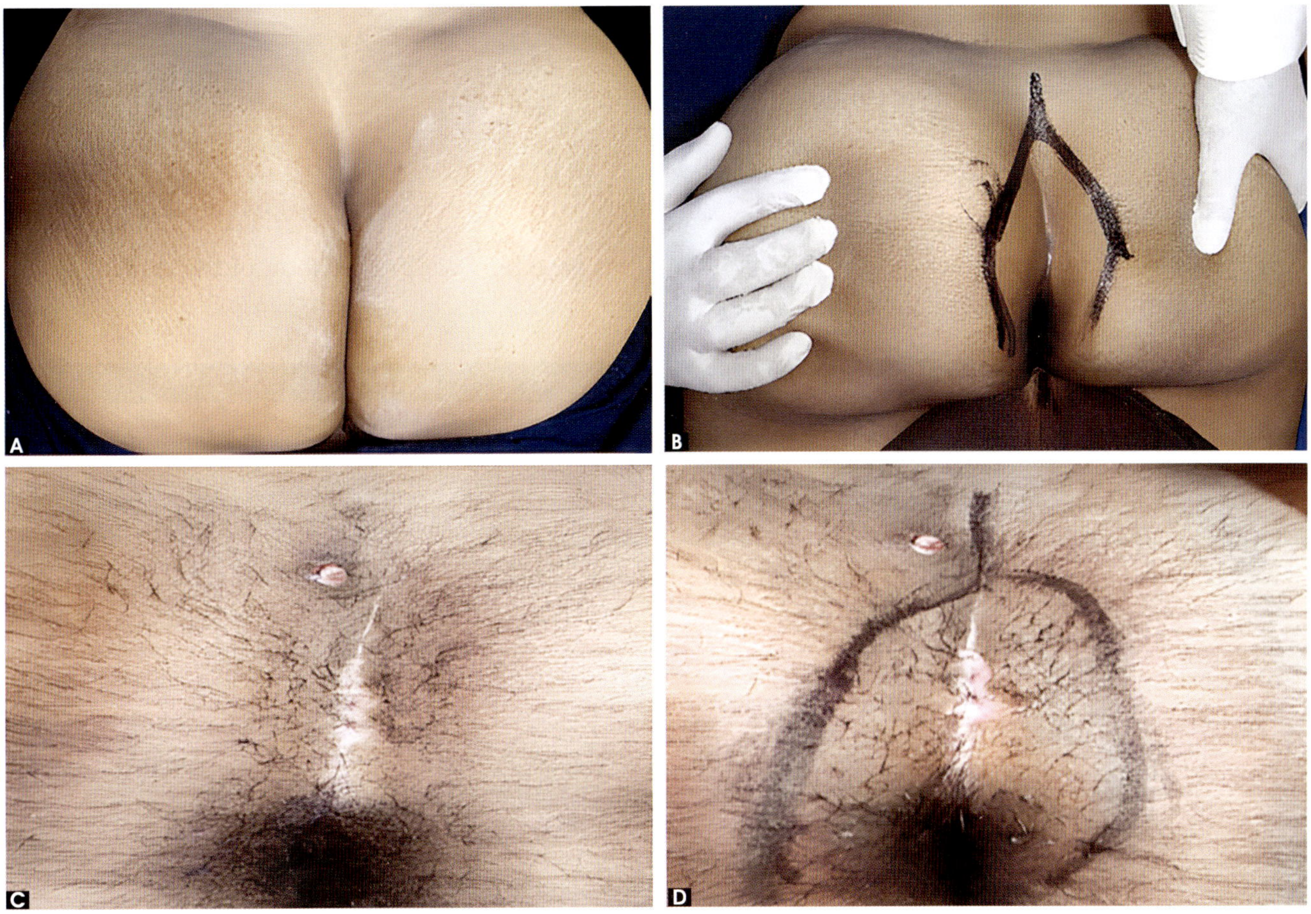

Fig. 7.3A-D: A, B) Marking the navicular area in a standing position. C, D) Marking of the navicular cleft showing the secondary opening outside the navicular area.

Classification of Pilonidal Sinus

Tezel proposed a new classification for the pilonidal sinus based on the presentation of the disease in the navicular area (Fig. 7.4A-E).

TABLE 7.1: TEZEL'S CLASSIFICATION OF PILONIDAL SINUS

Type of pilonidal sinus	*Presentation*	*Surgical recommendation*
Type 1	Asymptomatic pits with no history of drainage or abscess	• No surgical intervention • Removal of local hair • Maintain hygiene
Type II	Acute pilonidal abscess	• Drainage using a lateral incision
Type III	Pits in the navicular area with an abscess or prior drainage history	• Surgical procedure
Type IV	A severe condition in which one or more sinus openings are located outside the navicular region	• The Bascom treatment is coupled with separate excision of pits
Type V	Recurrent pilonidal sinus	• Bascom procedure

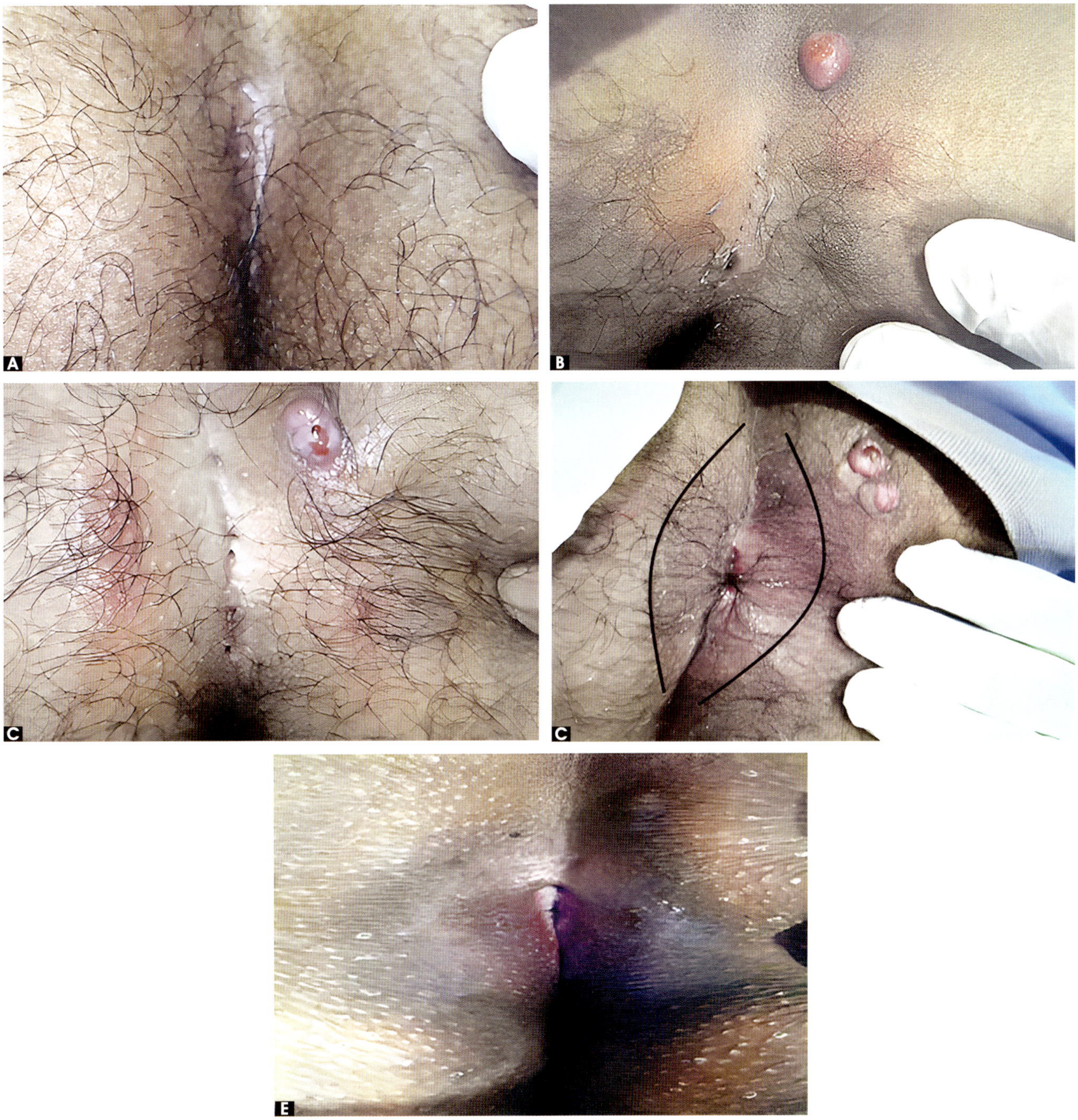

Fig. 7.4A to E: Tezel's classification. A) Type 1: Presence of pit (Asymptomatic). B) Type 2: Acute pilonidal abscess. C) Type 3: Pits in the navicular area with abscess drainage. D) Type 4: Extensive sinus disease with sinus opening outside the navicular area. E) Type 5: Recurrent pilonidal sinus disease after surgical treatment.

Surgical Procedures

- Karydakis procedure
- Bascom pit excision procedure
- Rhomboid excision (Limberg flap)
- Bascom Cleft lift procedure
- Z-Plasty (single/multiple)
- V-Y fascio-cutaneous flap
- Advancement flaps

A few popular surgical procedures like Karydakis, Bascom, Z Plasty and Limberg flap have been described.

Instrumentation (Fig. 7.5A, B)

- General surgical trolley
- Marker pen
- Skin hooks
- Monopolar diathermy
- Vacuum drainage set
- Suture materials: 3-0 Polyglactin/3-0 Nylon/Polypropylene/Skin cyanoacrylate glue
- Methylene blue ampoule

Indications

- Pilonidal disease with a deep natal cleft
- Recurrent disease
- Midline or paramedian disease
- Failure of minimally invasive techniques

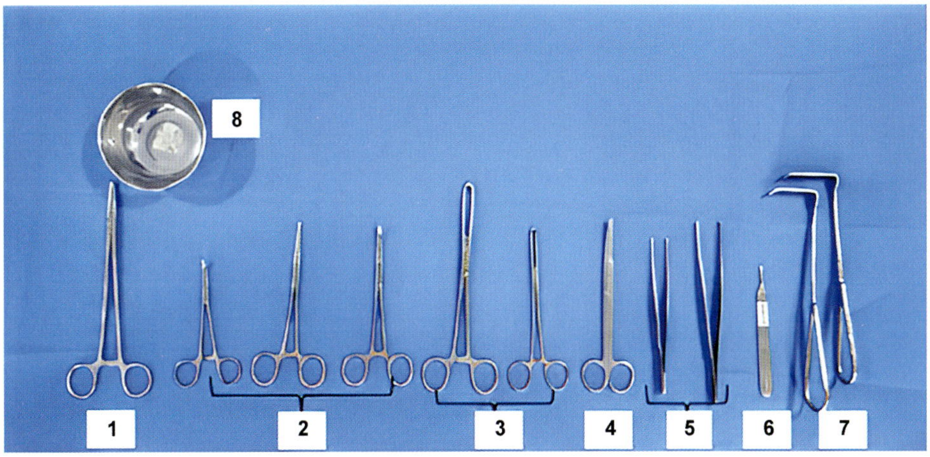

Fig. 7.5A: Surgical trolley.

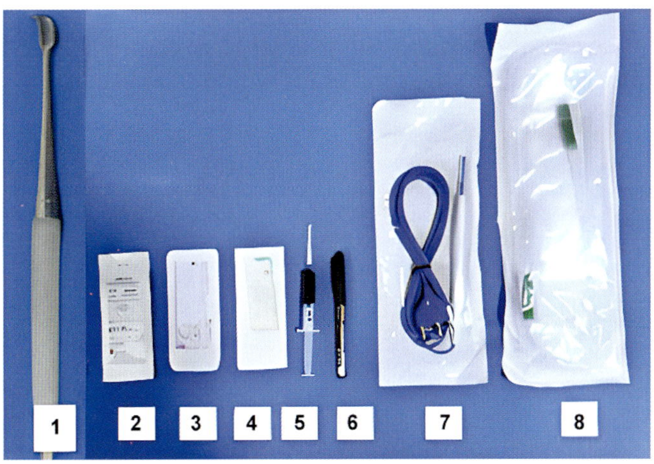

Fig. 7.5B: 1) Skin hook. 2, 3, 4) Sutures. 5) Methylene blue. 6) Marker. 7) Cautery. 8) Suction tube.

Karydakis Procedure (Fig. 7.6)

Position of the patient

Prone position with a small bolster under the hips and buttocks strapped apart after the skin markings.

Anesthesia

General with endotracheal intubation/Spinal/Epidural/Local infiltration with sedation.

Preparation

Trimming or shaving of the hair in and around the gluteal cleft before surgery. A single dose of Injection Amoxiclav 1.2 gm is given intravenously at the time of induction of anesthesia.

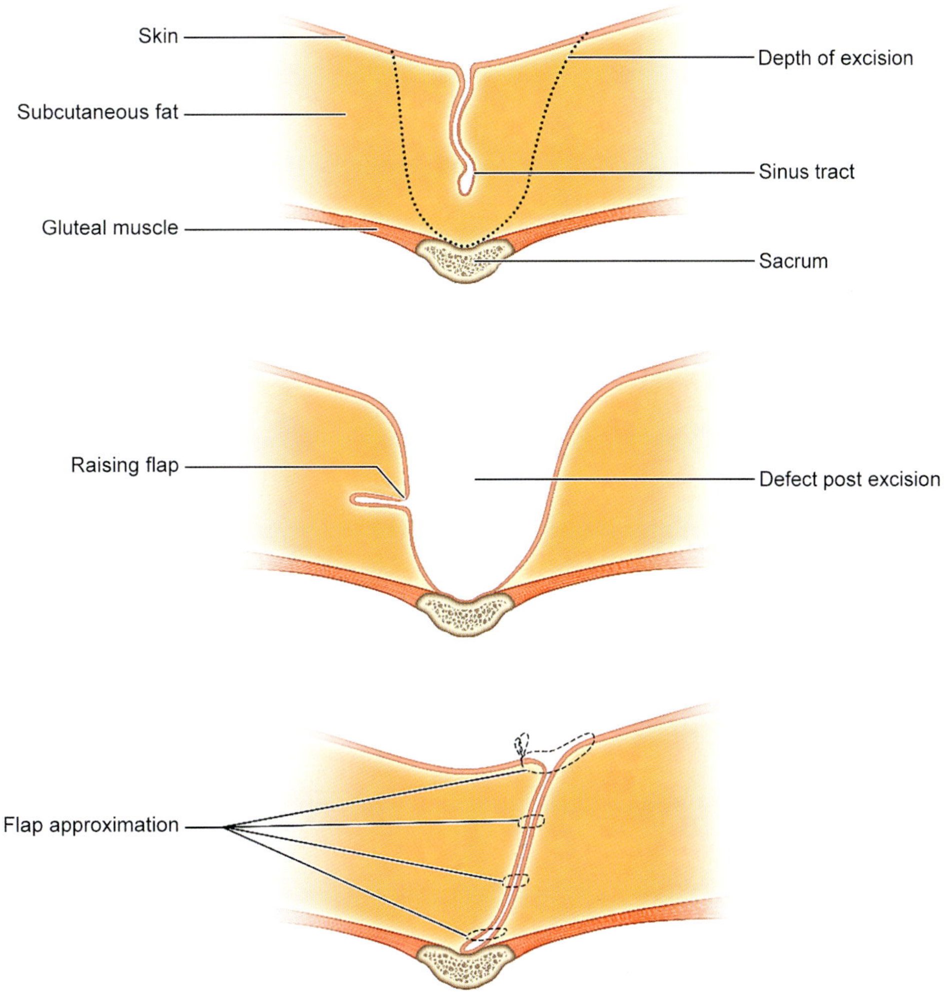

Fig. 7.6: Diagrammatic representation to show the excision of the pilonidal sinus with flap approximation.

Steps of the Procedure

Step 1: After cleaning the area with povidone iodine or chlorhexidine, an off-midline, elliptical skin marking is done. Methylene blue is instilled through the pits to delineate the tract. The upper and lower ends of the ellipse are placed 1 to 2 cm away from the midline (Fig. 7.7A).

Step 2: Off-midline excision of the tract is done. The excision is done vertically on the patient's right side and slanting on the left side. Hemostasis is achieved with monopolar diathermy (Fig. 7.7B). The clear margins of the excised tissue without methylene blue stains indicate complete removal of the diseased tract (Fig. 7.7C).

Step 3: The slanting left side flap is mobilized and carried across the midline to the right side. A negative suction drain is kept in the wound (Fig. 7.7D).

Step 4: Wound closure is performed in 2 to 3 layers, with the inner suturing done with 3-0 polyglactin, and the skin is approximated with 3-0 Nylon, Polypropylene, or Cyanoacrylate glue. The skin closure with Cyanoacrylate glue and a few interrupted skin sutures is shown in Fig. 7.7E, F. The drain is removed after 48 hrs, and the sutures after 10 to 14 days.

The final appearance of the wound after 14 days is shown in Fig. 7.7G.

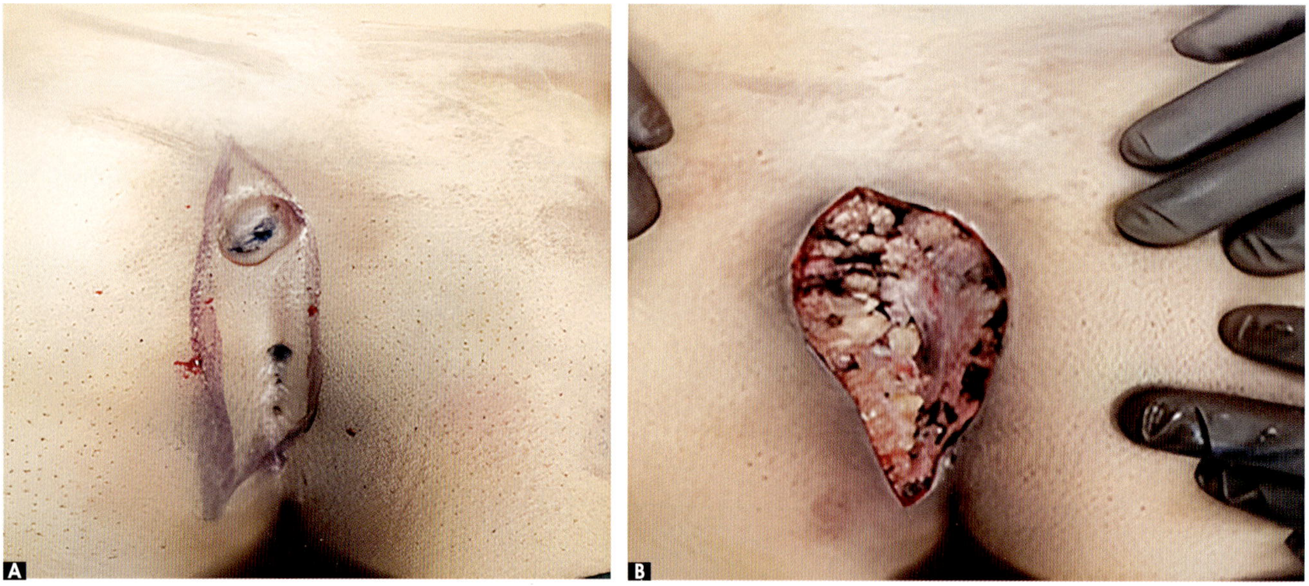

Fig. 7.7A-B: A) Preoperative picture: Primary and Secondary pits. B) Off-line excision of the tract.

Scan QR Code for Video on
Karydakis Procedure for Pilonidal Sinus

VIDEO 37

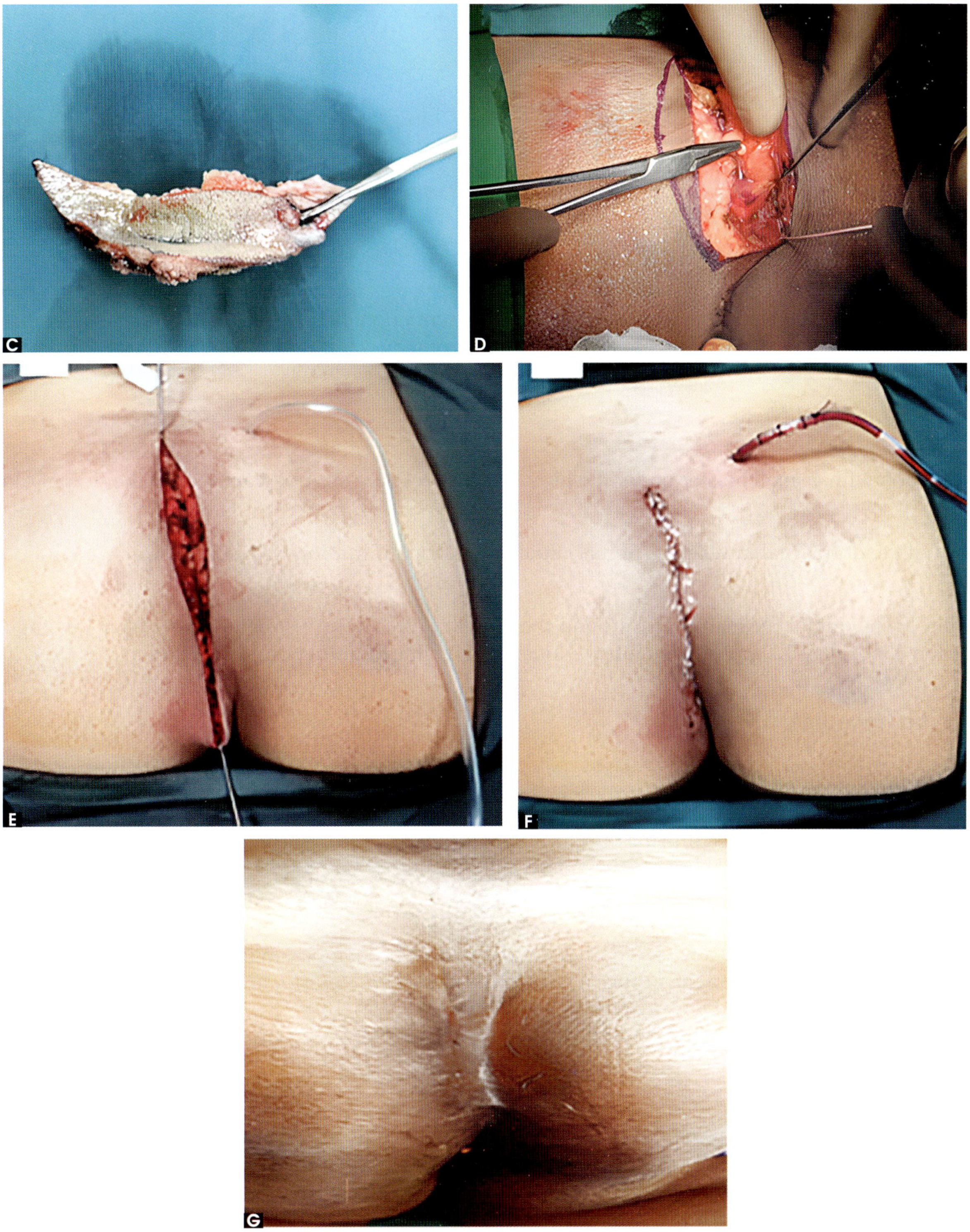

Fig. 7.7C-G: C) Excised specimen with methylene blue stained sinus tract. D) Closure of the wound in layers. E) Slanting edges carried out across the midline with placement of vacuum drain. F) Closure of wound with Cyanoacrylate and skin sutures. G) Complete healing of the wound.

LIMBERG'S (RHOMBOID) FLAP

The technique described was done on a patient with recurrent pilonidal disease. The primary pit is situated in the midline, and the secondary pit is superior and away from the midline (Fig. 7.8).

Instrumentation (Fig. 7.5A, B)

Position of the patient

Prone position with a small bolster under the hips. The buttocks are strapped apart after the skin markings.

Anesthesia

General with endotracheal intubation/Spinal/Epidural/Local infiltration with sedation.

Preparation

Trimming or shaving of the hair in and around the gluteal cleft is done just before the surgery. A single dose of Injection Amoxiclav 1.2 gm is given intravenously at the time of induction of anesthesia.

Steps of the Procedure

Step 1: The patient is placed in a prone jackknife position with a bolster under the hips and buttocks strapped with adhesive tapes (Fig. 7.9A).

Step 2: Methylene blue is instilled into the tract through the pit (Fig. 7.9B). The proposed incision site is infiltrated with saline and adrenaline.

Step 3: Midline is marked, and the excision length is measured (Fig. 7.9C).

Step 4: An off-midline (eccentrically placed) rhomboid is marked, encompassing the primary and the secondary pits. The rhomboid marking is done in such a way that superior and inferior angles are 60 degrees and lateral angles are 120 degrees (Fig. 7.9D).

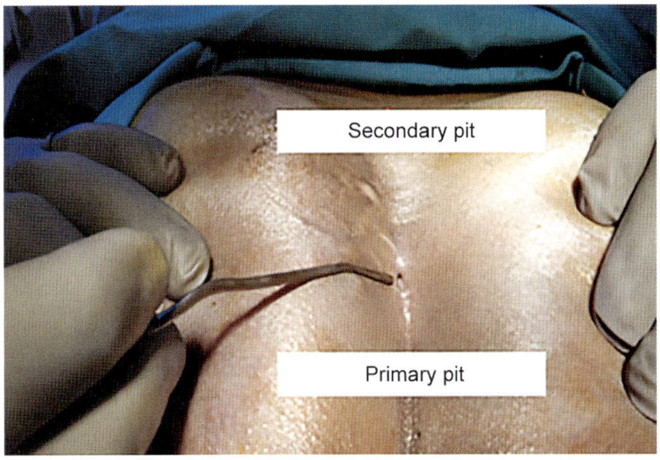

Fig. 7.8: Recurrent pilonidal sinus with primary and secondary pits.

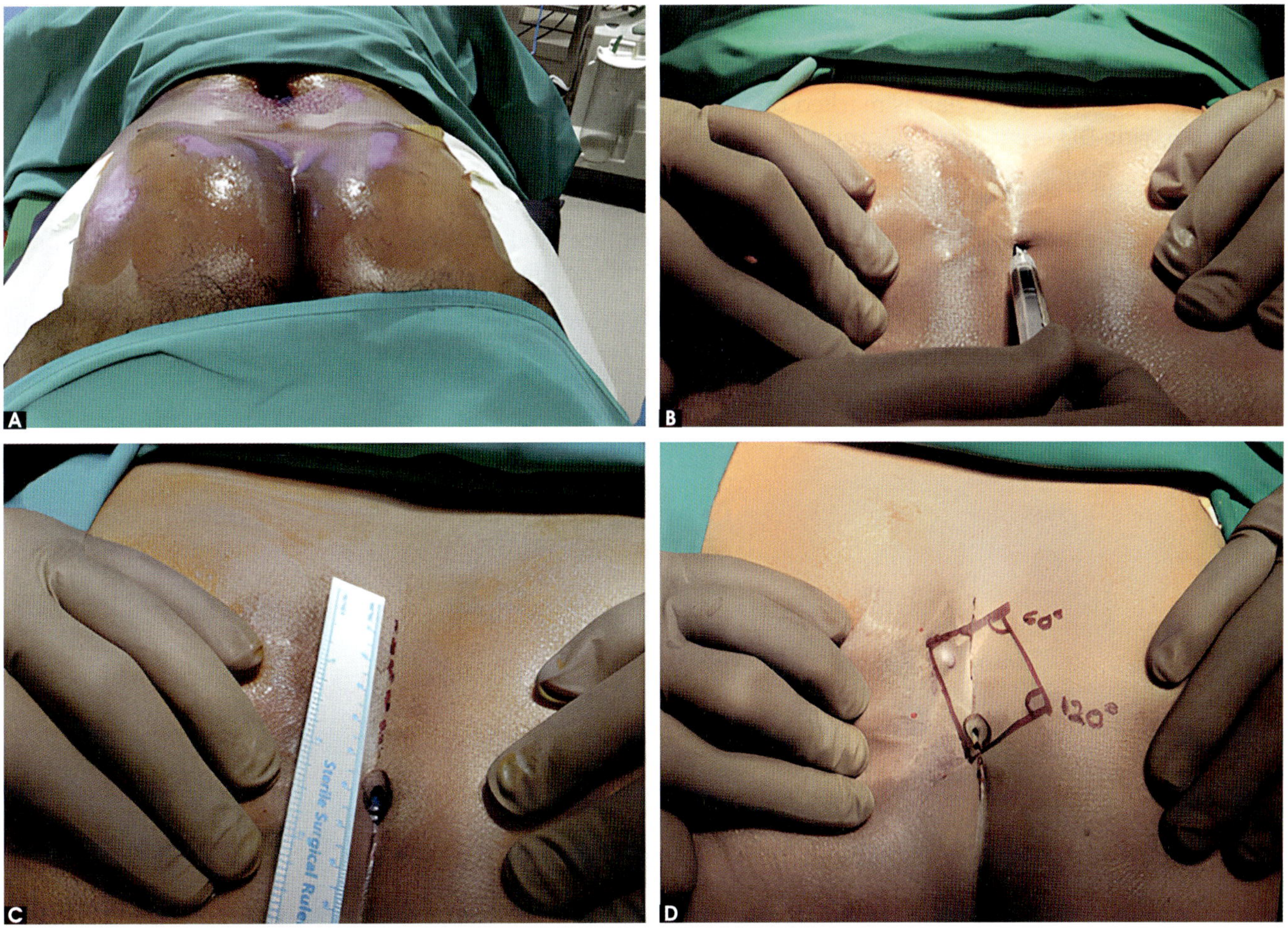

Fig. 7.9A-D: Technique of Limberg's (Rhomboid) Flap. A) Patient in a prone jackknife position. B) Instillation of methylene blue into the pit. C) Measurement of the tract to be excised. Since it is an off-centre rhomboid, the rotation is away from the anus. D). Marking of the rhomboid. Note that the angles marked give a rhomboid shape.

Step 5: An inferiorly-based flap is marked on the left side of the excision. An arrow shows the arc of rotation of the flap. Side BD is equal to BD′, and BC is equal and parallel to D′C′ (Fig. 7.9E).

Step 6: The sinus tract is excised, and hemostasis is achieved with the diathermy (Fig. 7.9F).

Step 7: The flap is harvested as a fascio-cutaneous flap and rotated into the defect. A negative suction drain is kept at the upper end, away from the wound and the midline (Fig. 7.9G).

Step 8: Final appearance at closure. The wound is closed in layers with 3-0 polyglactin. The skin is closed with 3-0 Nylon and Cyanoacrylate glue (Fig. 7.9H).

Scan QR Code for Video on
Limberg Flap (Rhomboid Flap)

VIDEO 38

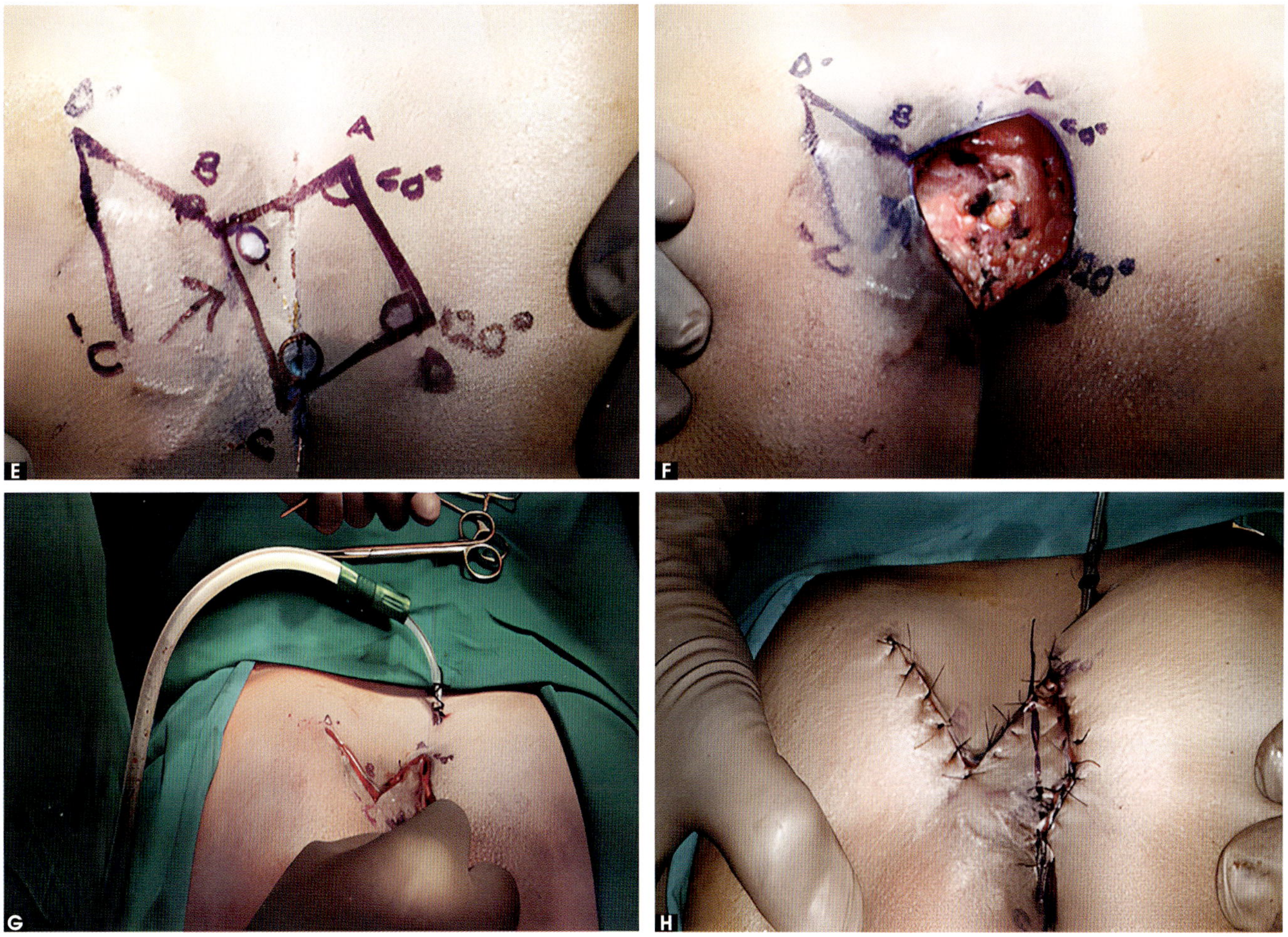

Fig. 7.9E-H: Technique of Limberg's (Rhomboid) Flap. E) Marking of the flap. F) Excision of the pilonidal sinus tract. G) Rotation of the flap and placement of the suction drain away from the midline. H) The final appearance of the wound at the end of the procedure.

BASCOM'S CLEFT CLOSURE TECHNIQUE

The schematic diagram of Bascom's procedure is shown in Fig. 7.10. The case discussed is of a patient operated on with a lay-open technique 6 months back with a resultant non-healing wound in the centre (Fig. 7.11).

Indications

In addition to the mentioned indications, the procedure can be done in non-healing wounds after Marsupialization/Saucerisation/Sinusotomy.

Instrumentation (Fig. 7.5A, B)

Position of the patient

Prone position with a small bolster under the hips of the patient and buttocks strapped apart after the skin markings.

Anesthesia

General with endotracheal intubation/Spinal/Epidural/Local infiltration with sedation.

Preparation

Trimming/shaving of the hair in and around the gluteal cleft before surgery. A dose of Injection Amoxiclav 1.2 gm is given intravenously at the time of induction of anesthesia.

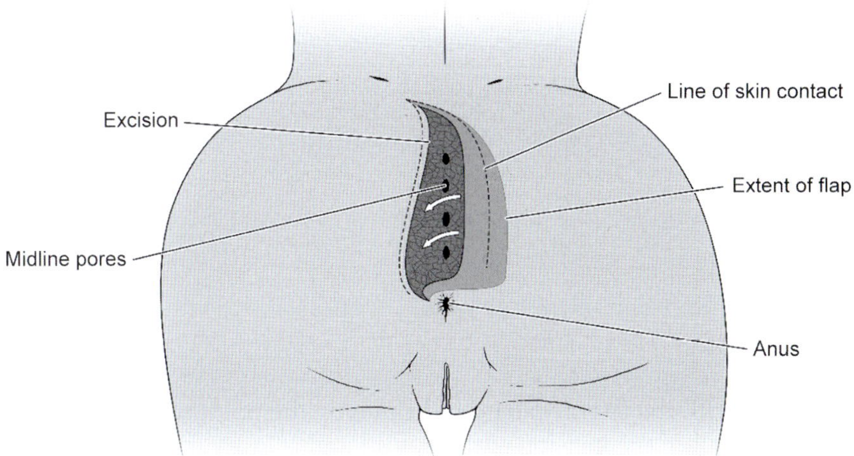

Fig. 7.10: Schematic diagram of Bascom's procedure.

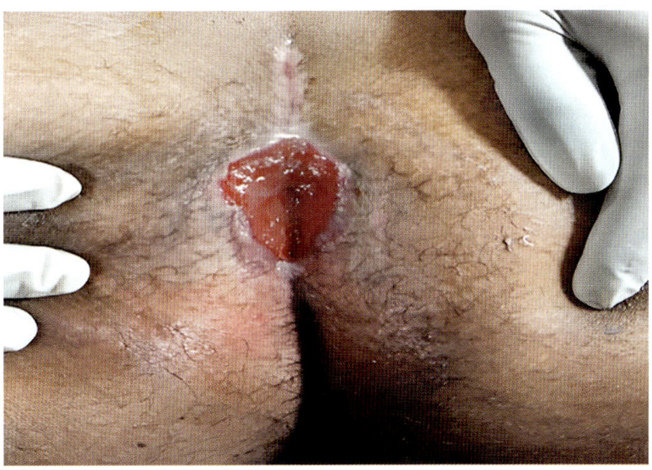

Fig. 7.11: Non-healing wound after a lay-open technique.

Steps of the Procedure

Step 1: The marking is done with the lateral extend indicated by the point where both buttocks meet without tension. Note that the lower end of the incision curls around and is away from the anus (Fig. 7.12A).

Step 2: The shaded area is de-epithelialized to allow the flap from the opposite side to slide across the midline to lie over the raw area (Fig. 7.12B).

Step 3: A full-thickness flap is raised on the patient's right side and undermined until the lateral markings. Skin hooks are used to aid the raising of the flap (Fig. 7.12C).

Step 4: Shaded area on the left side is de-epithelialized to prepare a natural area for the flap on the right side to inset. The straps on the buttocks are removed. The positioning of the flap towards the opposite side for overlapping is confirmed (Fig. 7.12D).

Step 5: The pilonidal sinus cavity demarcated by methylene blue is completely excised (Fig. 7.12E).

Step 6: The subcutaneous fat layer is approximated with interrupted 3-0 polyglactin to flatten the deep natal cleft (Fig. 7.12F).

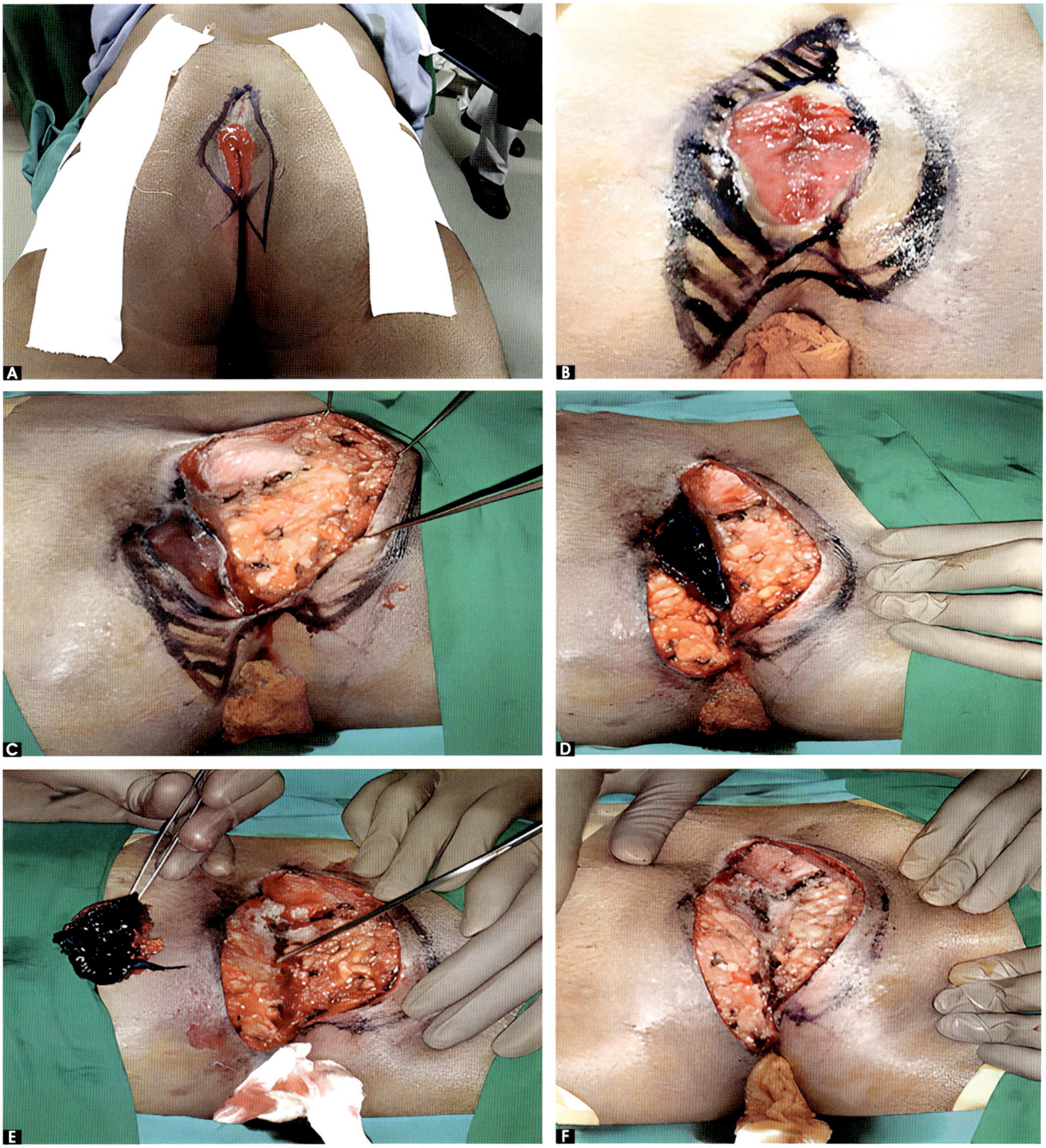

Fig. 7.12A–F: Bascom's cleft closure technique. A) Marking of the non-healing wound. B) Note the shaded area to be de-epithelialized. C) Skin hooks used to aid the raising of the flap. D) De-epithelialization of the shaded area and preparation of the area for the flap. E) Complete excision of pilonidal sinus. The methylene blue-stained tract can be seen. F) Approximation of subcutaneous fat.

Step 7: A negative suction drain is placed in the wound and brought out from the upper end, away from the midline (Fig. 7.12G).

Step 8: Skin is then approximated with interrupted sutures (Fig. 7.12H). Sometimes, post-operatively, the wound may break through (Fig. 7.12I).

The wound completely heals in 6 weeks (Fig. 7.12J). Another case of Bascom's cleft closure technique with good healing is shown in Fig. 7.12K.

Scan QR Code for Video on
Bascom Cleft Closure Technique
VIDEO 39

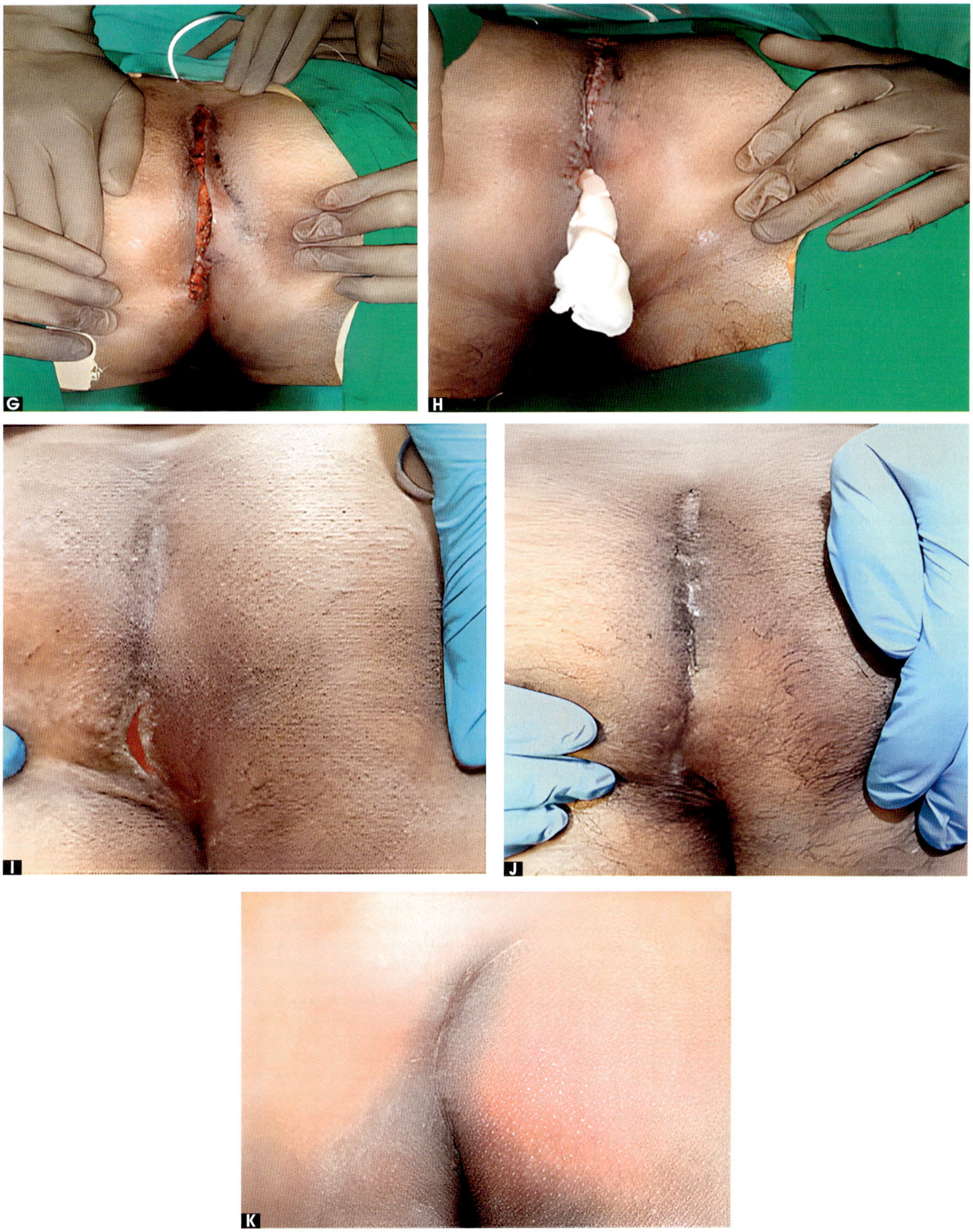

Fig. 7.12G–K: Bascom's Cleft closure technique. G) Placement of suction. Note that the suction has been taken out lateral to the midline. H) Approximation of skin to close the wound. I) Breakthrough of the wound during the healing period. J) Complete healing of the wound. K) Picture showing good healing with Bascom's cleft closure technique.

MULTIPLE Z PLASTY

The technique described is a modification of the Single Z Plasty, which requires general or regional anaesthesia and is associated with extensive denervation and disfigurement of the gluteal area.

Instrumentation (Fig. 7.5A, B)

Indications

- Pilonidal disease with a deep natal cleft
- Recurrent disease
- Midline or paramedian disease (close to midline)
- Failure of minimally invasive techniques

Position of the patient

Prone position with a small bolster under the hips of the patient and buttocks strapped apart after the skin markings.

Anesthesia

General with endotracheal intubation/Spinal/Epidural/Local infiltration with sedation.

Preparation

Trimming or shaving of the hair in and around the gluteal cleft before surgery. A single dose of Injection Amoxyclav 1.2 gm is given intravenously at the time of induction of anesthesia.

Steps of the Procedure

Step 1: The pits are excised in continuity by an elliptical incision. An elliptical incision also excises silent midline pits (Fig. 7.13A, B).

Step 2: The lateral cuts of Z plasty are made as per the principles of Z Plasty (Fig. 7.13C). The angle of the lateral cuts is 60 degrees, and the length of the lateral cuts is equal to the distance between each cut (Fig. 7.13D). The cuts are of full thickness and up to the subcutaneous fatty layer (Fig. 7.13E).

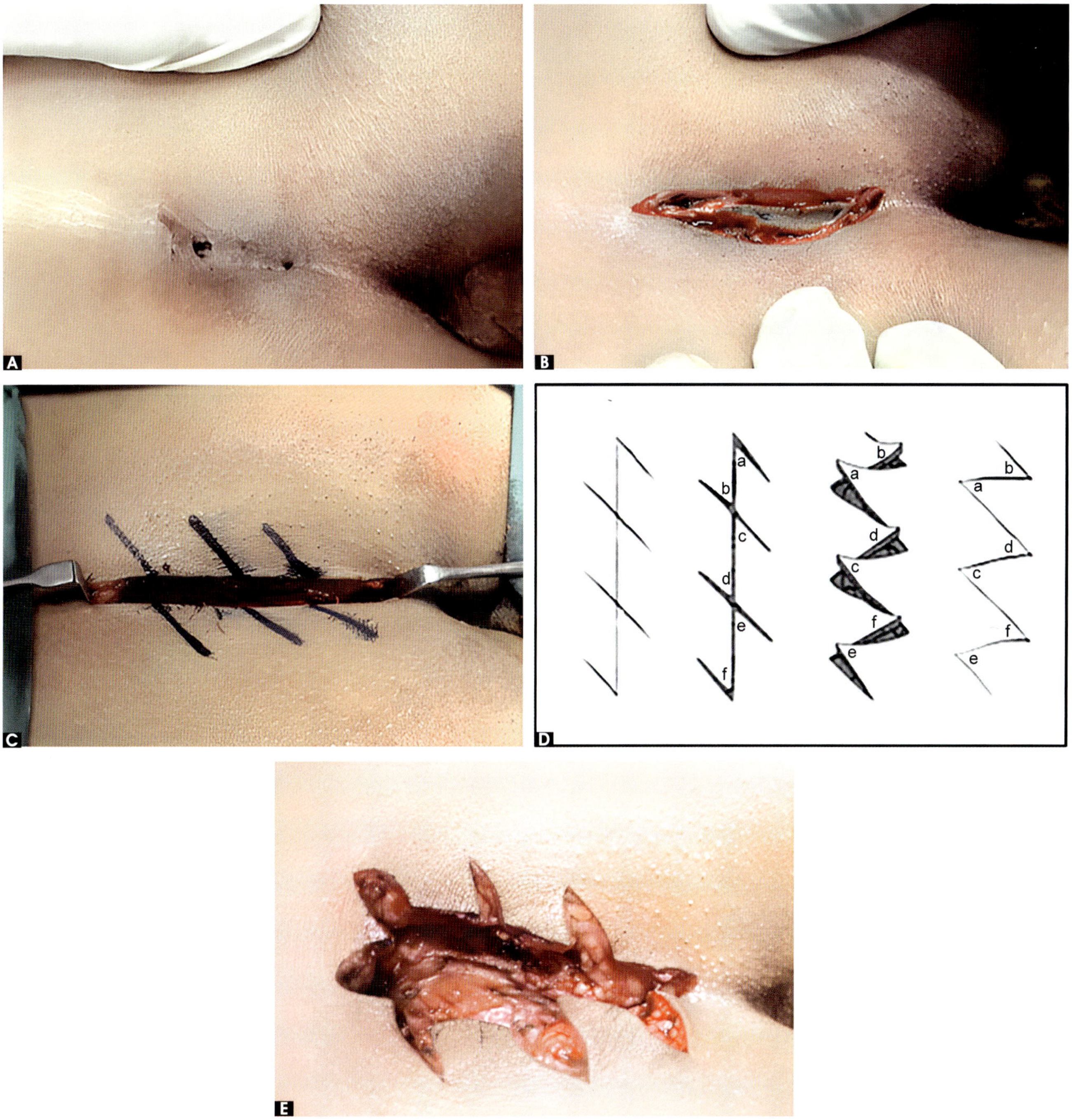

Fig. 7.13A-E: A) Preoperative picture showing both the primary and secondary pits in the midline. B) Excision of the pits by an elliptical incision. C, D) The lateral cuts of Z plasty as per the principles of Z Plasty. E) Full-thickness cuts upto the subcutaneous fatty layer. Skin approximation after keeping a subcutaneous suction drain.

Step 3: The flaps are moved to interdigitate with each other (Fig. 7.13F). The flaps are sutured in layers, the subcutaneous layer with PDA 3-0, and the skin is approximated with 4-0 Nylon, Polypropylene or Glue (Fig. 7.13G, H).

The completely healed wound at 4 weeks and 6 months is shown in Fig. 7.13I, J.

Scan QR Code for Video on
Multiple Z-Plasty for Pilonidal Sinus

VIDEO 40

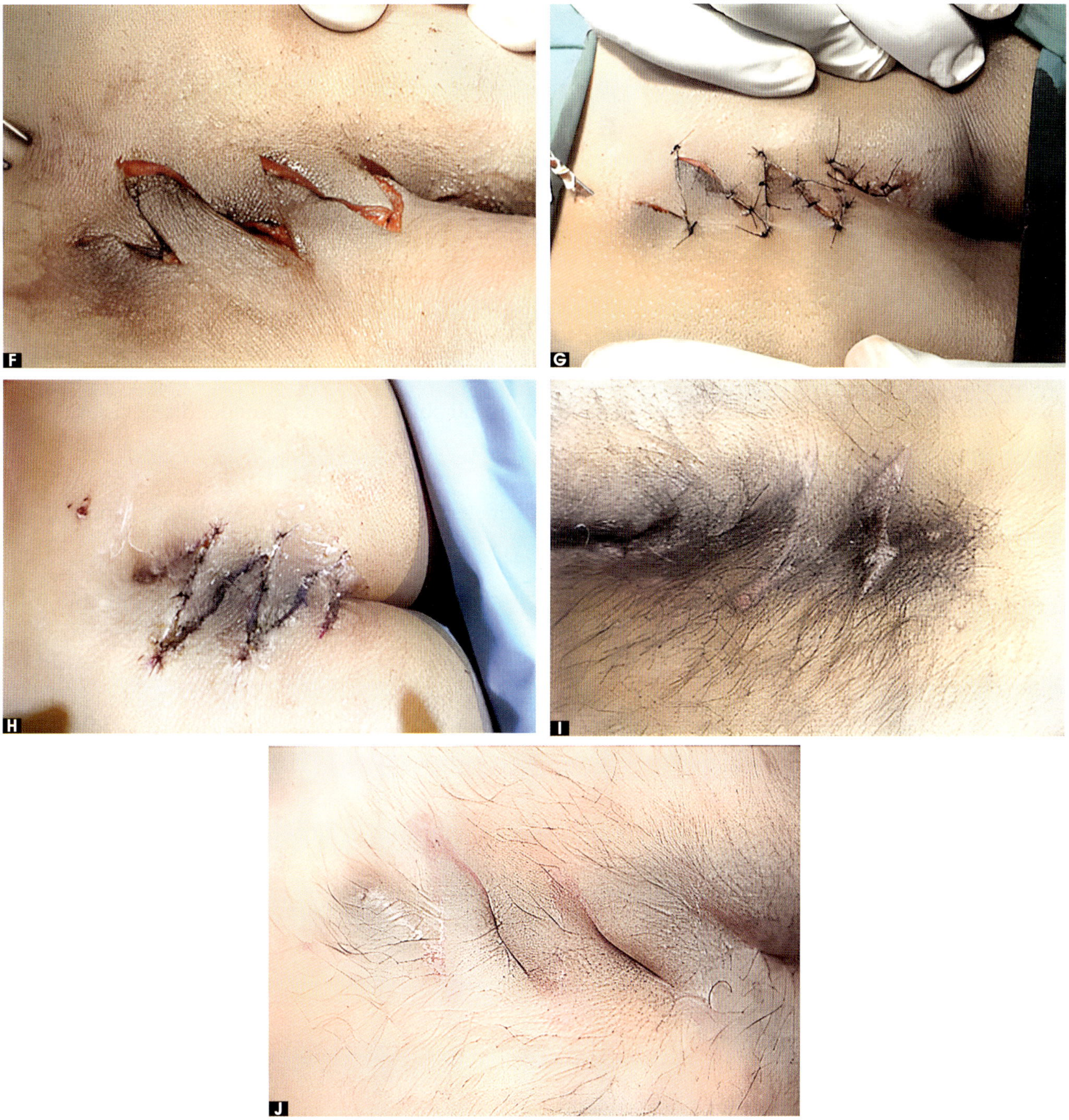

Fig. 7.13F-J: F) Interdigitating of the flaps. G, H) Closure with Nylon or Cyanoacrylate glue. I) Complete healing at 4 weeks. J) Appearance at 6 months.

MINIMALLY INVASIVE PROCEDURE FOR THE MANAGEMENT OF PILONIDAL SINUS

Video-Assisted Laser Ablation of the Pilonidal Sinus (VALAPS)

Principle

Laser ablation of the sinus cavity to destroy the epithelium and obliterate the tract under direct vision.

Instrumentation

Device for video-assisted endoscopy

- Fistuloscope 8-degree with angled eyepiece, outer diameter 3.3 × 4.7 mm, working length handle 18 cm (Fig. 7.14)
- Obturator
- Handle
- Endoscopic seal for working channel
- Wire tray for cleaning, storage, and sterilization
- Coagulation electrode
- Brush
- Grasping forceps 2 mm diameter, length 30cm with double action jaws
- Plastic handle
- Outer sheath
- Camera
- Fibre optic cable
- Light source

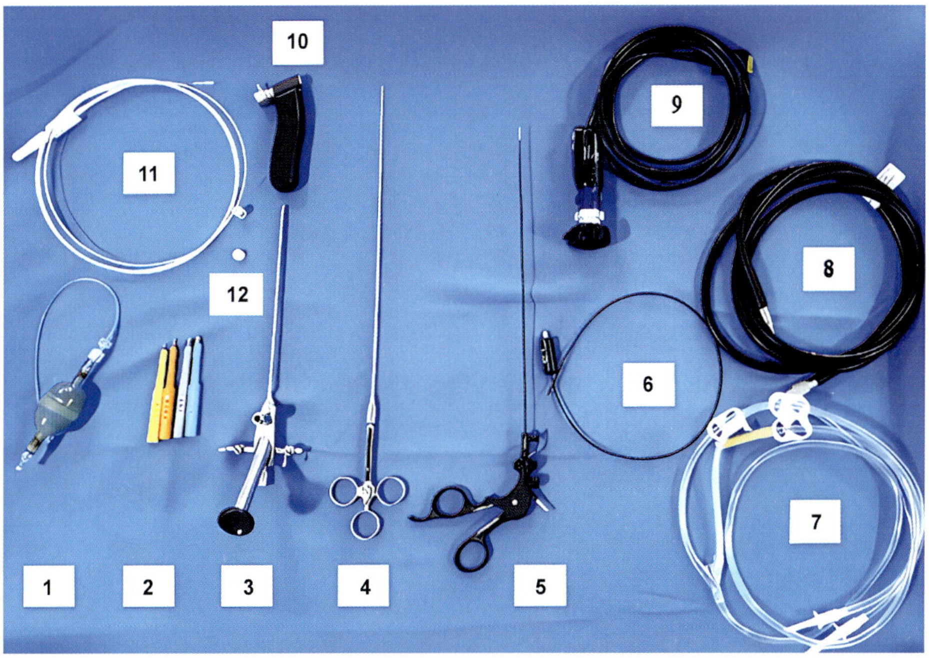

Fig. 7.14: Instrumentation for VALAPS. 1) Path finder. 2) Punch Biopsy forceps. 3) Fistuloscope. 4) Brush with handle. 5) Grasper forceps. 6) Cautery lead. 7) Irrigation tube (TUR set). 8) Light Source. 9) Camera. 10) Handle. 11) Laser fibre. 12) Stopper.

Device for pit excision

- Dermatology biopsy forceps (Fig. 7.15A, B). Different sizes are available.

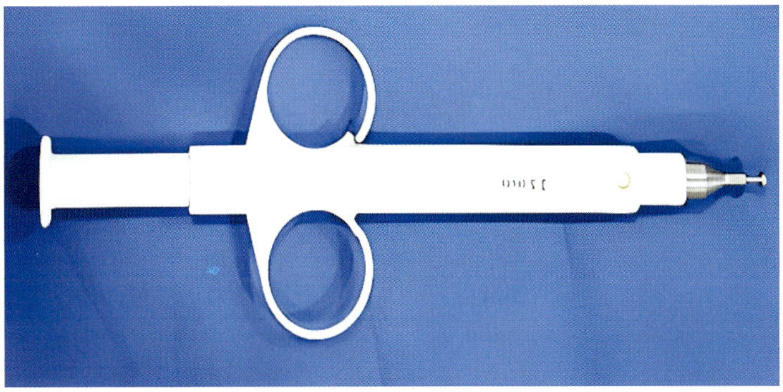

Fig. 7.15A: Pit excision forceps.

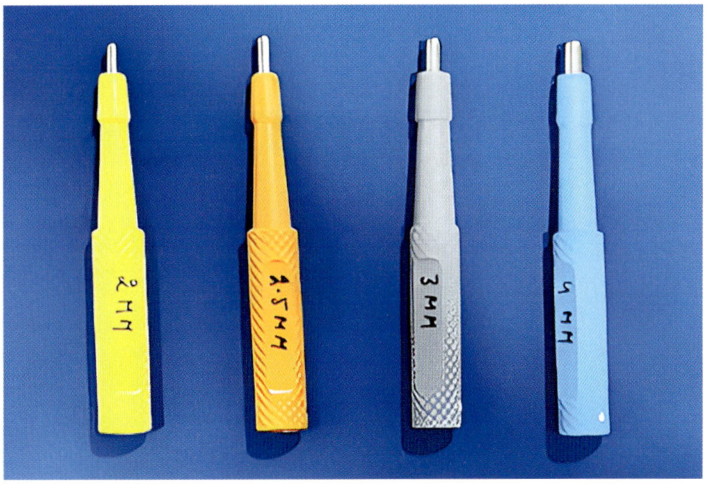

Fig. 7.15B: Pit biopsy forceps (available from 1 to 10 mm sizes).

Assembling the Fistuloscope

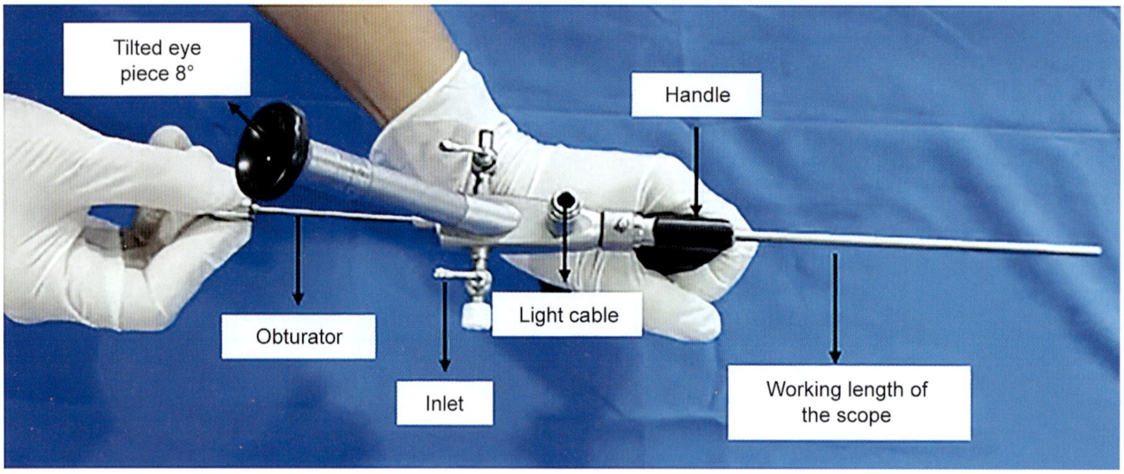

Fig. 7.16: Fistuloscope.

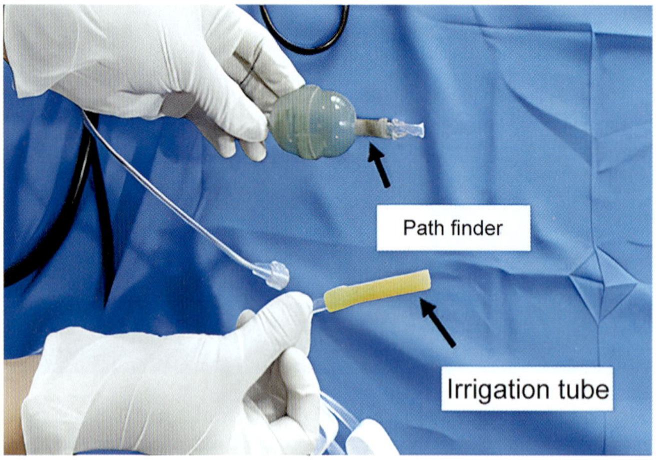

Fig. 7.17: Path finder with irrigation tube.

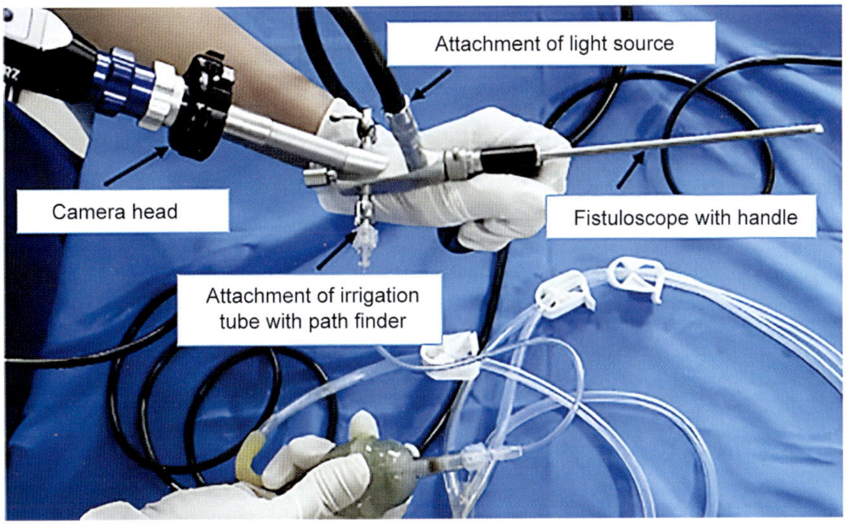

Fig. 7.18: Assembled fistuloscope.

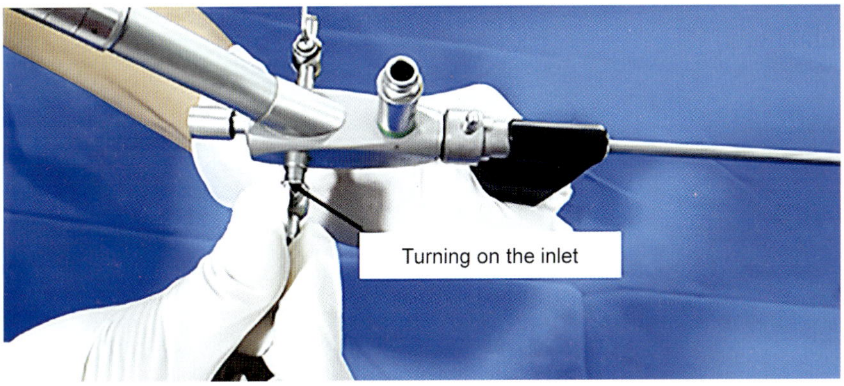

Fig. 7.19: Turning on the irrigation channel.

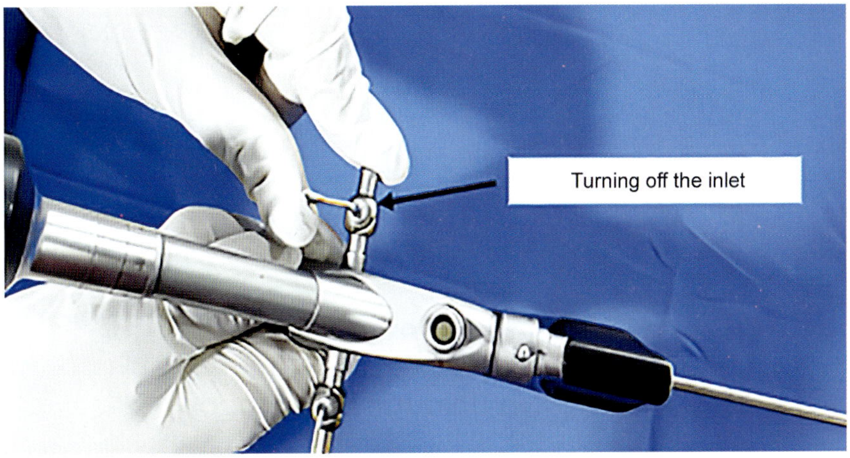

Fig. 7.20: Turning off the irrigation channel.

Scan QR Code for Video on
Assembling Video Endoscope for VALAPS
VIDEO 41

Device for Laser Ablation (Fig. 7.21A-E)

Wavelength: 1470 nm wavelength.

Fibre: 360-degree radial fibre.

Dosage! Energy! Fiber!

Dosage: 12 W per second per mm (Fig. 7.21)

Mode: Continuous mode

Energy: Total energy delivered depends on the length of the tract.

Position of the patient: Prone position with buttocks strapped apart.

Type of anesthesia: Spinal/Local infiltration of lidocaine.

Preparation: Shave a circular area of 6–10 inches around the opening of the sinus.

Scan QR Code for Video on
Use of Laser Fibre through Fistuloscope
VIDEO 42

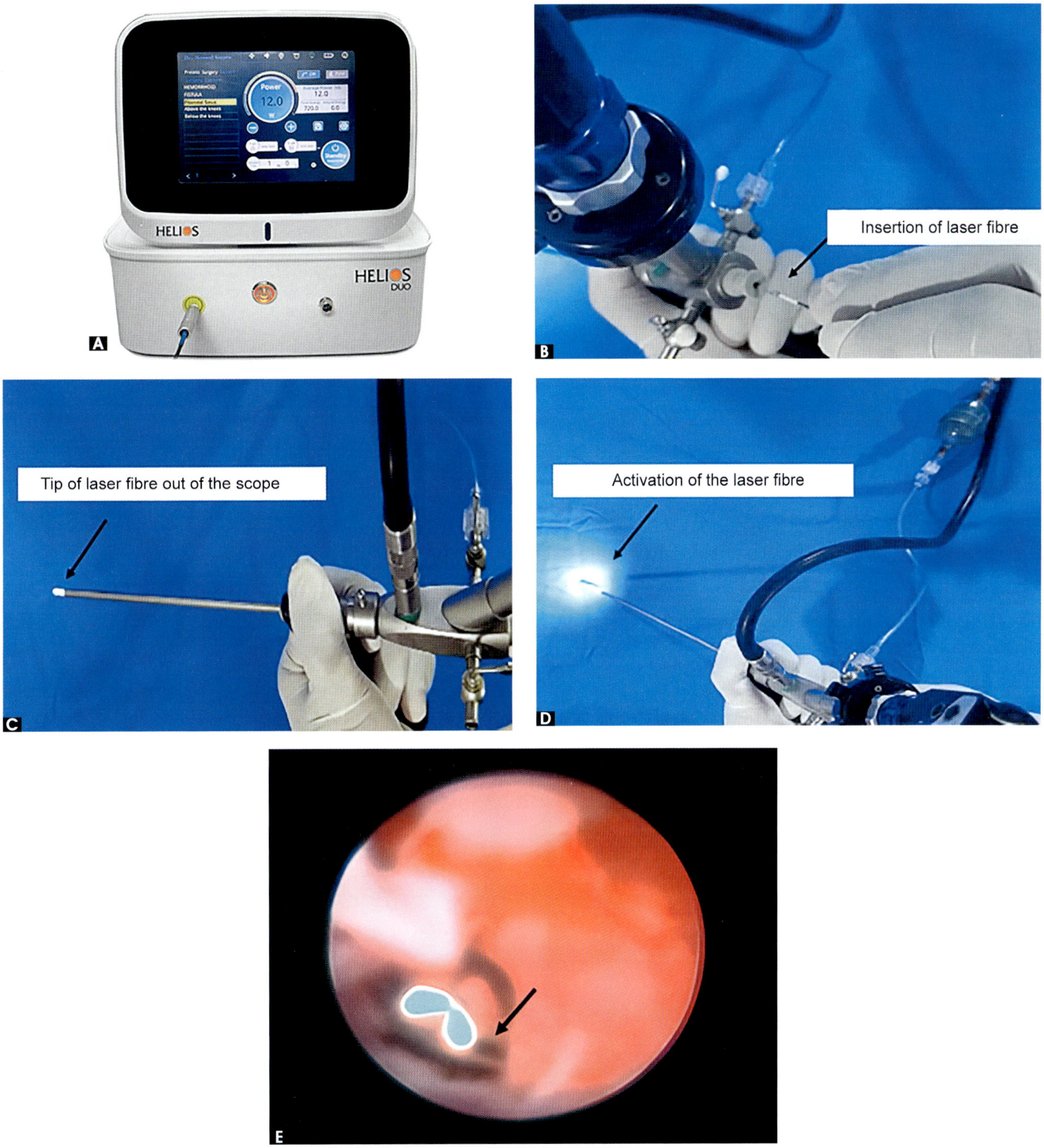

Fig. 7.21A–E: Laser ablation equipment. A) Laser machine 1470 nm. B) Insertion of radial laser fibre through the working channel. C) Laser fibre tip outside fistuloscope lumen. D) Fibreoptic light and laser beam as seen before activation. E) Laser fibre as seen inside the sinus. The black color rings are of radial fibre.

Steps of the Procedure

Step 1: The first step involves excision of the pits using punch biopsy forceps (Fig. 7.22A).

Step 2: If there is no secondary opening away from the midline, convert the sinus tract into a tunnel by creating an iatrogenic opening 3–4 mm wide and 1–1.5 cm lateral to the midline (Fig. 7.22B). This helps in easy cleaning of the tract.

Step 3: Insert the fistuloscope through this tunnel to visualize the entire tract (Fig. 7.22C). Identify the hair and necrotic material and remove them with sharp curetting followed by irrigation of the sinus tract (Fig. 7.22D, E, F).

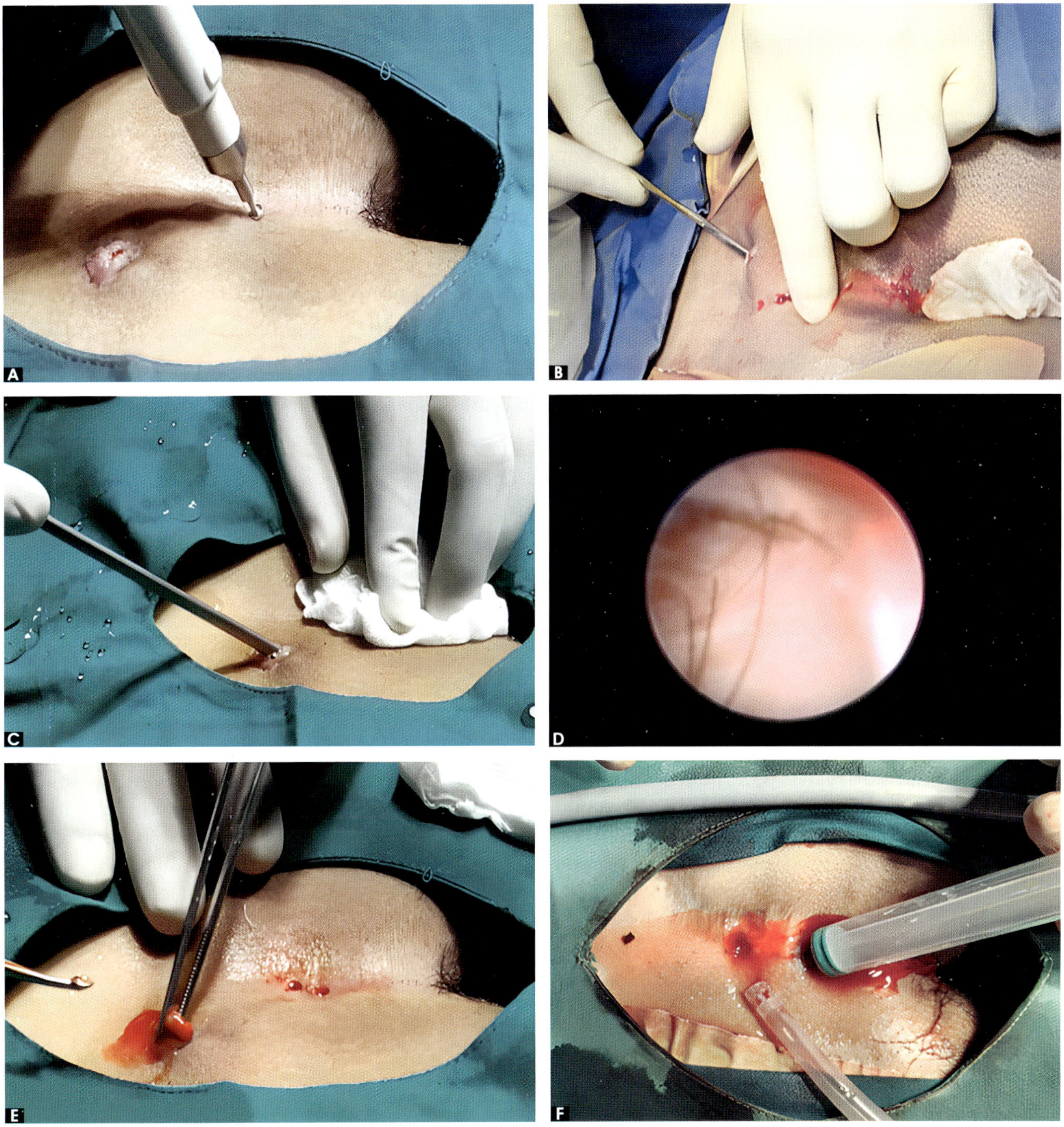

Fig. 7.22A to F: Steps of Video-Assissted laser ablation of pilonidal sinus technique. A) Excision of pits using pit excision forceps. B) Creation of an iatrogenic opening 1 to 1.5 cm away from the midline. C) Insertion of the fistuloscope through the secondary opening of the pilonidal sinus. D) Presence of necrotic material and hair as seen under video endoscope. E) Curetting of the sinus tract. F) Tuft of hair removed after curetting the sinus tract.

Step 4: Introduce Corona, 360° radial laser 600 µm with distal and outer diameters of 1800 µm into the sinus through the working channel of the video endoscope. Always keep the tip of the laser fibre 1 cm away from the lens of the fistuloscope to avoid damage to the lens (Fig. 7.22G).

Step 5: Ablate the entire tract using laser equipment of 1470 nm wavelength. The energy given is 12 watts per second per mm in continuous mode (Fig. 7.22H).

Step 6: Again curette and irrigate the tract to remove the burnt-out necrotic material. The pits may be closed with a skin suture (Fig. 7.22I).

Step 7: To review the tract, the fistuloscope scope is reinserted in the pilonidal sinus cavity (Fig. 7.22J).

Step 8: The secondary opening is widened, and the wound is dressed using an antiseptic ointment (Fig. 7.22K, L).

Tips and Tricks

- While releasing the energy, ensure a distance of at least 1 cm between the laser fibre tip and the video endoscope lens. Otherwise, the tip of the scope can be damaged by thermal energy.
- At the time of discharge of the patient, saline irrigation of the wound is carried out to remove any leftover debris.

Conclusion

While minimally invasive techniques are gaining popularity in managing pilonidal sinus disease, conventional methods like Karydakis, Bascom and Limberg's flap should not be overlooked. The Video-assisted laser ablation of pilonidal sinus (VALAPS) technique allows direct examination of the sinus tract and enables removal of hair and the necrotic material under vision. The laser also helps ablate and shrink the tract. This technique offers the advantages of low postoperative discomfort and a quick return to work for the patients. Hence, minimally invasive procedures are a valuable option in the armamentarium of treatment for pilonidal sinus disease.

Scan QR Code for Video on
VALAPS

VIDEO 43

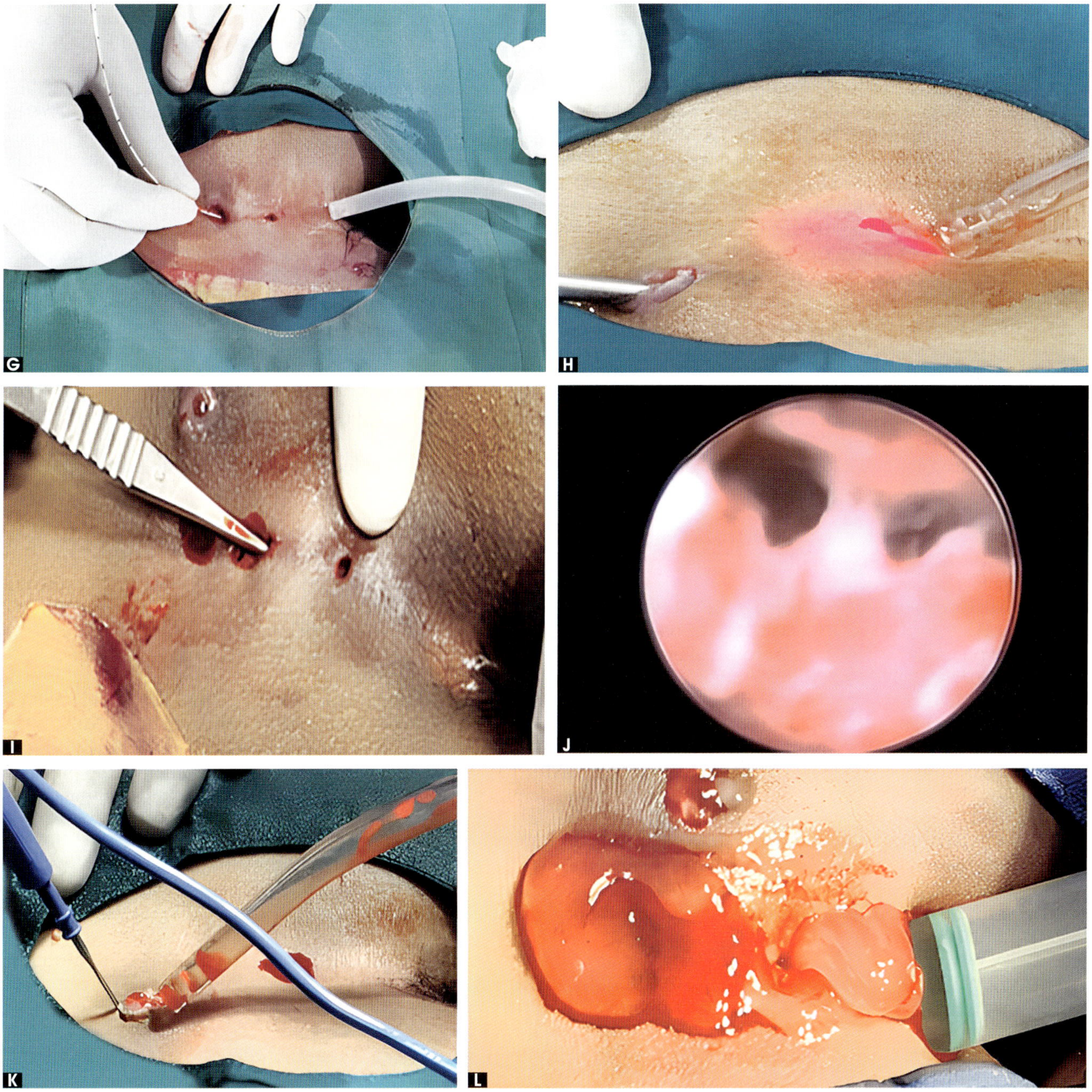

Fig. 7.22G to L: Steps of Video-Assissted laser ablation of pilonidal sinus technique. G) Irrigation of the tract. H) Laser ablation of the sinus tract using radial fibre. I) Curetting of the sinus cavity. J) Visualizing the charred tissue in the tract. K) Widening of the secondary opening. L) Dressing with antiseptic ointment.

FURTHER READING

- Aithal SK, Rajan CS, Reddy N. Limberg flap for sacrococcygeal pilonidal sinus a safe and sound procedure. Indian J Surg. 2013 Aug;75(4):298–301. doi: 10.1007/s12262-012-0489-5. Epub 2012 May 6. PMID: 24426457; PMCID: PMC372680
- Dahl HD, Henrich MH. [Light and scanning electron microscopy study of Tezel E. A new classification according to the navicular area concept for sacrococcygeal pilonidal dis- ease. Colorectal Dis. 2007;9(6):575–6. https://doi. org/10.1111/j.1463-1318.2007.01236.x.
- Dönmez M, Uludag M. Evaluation of the Early Outcomes of Laser-Endoscopic Pilonidal Sinus Treatment Combination and Comparison With the Combination of Cautery-Phenol-Endoscopic Pilonidal Sinus Treatment. Cureus. 2022 Jul 17;14(7):e26948. doi: 10.7759/cureus.26948. PMID: 35989794; PMCID: PMC9378937.
- Giarratano G, Toscana C, Shalaby M, Buonomo O, Petrella G, Sileri P. Endoscopic pilonidal sinus treatment: long-term results of a perspective series. J Soc Laparoendosc Surg. 2017;21(3):e2017.00043. https:// doi.org/10.4293/JSLS.2017.00043.
- Gupta K, Mital K, Gupta R. Video-assisted laser ablation of pilonidal sinus VALAPS—a combined mini- mally invasive approach for management of pilonidal sinus. IJCAR. 2019;8(09):19789–93.
- Harlak A, Mentes O, Kilic S, Coskun K, Duman K, Yilmaz F. Sacrococcygeal pilonidal disease: analysis of previously proposed risk factors. Clinics (Sao Paulo, Brazil). 2010;65(2):125–31. https://doi. org/10.1590/S1807-59322010000200002.
- Hove CR, Williams EF 3rd, Rodgers BJ. Z-plasty: a concise review. Facial Plast Surg. 2001 Nov;17(4):289–94. doi: 10.1055/s-2001-18828. PMID: 11735063.
- Imam A, Khalayleh H, Pines G, Khoury D, Mavor E, Pelta A. Pilonidal Sinus Management; Bascom Flap Versus Pilonidal Pits Excision: A Single-Center Experience. Ann Coloproctol. 2021 Apr;37(2):109–114. doi: 10.3393/ac.2019.11.19.2. Epub 2020 Nov 6. PMID: 33171038; PMCID: PMC8134928.
- Immerman SC. The Bascom Cleft Lift as a Solution for All Presentations of Pilonidal Disease. Cureus. 2021 Feb 1;13(2):e13053. doi: 10.7759/cureus.13053. PMID: 33552799; PMCID: PMC7854339.
- Karydakis GE. Easy and successful treatment of pilonidal sinus after explanation of its causative process. Aust N Z J Surg. 1992;62(5):385–9.
- Khanna A, Rombeau JL. Pilonidal disease. Clin ColonRectal Surg. 2011;24:46–53.
- Kumar NA, Sutradhar P. Karydakis procedure for sacrococcygeal pilonidal sinus disease: Our experience. Indian J Plast Surg. 2014 Sep-Dec;47(3):402–6. doi: 10.4103/0970-0358.146615. PMID: 25593428; PMCID: PMC4292120.
- Matsumoto EA, Liang H, Mahadevan L. Topology, Geometry, and Mechanics of Z-Plasty. Phys Rev Lett. 2018 Feb 9;120(6):068101. doi: 10.1103/PhysRevLett.120.068101. PMID: 29481240.
- Meinero P, La Torre M, Lisi G, Stazi A, Carbone A, Regusci L, Fasolini F. Endoscopic pilonidal sinus treatment (EPSiT) in recurrent pilonidal dis-ease: a prospective international multicenter study. Int J Colorectal Dis. 2019;34(4):741–6. https://doi. Org/10.1007/s00384-019-03256-8.
- Milone M, Musella M, Di Spiezio Sardo A, Bifulco G, Salvatore G, Sosa Fernandez LM, Bianco P, Zizolfi B, Nappi C, Milone F. Video-assisted ablation of pilonidal sinus: a new minimally invasive treatment—a pilot study. Surgery. 2014;155(3):562–6. https://doi. org/10.1016/j.surg.2013.08.021.
- Milone M, Velotti N, Manigrasso M, Milone F, Sosa Fernandez LM, De Palma GD. Video-assisted ablation of the pilonidal sinus (VAAPS) versus sinuses- tomy for treatment of chronic pilonidal sinus disease: a comparative study. Update Surg. 2019;71(1):179–83. https://doi.org/10.1007/s13304-018-00611-2.
- Nixon AT, Garza RF. Pilonidal cyst and sinus. StatPearls; 2020.
- Patey DH, Scarff RW. Pathology of the postanal pilonidal sinus; it's bearing on treatment. Lancet. 1946;2(6423):484–6. https://doi.org/10.1016/ s0140-6736(46)91756-4.
- Rohrich RJ, Zbar RI. A simplified algorithm for the use of Z-plasty. Plast Reconstr Surg. 1999 Apr;103(5):1513–7; quiz 1518. PMID: 10190452.
- Shockley WW. Scar revision techniques: z-plasty, w-plasty, and geometric broken line closure. Facial Plast Surg Clin North Am. 2011 Aug;19(3):455-63. doi: 10.1016/j.fsc.2011.06.002. PMID: 21856534.
- Sion-Vardy N, Osyntsov L, Cagnano E, Osyntsov A, Vardy D, Benharroch D. Unexpected location of pilonidal sinuses. Clin Exp Dermatol. 2009;34(8):e599–601. https://doi.org/10.1111/j.1365-2230.2009.03272.x.
- Stelzner F. Die Ursache des pilonidal sinus und der Pyodermia fistulans sinifica [Causes of pilonidal sinus and pyoderma fistulans sinifica]. Langenbecks Arch Chir. 1984;362(2):105–18. German. https://doi. org/10.1007/BF01254185.
- Svarre KJ, Serup CM, Kanstrup CT, Kleif J, & Bertelsen CA. (2023). Long-term outcome after Bascom's cleft-lift procedure under tumescent local analgesia for pilonidal sinus disease: a cohort study. Colorectal Disease, 25(4), 707–716.
- Yildiz MK, Ozkan E, Odaba ı HM, Kaya B, Eri C, Abuo lu HH, Günay E, Fersahoglu MM, Atalay S. Karydakis flap procedure in patients with sacrococcygeal pilonidal sinus disease: experience of a single centre in Istanbul. ScientificWorldJournal. 2013 May 14;2013:807027. doi: 10.1155/2013/807027. PMID: 23766710; PMCID: PMC3666289.
- Zito PM, Jawad BA, Hohman MH, Mazzoni T. Z-Plasty. 2023 Mar 7. In: StatPearls [Internet]. Treasure Island (FL): StatPearls Publishing; 2023 Jan–. PMID: 29939552.

Chapter

8

Surgical Management of Anal Fissure

An anal fissure is a painful tear in the anal canal that may extend from the mucocutaneous junction to the dentate line. An acute anal fissure usually heals within six weeks. A fissure is known as a chronic fissure if it is present for more than 6 weeks.

Most anal fissures lie either anteriorly or posteriorly in the midline. Approximately 90% of the fissures are located posteriorly. Anterior fissures are more common in females. Sometimes, a patient may present with both an anterior and a posterior fissure (Fig. 8.1). A lateral fissure may be associated with conditions like Crohn's, tuberculosis, HIV or syphilis.

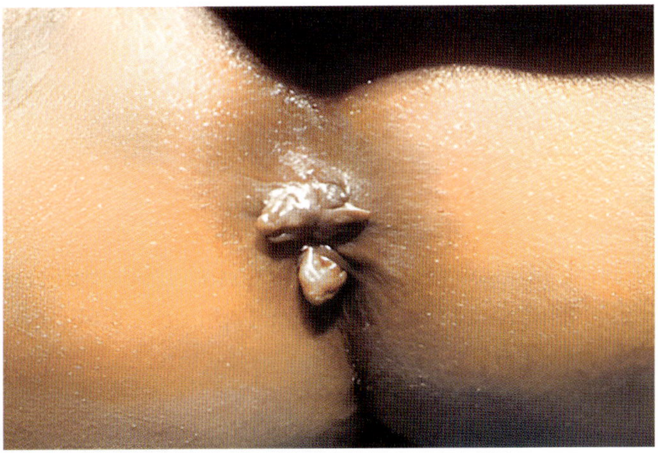

Fig. 8.1: Presence of anterior and posterior anal fissures with sentinel piles.

Classification of Anal Fissure

Fissures are graded as follows:

- Grade 1: Superficial linear tear
- Grade 2: A deep linear tear associated with a small sentinel pile
- Grade 3: Deep linear tear having fibrosed margins and an associated sentinel pile
- Grade 4: A wide tear with visible fibres of the internal anal sphincter and an associated sentinel pile
- Grade 5: A wide pear-shaped tear having visible fibres of the internal anal sphincter and associated with hypertrophic anal papillae with sentinel piles (Fig. 8.2A–E).

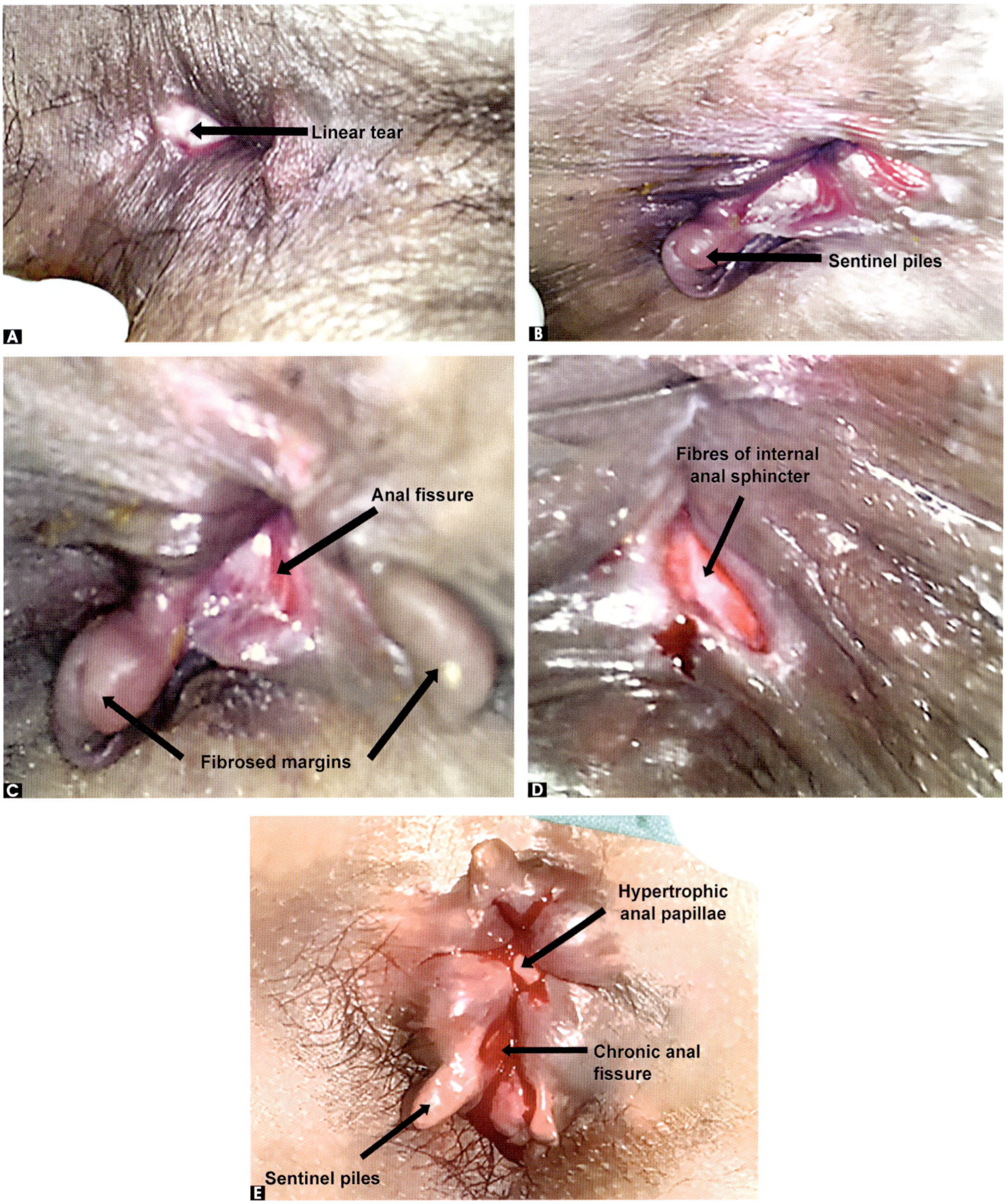

Fig. 8.2A-E: Classification of anal fissures. A) Superficial linear tear. B) Deep linear tear with sentinel piles. C) Deep linear tear having fibrosed margin and associated sentinel piles. D) Linear tear with visible fibres of IAS. E) Anal fissure triad showing chronic anal fissure, hypertrophic anal papillae and sentinel piles.

Surgical Management of Anal fissure

Failure of medical management is an indication of surgery. Manual anal dilation should not be done as it may rupture the internal and external anal sphincter fibres. Once the muscle fibres are ruptured, there is fibrosis which decreases the elasticity of the sphincter, leading to anal incontinence in some patients.

In a high-pressure anal fissure, the anal tone increases, leading to a spasm of the internal anal sphincter (IAS). The surgical intervention aims to remove the spasm by cutting the IAS. The IAS is always cut from its lower end to the dentate line, irrespective of the fissure length. As the IAS relaxes, the fissure heals due to increased blood supply.

The surgical procedures performed for anal fissures are:

1. Internal Sphincterotomy

Lateral internal sphincterotomy (LIS) – closed or open method. LIS is a procedure of choice with high-pressure fissures where the anal tone is markedly increased.

Indications

- Failed conservative treatment
- Fissures associated with high pressure (increased anal tone)

Contraindications

- Fissures associated with low pressure (laxed anal tone)

2. Anal Advancement Flap (AAF)

Indications

- Low-pressure fissures where the anal tone is reduced.

In an anal fissure triad, a fissurectomy can be done, and the associated skin tag, hypertrophic papilla and rolled-out fissure margins can be excised. One should never do posterior sphincterotomy, which may lead to a keyhole deformity, pruritis ani and fecal soiling.

Closed Lateral Internal Sphincterotomy

Instrumentation: Figure 8.3A, B

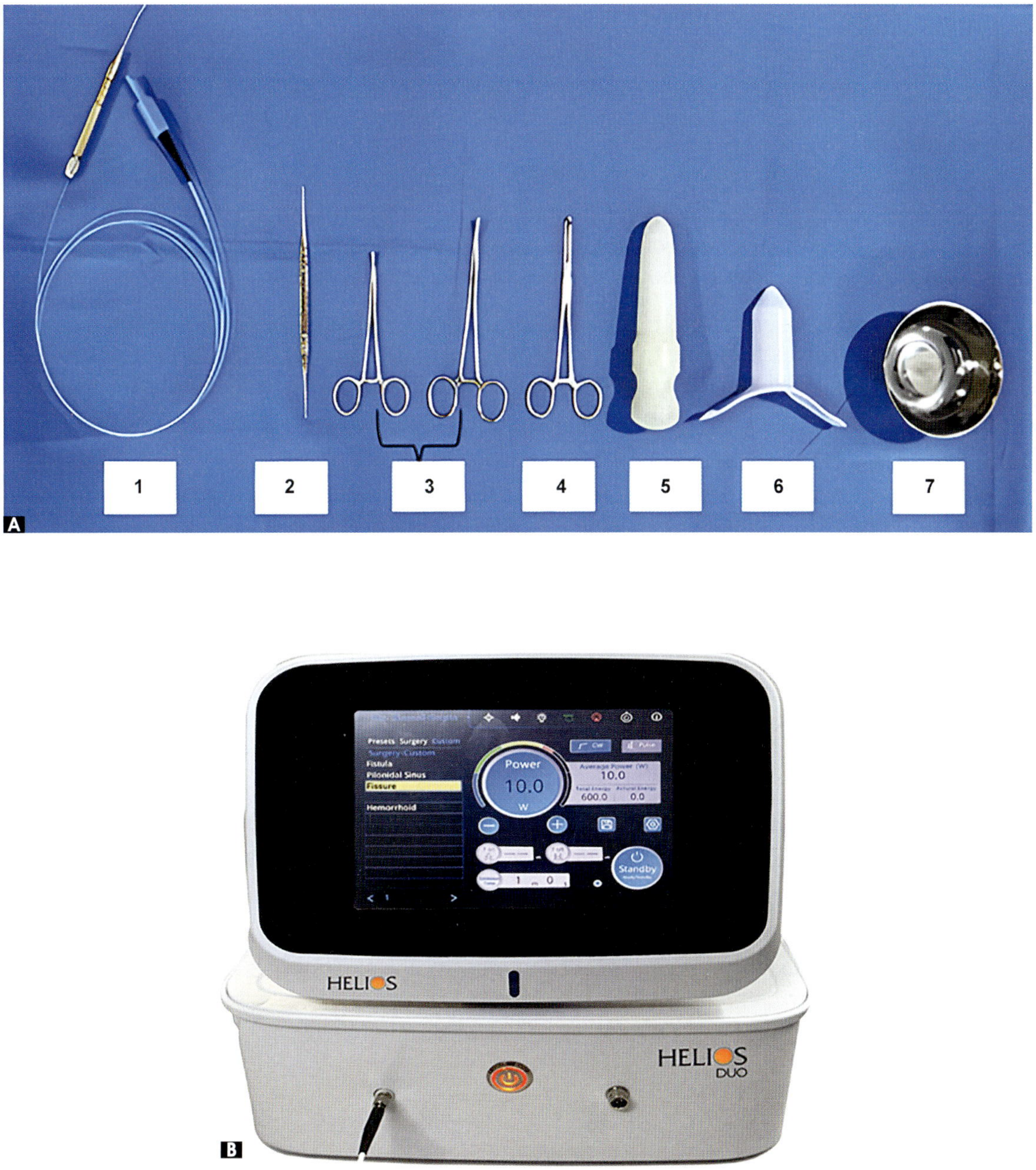

Fig. 8.3A, B: Instrumentation. A) 1) Bare laser fibre with handle. 2) Fine curette. 3) Mosquito and artery forceps. 4) Allis. 5) Anal dilator. 6) Half-cut proctoscope. 7) Lidocaine jelly. B) Diode laser 1470.

Scan QR Code for Video on
Sharpening of Laser Fibre

VIDEO 44

Anesthesia: Spinal/General/Pudendal nerve block.

Position of the patient: Lithotomy

Steps of the Procedure

Step 1: The local area at the fissure site is palpated. Sim's speculum (one-sided) is inserted into the anal canal. Traction is given directly opposite to the site of the incision. For a right-handed surgeon, the traction is given towards 9 o'clock; for a left-handed surgeon, the traction is given towards 3 o'clock. The sphincters stand out with traction, and the intersphincteric groove becomes easily identifiable (Fig. 8.4A).

Step 2: The left forefinger is inserted into the anal canal up to the dentate line for guiding the blade. The left thumb is placed lateral to the incision site to push the external anal sphincter away. A 15-number blade on the handle is inserted in the intersphincteric groove between 3 and 5 o'clock, up to the dentate line. Alternatively, an 11-number blade or an ophthalmic knife can be inserted (Fig. 8.4B).

Step 3: The blade is turned 90 degrees to face the internal anal sphincter, and the fibres are cut in a single stroke. Since it is a blind procedure, sometimes a few fibres of IAS may be missed due to angulation of the blade leading to partial sphincterotomy. The fibres can be broken by pressing them (Fig. 8.4C).

Step 4: Sometimes, the patient may have bleeding from the surgery site. Pressing the operative site like a pinchcock for 5–10 minutes will stop the bleeding. If the bleeding persists, a deep purse string suture can be taken at the incision site.

The post-operative wound at the end of the procedure is shown in Fig. 8.4D.

Tips and Tricks

- If a wide area is present after the skin tag excision, the edges can be approximated with horizontal mattress sutures using 4/0 rapid Polyglactin.
- A gauze wick can be kept inside to maintain the hemostasis.
- A diclofenac suppository can be inserted into the anal canal at the end of the procedure to reduce post-operative pain.
- Post-operatively osmotic laxatives should be used to prevent constipation.

Advantages of Closed LIS

- No large wound or raw area is created.

Disadvantages of Closed LIS

- Sometimes severe bleeding can occur. Complete hemostasis has to be maintained.
- If the mucosa is punctured while doing closed LIS, an intersphincteric fistula may form if the wound gets infected.

Scan QR Code for Video on
Closed LIS

VIDEO 45

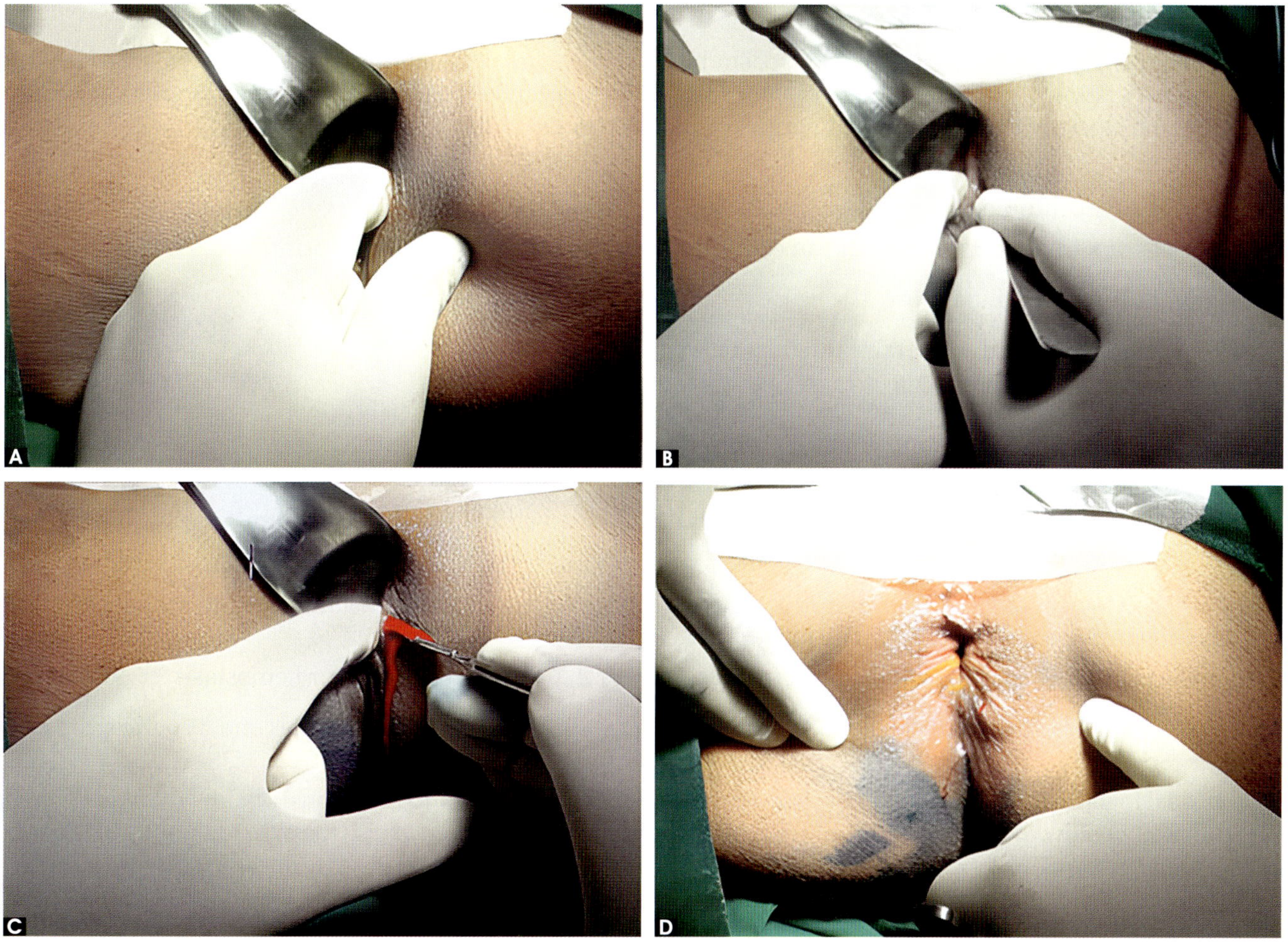

Fig. 8.4A-D: The technique of closed lateral internal sphincterotomy. A) Palpation of intersphincteric groove after insertion of Sim's speculum. B) Insertion of the blade in the intersphincteric groove. C) Rotation of scalpel medially towards the IAS to cut the muscle. D) Post-operative wound as seen after the surgical procedure.

Open Lateral Internal Sphincterotomy

This technique relieves the anal sphincter spasm by cutting the internal anal sphincter under vision. Healing rates and results are the same for open and closed lateral inter sphincterotomy. The open lateral sphincterotomy is done at 3 o'clock by the right-handed surgeon and at 9 o'clock by the left-handed.

Preoperative Preparation

Preparation for surgery includes giving an osmotic or a stimulant laxative a night prior.

Position of the patient: Lithotomy

Type of anesthesia: Spinal/General/Pudendal nerve block.

Steps of the Procedure

Step 1: Anoscope is introduced into the anal canal, and the intersphincteric groove is identified (Fig. 8.5A, B).

Step 2: A horizontal incision crossing both IAS and EAS or a vertical incision 5–10 mm long is given in the intersphincteric groove.

Step 3: With mosquito forceps, the fibres of the IAS are separated from the mucosa and cut with scissors, cautery or laser. The IAS is cut up to the dentate line (Fig. 8.5C).

Hemostasis is maintained with the cautery. Vicryl 3/0 or 4/0 can also be used for hemostasis.

Step 4: The next step is to manage the associated conditions like skin tags, sentinel piles and hypertrophic anal papillae (8.5D).

It is ideal to inject saline adrenaline (1 drop adrenaline in 10 ml saline) subcutaneously below the skin tag and submucosally below the hypertrophic papilla. Wait for 5 minutes and then excise the skin tag with a blade or a cautery. The hypertrophic papilla is cauterized. The rolled-out margins of the fissure and the floor are curetted for faster healing. Complete hemostasis is maintained using cautery. The final image after open lateral internal sphincterotomy is shown in Fig. 8.5E. The use of cautery for open lateral internal sphincterotomy is shown in Fig. 8.5F.

Scan QR Code for Video on

Open LIS

VIDEO 46

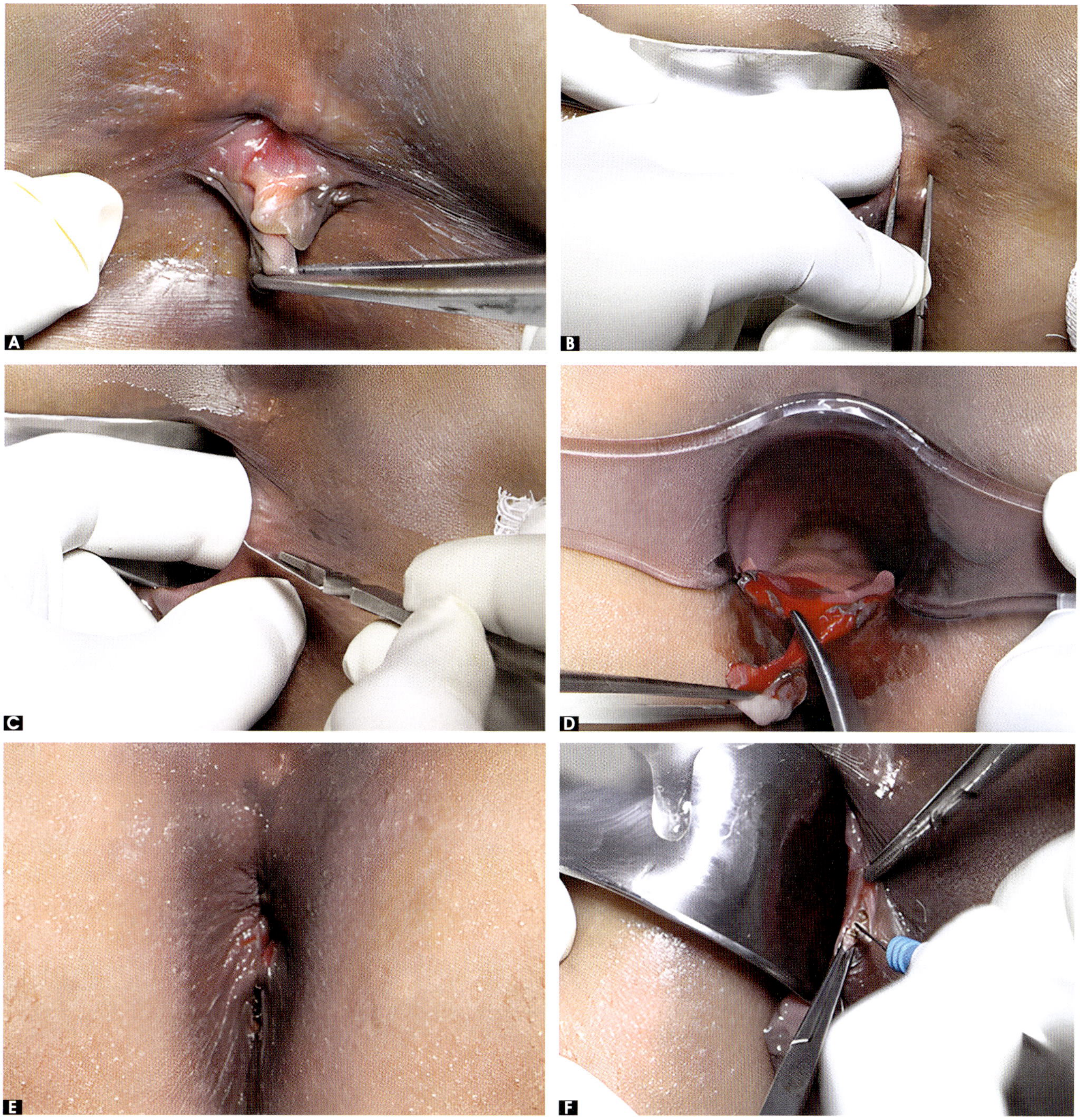

Fig. 8.5A-F: The technique of open lateral internal sphincterotomy. A) Anal fissure with sentinel piles. B) Insertion of Sim's speculum and palpation of the intersphincteric groove. C) Cutting of the IAS fibres horizontally. D) Excision of posterior sentinel piles with the blade. E) Post-operative wound. F) Demonstration of incision with a cautery.

Use of Laser for Lateral Internal Sphincterotomy

The principle and approach for LIS remains the same as in open and closed techniques. The only distinction lies in the energy source used to divide the sphincter. Instead of scissors or cautery, a bare laser fibre is used for LIS.

Instrumentation: Same as shown in Fig. 8.3A, B

Position of the patient: Lithotomy

Type of anesthesia: Spinal/General/Pudendal nerve block

Type of fibre: Bare

Dosage: 10 W

Mode: Continuous mode

Steps of the Procedure

Step 1: A bivalve proctoscope is inserted into the anal canal. Once stretched, the intersphincteric groove can easily be seen (Fig. 8.6A).

Step 2: A bare fibre is used to make an incision through the intersphincteric space at 3 o'clock (Fig. 8.6B). The energy released is 10 W per sec in a continuous mode. The sphincter is cut gradually after rotating the tip of the laser fibre from lateral to medial (Fig. 8.6C).

Step 3: As it is a blind procedure, sometimes a few fibres of IAS are left undivided, leading to partial sphincterotomy. A mosquito forceps is introduced, and the uncut fibres, if any, are brought out and divided (Fig. 8.6D). Hemostasis is maintained by spraying the laser beam on the tissue 1 mm away from the bleeding site.

Step 4: The base of the fissure is curetted (Fig. 8.6E).

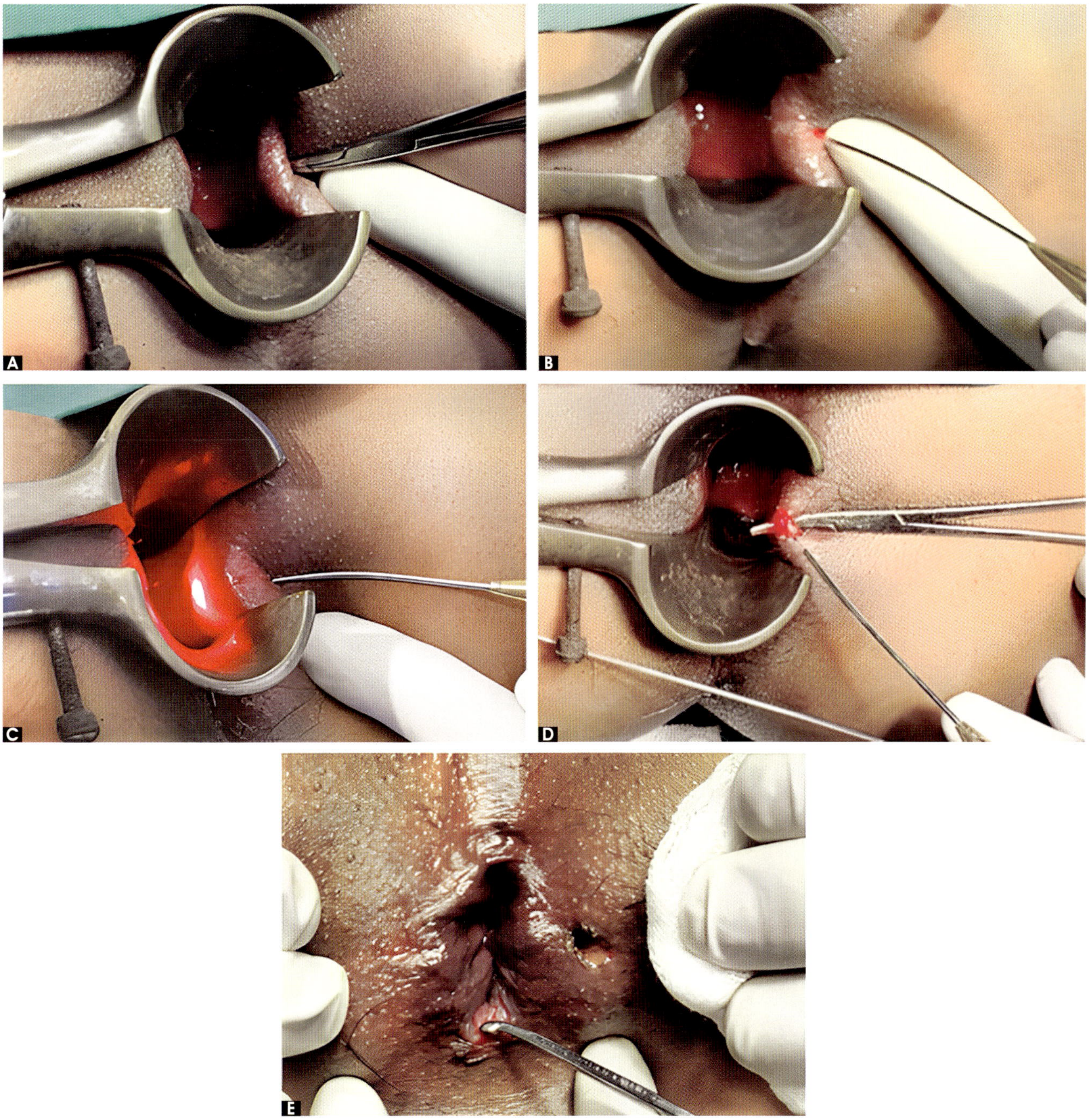

Fig. 8.6A-F: The technique of closed lateral internal sphincterotomy using laser. A) Intersphincteric groove as seen after insertion of bivalve proctoscope. B) Insertion of bare laser fibre into the intersphincteric groove. C) Light of laser fibre as seen while cutting the IAS up to the dentate line. D) Insertion of mosquito in the intersphincteric groove to check the fibres uncut with laser. E) Curetting of the base of the anal fissure.

Step 5: Bupivacaine 0.5% is infiltrated locally at the wound site, followed by pudendal nerve block (Fig. 8.6F, G, H).

The post-operative wound is shown in Fig. 8.6 I.

Scan QR Code for Video on
Closed laser LIS (1)
VIDEO 47

Scan QR Code for Video on
Closed laser LIS (2)
VIDEO 48

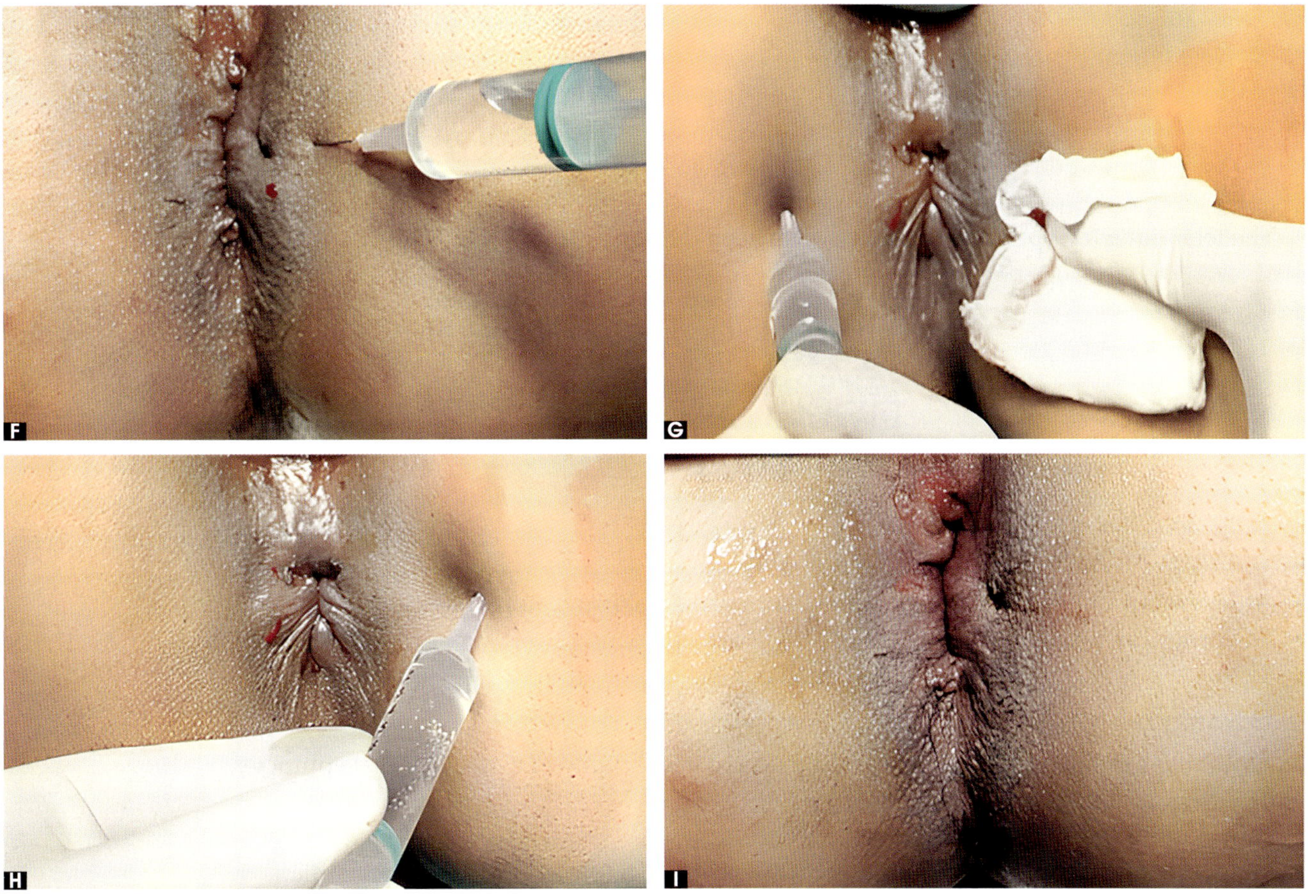

Fig. 8.6G-I: The technique of closed lateral internal sphincterotomy using laser. F) Local infiltration of bupivacaine at the operated site. G and H). Pudendal nerve block to reduce post-operative pain. I). Final wound after the surgery.

The technique for open LIS using laser has been demonstrated in Fig. 8.7A-D.

Scan QR Code for Video on
Open LIS with Laser

VIDEO 49

Advantages of Open LIS

- As IAS is cut under vision, the likelihood of partial sphincterotomy is negligible.
- The procedure is easily reproducible.

Disadvantages

- Mistaking the subcutaneous part of the external anal sphincter as the internal sphincter.
- Bleeding can be troublesome.
- Pain is more as compared to closed LIS.
- Infection of the incision wound may occur, leading to a low intersphincteric fistula.

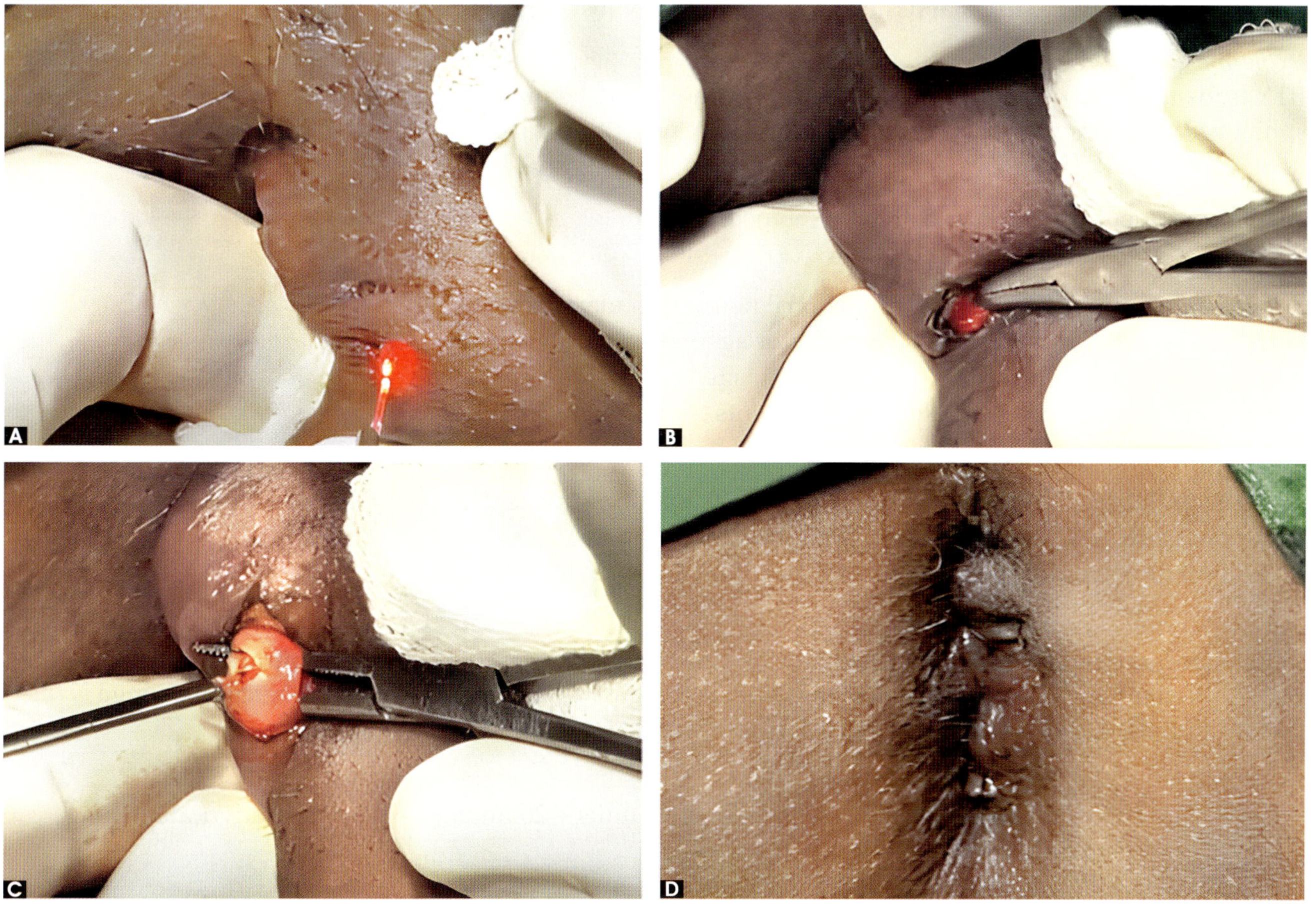

Fig. 8.7A-D: The technique of open lateral internal sphincterotomy using laser. A) Incision is given by bare laser fibre in the intersphincteric groove. B, C) IAS is brought out through the incision using mosquito forceps and cut with the laser. D) Post-operative wound.

Botulinum Toxin Sphincter Spasmolysis (BoSS)

Botulinum Toxin (BTX) for anal fissures was first used by Jost & Schimrigh.

Principle

BTX leads to temporary reversible sphincter spasmolysis (Chemical Sphincterotomy) to relieve internal anal sphincter (IAS) spasm induced by anal fissures. Since no cutting is involved, there is no anatomical destruction.

Indication

Anal fissure (acute or chronic) with anal sphincter spasm.

Contra-indications

- Peripheral motor neuropathy or functional neuromuscular disorders
- Co-administration with aminoglycosides or agents interfering with neuromuscular transmission
- Inflammatory skin disorders at the injection site
- Pregnancy, lactating females, pediatric patients.

Material

- Injection Botulinum Toxin (Fig. 8.8A) – 50 IU (available as freeze-dried powder).
- 5cc syringe + 20G needle + sterile distilled water (Fig. 8.8B)
- 3 × 1 ml tuberculin syringe + 26G small needle (1.25 cm) (Fig. 8.9)

Reconstitution

2.5 ml of sterile distilled water is injected into the vacuum-packed vial of BTX, and a uniform solution is formed by thorough mixing. The solution formed is in the strength of 0.1 ml = 2 units. The tuberculin syringe is filled as 1 ml = 20 units + 1 ml = 20 units and 0.5 ml = 10 units.

Dose

An average of 40 IU (30 to 50 IU) in divided doses of 20 units + 20 units +/– 10 units is advocated.

Site

The injection is given in the belly of the IAS muscle distal to the dentate line away from the fibrosed edges of the anal fissure, i.e. 5 o'clock and 8 o'clock position with the patient in the lithotomy position.

Anesthesia: Spinal/General/Pudendal nerve block.

Position: Lithotomy/Jack-knife.

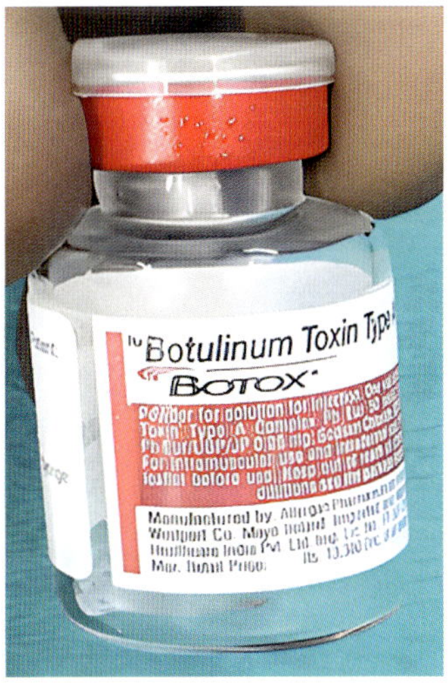

Fig. 8.8A: Botox

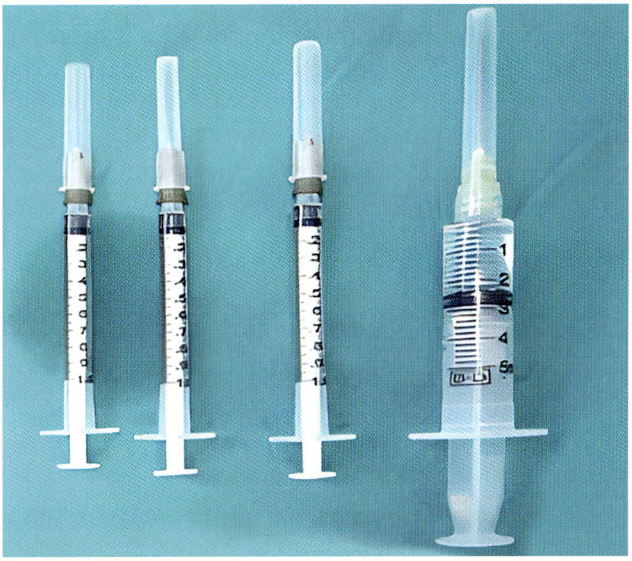

Fig. 8.8B: Tuberculin and 5 ml syringes

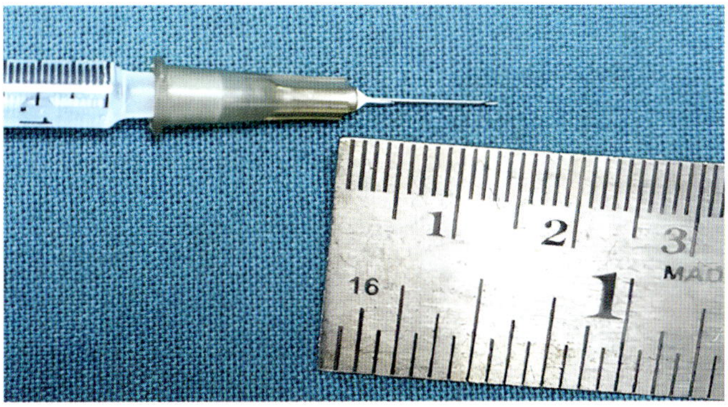

Fig. 8.9: Length of the needle.

Steps of the Procedure

Step 1: The area is cleaned with an antiseptic solution, and draping is done. Digital rectal examination and proctoscopy is done.

Step 2: A bivalve anal speculum or a Sim's speculum is inserted into the anal canal to make the IAS taut. The lower border of IAS is palpated to identify the intersphincteric groove.

Step 3: The needle of the first syringe containing 1 ml of the solution is inserted through the intersphincteric groove at 5 o'clock (Fig. 8.10A). The needle is angulated at 30 to 45 degree to enter the IAS upto the dentate line. One should confirm that the needle is neither in the external anal sphincter nor in the puborectalis sling. The solution is released, making sure to avoid any mucosal wheal.

Pressure is given for 2 minutes at the injection site to avoid hematoma and subsequent perianal abscess if it gets infected.

Step 4: The same procedure is repeated at 8 o'clock using the second syringe containing 1 ml of solution (Fig. 8.10B).

In the case of hypertrophic IAS, the third syringe containing 0.5 ml of solution can be injected at 1 o'clock.

Step 5: Hypertrophied anal papillae and sentinel pile masses are handled appropriately.

Tips and Tricks

- Complete haemostasis must be maintained. Otherwise, a hematoma may form and lead to perianal abscess. A small external sterile gauze dressing is applied for up to 2 hours post operatively.
- As the systemic absorption of BTX can lead to dyspnoea, dysphagia, atrial fibrillation and ectopics, the patient should be kept under observation for 12 hours.

Scan QR Code for Video on
BOTOX

VIDEO 50

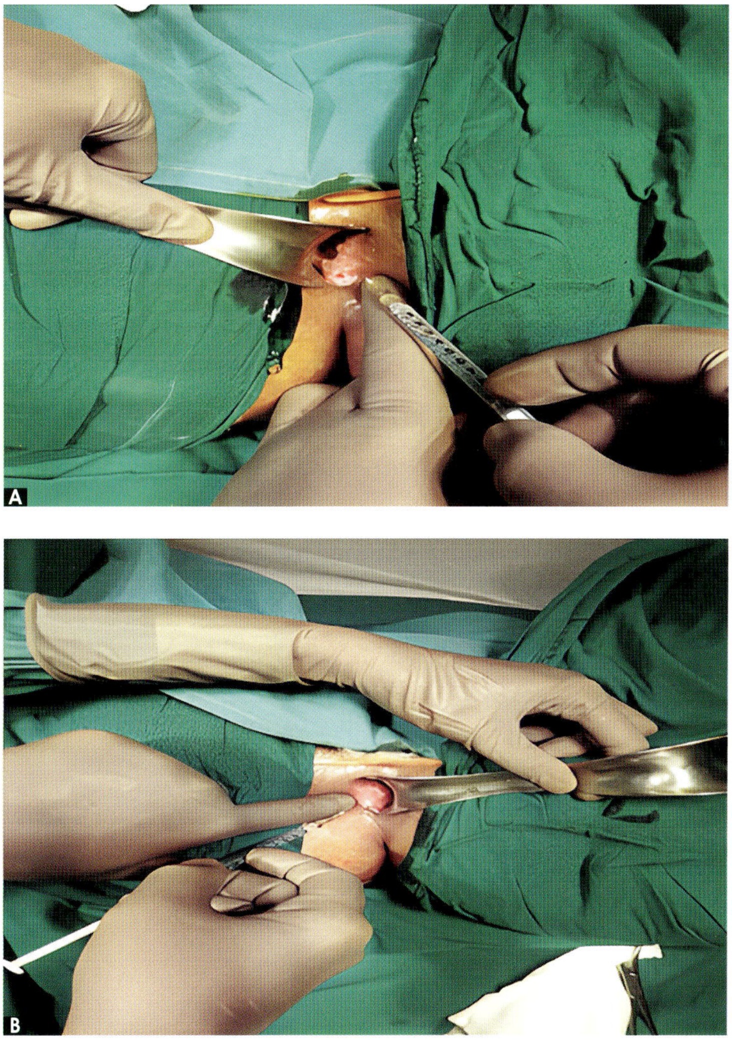

Fig. 8.10A, B: The technique of Botox: A) Injection of Botox at 5 o'clock. B) Injection of Botox at 8 o'clock (Procedure, images and video Courtesy: Dr Pravin Gore, Mumbai).

MUCOSAL ADVANCEMENT FLAPS FOR CHRONIC FISSURE IN ANO

Indication

- Chronic fissure in ano with decreased anal tone

Anesthesia: Spinal/General

Position: Lithotomy

Steps of the Procedure

Step 1: Open the anal canal gently by inserting a well-lubricated index finger.

Step 2: Rotate the finger clockwise and insert another finger to open the anal canal further.

Step 3: Gently insert an operating proctoscope. The scope used in MIPH is most appropriate.

Step 4: Refresh both the upper and the lower margins of the fissure. Remove any sentinel piles or hypertrophic papillae if present (Fig. 8.11A, B, C).

Step 5: Raise the mucosal flap, including mucosa, submucosa, and a few fibres of the internal sphincter. The flap should be almost double the size of the fissure wound to avoid tension on the flap and to prevent flap necrosis (Fig. 8.11D).

Step 6: Secure hemostasis using bipolar cautery.

Step 7: Suture the flap with the lower margin of the fissure by interrupted 3-0 Vicryl (Fig. 8.11E).

Step 8: Excise the small dog ears at the margins of the flap if formed.

Place a gauge as a dressing. Postoperatively, prophylactic antibiotic cover for 5 days, mild laxative, analgesics as per requirement and finger application of betadine ointment at the anal verge is recommended. While applying the ointment, the patient should be advised not to use any applicator as it may damage the flap.

Conclusion

Lateral internal sphincterotomy is considered the gold standard for anal fissures. The choice between closed or open techniques is left to the surgeon's discretion. The posterior sphincterotomy should always be avoided.

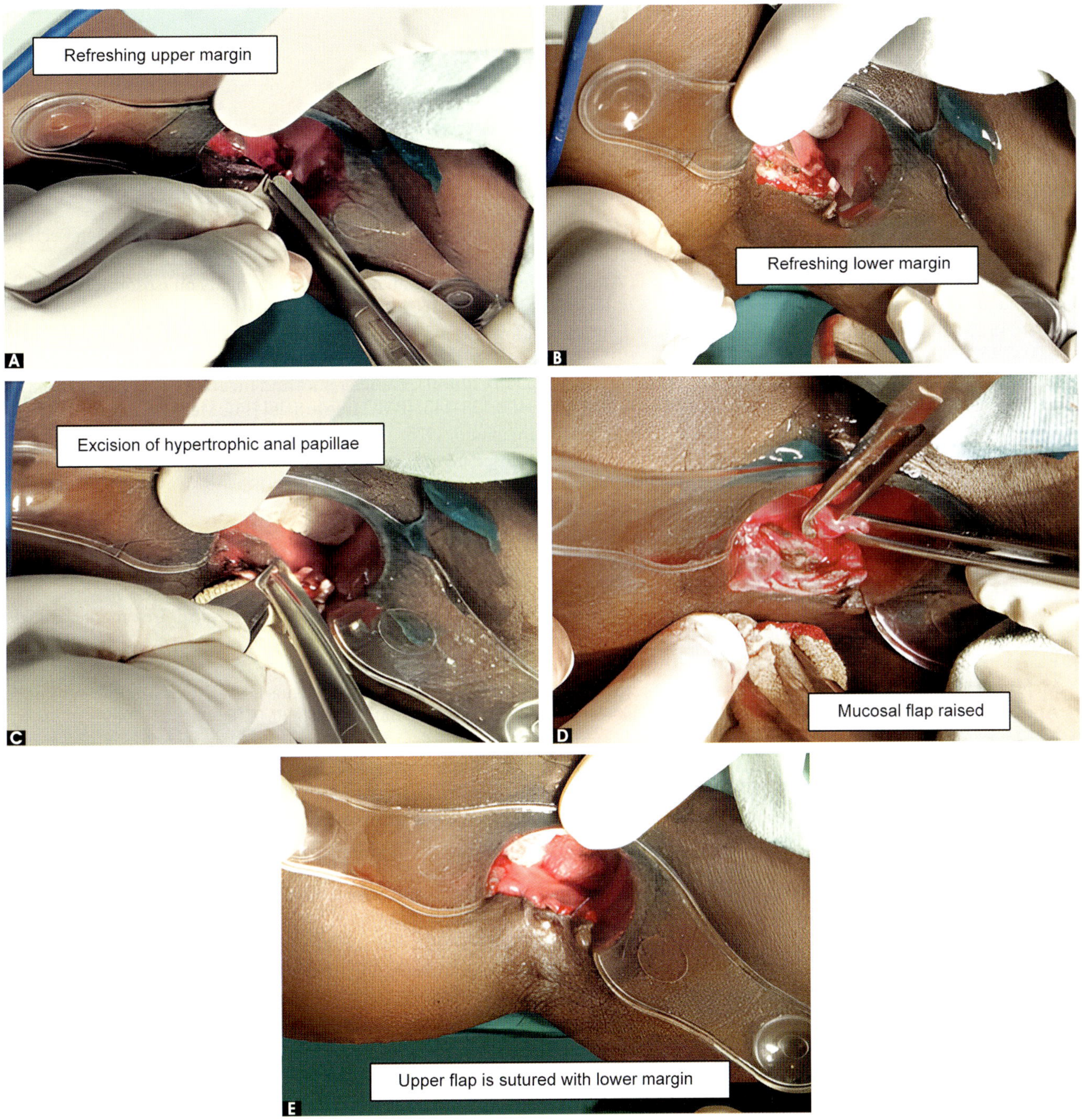

Fig. 8.11A-E: Technique of mucosal advancement flap for chronic anal fissures. A, B) Refreshing upper and lower margins of the fissure. C) Excision of the hypertrophic anal papilla. D) Raising mucosal advancement flap from the upper excised margin of the fissure. E) Suturing of the raised mucosal flap with the lower margin of the excised anal fissure. (Procedure and images courtesy: Dr SK Nigam, Bhopal).

FURTHER READING

- Abcarian H, Lakshmanan S, Read DR, Roccaforte P. The role of the internal sphincter in chronic anal fissures. Dis Colon Rectum. 1982 Sep;25(6):525–8. DOI: 10.1007/BF02564159. PMID: 7117055.
- Arslan K, Ereno lu B, Do ru O, Kökçam S, Turan E, Atay A. Effect of chronic anal fissure components on isosorbide dinitrate treatment. World J Surg. 2012 Sep;36(9):2225–9. DOI: 10.1007/s00268-012-1604-2. PMID: 22526048.
- Beaty JS and Shashidharan M (2016). Anal Fissure. Clinics in colon and rectal surgery, 29(1),30–37. https://doi.org/10.1055/s-0035-1570390
- Choi YS, Kim DS, Lee DH, Lee JB, Lee EJ, Lee SD, Song KH, Jung HJ. Clinical Characteristics and Incidence of Perianal Diseases in Patients with Ulcerative Colitis. Ann Coloproctol. 2018 Jun;34(3):138–143. [PMC free article] [PubMed] [Reference list].
- Goligher J Surgery of anus, rectum, and colon, chapter on fissure in ano, 1975.
- Gupta V, Rodrigues G, Prabhu R and Ravi C (2014). Open versus closed lateral internal anal sphincterotomy in the management of chronic anal fissures: A prospective randomized study. Asian journal of surgery, 37(4), 178–183.
- Jahnny B and Ashurst JV. (2020). Anal fissures. In StatPearls [Internet]. StatPearls Publishing.
- Jonas M and Scholefield JH (2001). Anal fissure. Gastroenterology Clinics of North America, 30(1), 167–181.
- Klosterhalfen B, Vogel P, Rixen H, Mittermayer C (1989). "Topography of the inferior rectal artery: a possible cause of chronic, primary anal fissure." Dis. Colon Rectum. 32 (1): 43–52. PMID 2910660.
- Lockhart-Mummery J P. London: Baillere; 1934. Diseases of the Rectum and Colon and Their Surgical Treatment. [Google Scholar] [Ref list].
- Lu Y, Lin A. Lateral Internal Sphincterotomy. JAMA. 2021;325(7):702. doi:10.1001/jama.2020.16708
- McNamara MJ, Percy JP, Fielding IR. A manometric study of anal fissure treated by subcutaneous lateral internal sphincterotomy. Ann Surg. 1990 Feb;211(2):235–8. DOI: 10.1097/00000658-199002000-00017. PMID: 2302000; PMCID: PMC1357969.
- Nelson RL (2014). Anal fissure (chronic). BMJ clinical evidence, 2014, 0407.
- Nessar G, Topbas M. Lateral Internal Partial Sphincterotomy Technique for Chronic Anal Fissure. Indian J Surg. 2017 Jun;79(3):185–187. doi: 10.1007/s12262-016-1467-0. Epub 2016 Mar 12. PMID: 28659668; PMCID: PMC5473792.
- Popat A, Pandey CP, Agarwal K, Srivastava VP, Sharma SM, Dixit A, A comparative study of the role of topical diltiazem 2% organic gel and lateral internal sphincterotomy for the management of chronic fissure in ano Int J Contemporary Med Res 2016 3(5):1363–65. [Google Scholar]
- Schouten WR, Briel JW, Auwerda JJ. Relationship between anal pressure and anodermal blood flow. The vascular pathogenesis of anal fissures. Dis Colon Rectum 1994;37:664–669 27 QEW5WS.
- WH Jost, K Schimrigk Dis Colon Rectum1993 Oct;36(10):974. PMID: 8404394. doi: 10.1007/BF02050639
- Wienert V, Raulf F and Mlitz H. (2017). Historical Aspects of Anal Fissure Pathology. In Anal Fissure (pp 91–98). Springer, Cham.
- Zaghiyan KN, Fleshner P. Anal fissure. Clin Colon Rectal Surg. 2011 Mar;24(1):22-30. doi: 10.1055/s-0031-1272820. PMID: 22379402; PMCID: PMC3140330.

Chapter

9

Postoperative Wound Care After Anorectal Surgery

Management of anorectal wounds after surgery play an important role in healing.

The materials and methods for wound management depend upon the type of procedure performed. These include:

- Ice pack
- Sitz bath
- Topical ointments
- Cleaning and dressings of fistula wounds
- Managing wound after video-assisted laser ablation of the pilonidal sinus (VALAPS).

The commonly used ointments and cleansing agents are shown in Fig. 9.1.

POSTOPERATIVE CARE AFTER EXCISIONAL HEMORRHOIDECTOMY

Sitz Bath

The water must be lukewarm, ideally at 40 to 42 degrees. Hot water can cause perianal burns and excoriation of the perineal skin (Fig. 9.2). Sitz bath is recommended twice a day for 10 to 15 minutes.

Principle

Relieves pain by promoting blood flow, eliminates wound soiling, and relaxes the internal anal sphincter to expedite wound healing.

Topical Ointments

The patient is advised to apply the ointment after defecation. A combination of metronidazole, sucralfate and lidocaine is preferred. The patient is also advised to apply lidocaine jelly 10 minutes before defecation.

Scan QR Code for Video on

Sitz Bathtub

VIDEO 51

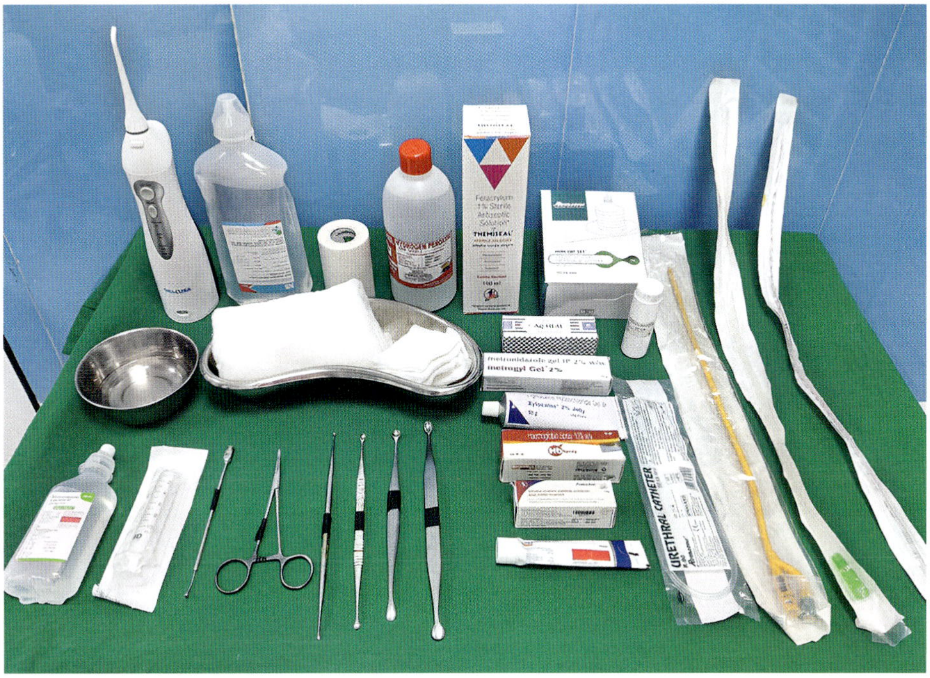

Fig. 9.1: Wound care trolley

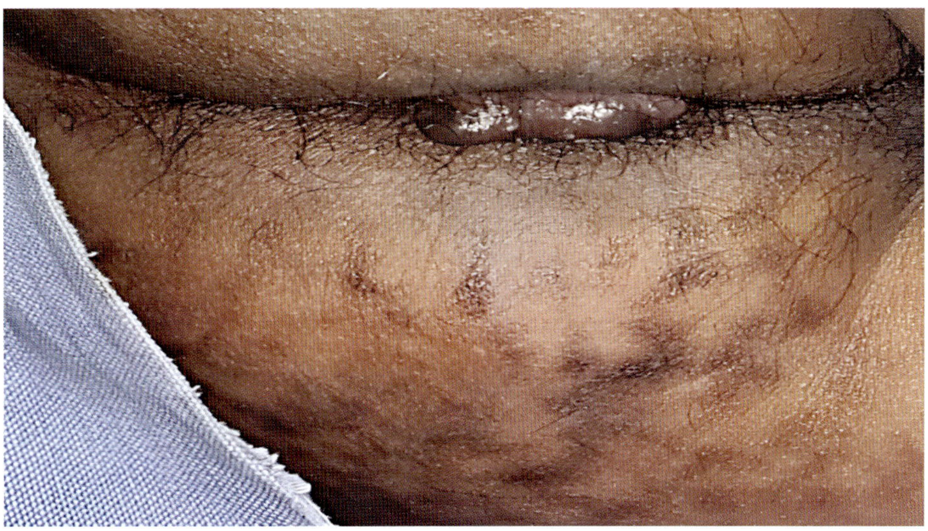

Fig. 9.2: Burns in the perianal area after a hot sitz bath

WOUND CARE AFTER LASER HEMORRHOIDOPLASTY

Ice Packs

Immediately after LHP, an ice finger is placed in the anal canal for 8-10 minutes. The ice finger should not be kept directly in contact with the mucosa as it can lead to crystallization in the capillaries giving a frostbite-like condition (Fig. 9.3).

Principle

To reduce edema resulting from the cellular damage caused by laser energy.

Scan QR Code for Video on
How to Prepare an Ice Finger and How to Insert it at the End of the Procedure
VIDEO 52

WOUND CLEANING AFTER FISTULA SURGERY (FISTULOTOMY/FISTULECTOMY)

Keeping the wound area clean after fistula surgery is essential. Fecal matter can cause contamination of the wound. Simple tap water can be used. The normal saline solution can also be used as it is an isotonic solution, non-cytotoxic and does not change the normal bacterial flora.

Instructions to the Patient

- Patients must be guided to do proper cleaning of the anal region by using a hand faucet.
- Alternatively, a plastic bottle can be used. The bottle is filled with water, and multiple holes are made at the top of the cap (Fig. 9.4). The bottle is then pressed, and the area is cleaned with significant pressure. One can also use spray bottles with water to clean the area (Fig. 9.5). Cotton balls should not be used to clean the area, as the lint may get stuck in the wound margins and cause irritation and itching. Further, it may lead to foreign body granuloma formation.
- Using a sterile dressing pad after application of the ointment can avoid soiling and contamination of the clothes.

Scan QR Code for Video on
Managing Fistula Wounds
VIDEO 53

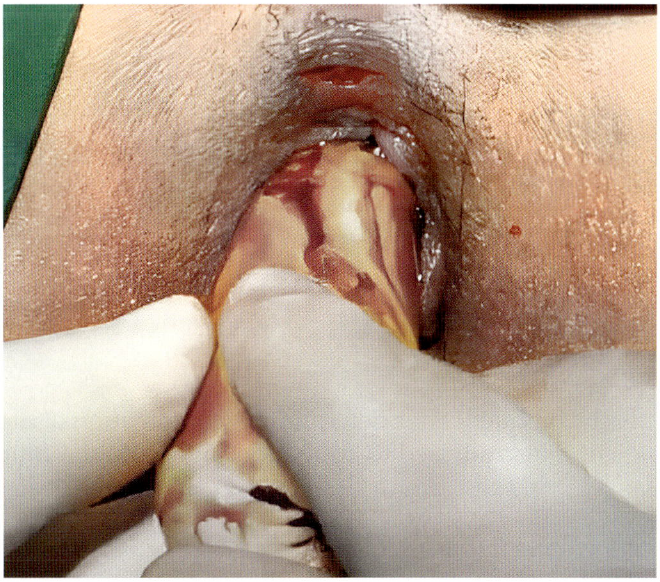

Fig. 9.3: Insertion of ice finger after laser hemorrhoidoplasty

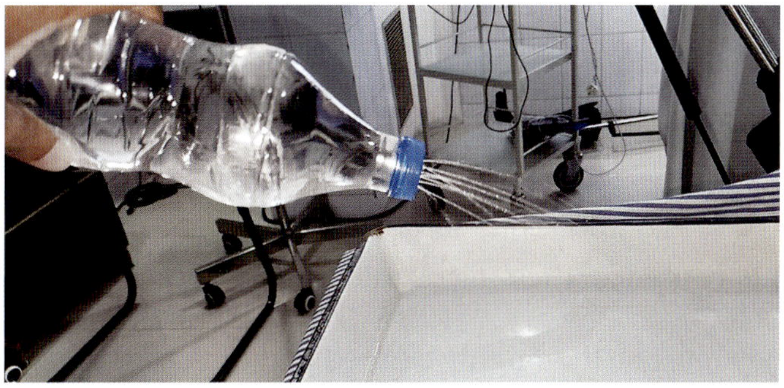

Fig. 9.4: Plastic bottle with multiple holes made in the cap

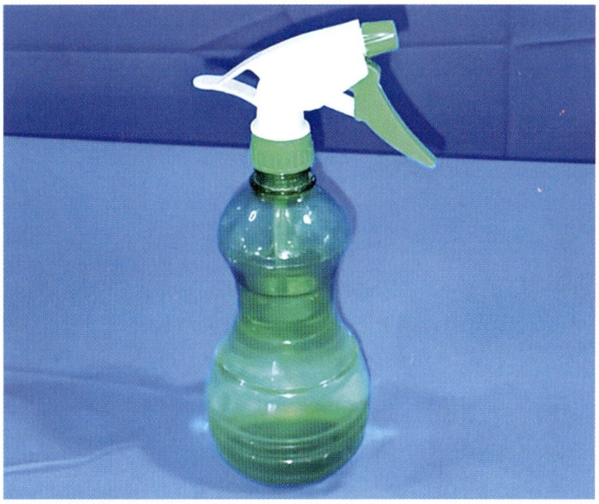

Fig. 9.5: Spray bottle used for irrrigation

- The tunnelling fistula wounds created after coring can be washed using an irrigation cannula (Fig. 9.6).
- Fistula wounds with drains have to be carefully managed. The drains have to be irrigated thoroughly and cautiously.

Scan QR Code for Video on
Managing Drain in the Abscess Cavity
VIDEO 54

Topical Ointments After Fistula Surgery

The patient is advised to apply the ointment after defecation. A combination of metronidazole, sucralfate and lidocaine is preferred. The patient is also advised to apply lidocaine jelly 10 minutes before defecation.

CLEANSING OF WOUNDS AFTER PILONIDAL SINUS

Educating the patient to manage the wound and peri-wound area is crucial. The following must be explained to the patient and the attendants.

- Cleansing of the wound
- Change of dressings
- Hair removal – once in 2 weeks
- Decontamination

Dressings Commonly used After Pilonidal Sinus Surgery

- Octenidiene is most commonly used for dressing pilonidal sinus wounds. It has antifungal and antimicrobial effects.
- The pilonidal sinus wounds must be thoroughly cleaned and dressed with antiseptic ointments, Hb spray and micronized PHMB granules.

Scan QR Code for Video on
Pilonidal Sinus with Irrigation
VIDEO 55

Topical Ointment in An Anal Fissure

A combination of lidocaine and Nifedipine or Diltiazem is preferred.

Scan QR Code for Video on
Application of Ointment
VIDEO 56

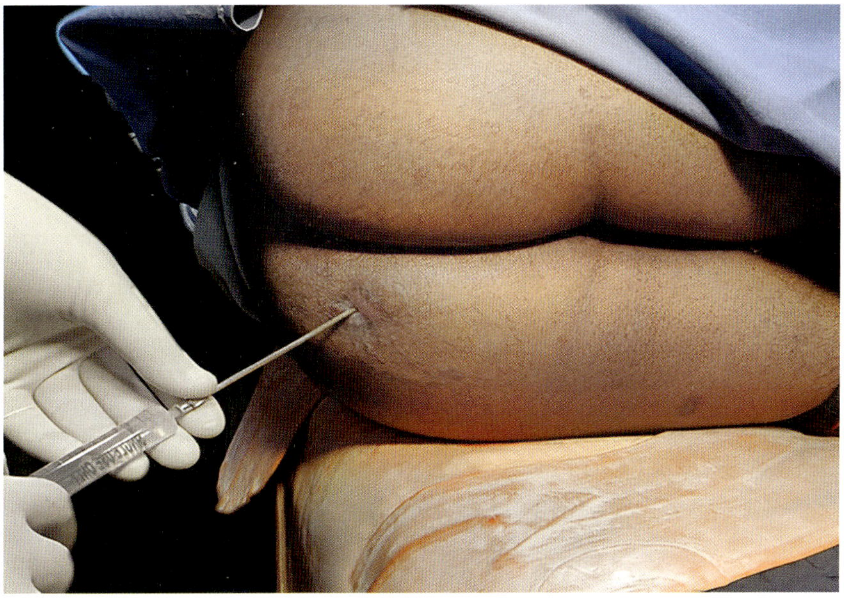

Fig. 9.6: Irrigation of fistula wounds using an irrigation cannula

Conclusion

Wounds recover fast after minimally invasive procedures as the raw area created is very small. Timely and proper wound management, appropriate cleansing, and dressings can prevent the wound from becoming infected.